T0295410

HYSTERESIS AND NEURAL MEMORY

HYSTERESIS AND NEURAL MEMORY

Isaak Mayergoyz
University of Maryland, USA

Can Korman
George Washington University, USA

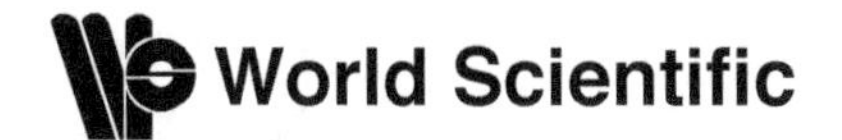

NEW JERSEY • LONDON • SINGAPORE • BEIJING • SHANGHAI • HONG KONG • TAIPEI • CHENNAI • TOKYO

Published by

World Scientific Publishing Co. Pte. Ltd.
5 Toh Tuck Link, Singapore 596224
USA office: 27 Warren Street, Suite 401-402, Hackensack, NJ 07601
UK office: 57 Shelton Street, Covent Garden, London WC2H 9HE

British Library Cataloguing-in-Publication Data
A catalogue record for this book is available from the British Library.

HYSTERESIS AND NEURAL MEMORY

ISBN 978-981-120-950-5

For any available supplementary material, please visit
https://www.worldscientific.com/worldscibooks/10.1142/11532#t=suppl

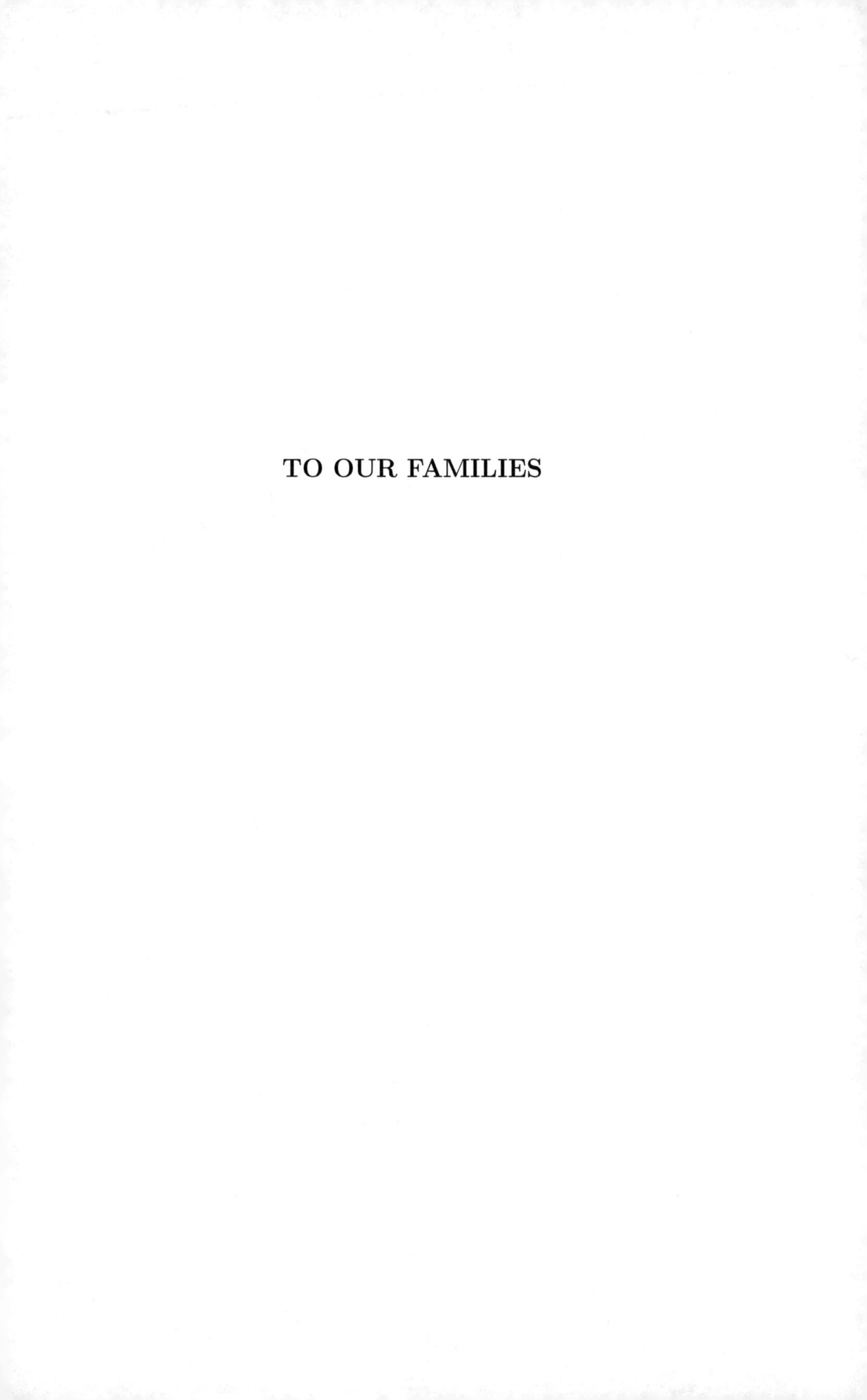

TO OUR FAMILIES

Preface

This book deals with mathematical models of hysteresis phenomena and their applications to the modeling of neural memory. The immediate question can be asked as to why hysteresis models are relevant to neural memory. The reason is that hysteresis and its models are endowed with memory. This memory is selective and distributed in nature with many properties similar to those observed in neural memory. The related question is where the physical phenomena of hysteresis occur in neural systems. It turns out that ion channels of neurons exhibit hysteresis. This hysteresis is due to the multiplicity of metastable (i.e., conformational) states of channel proteins. These proteins control the conduction of ion channels, which are involved in the two most fundamental signal processing aspects of neural memory, such as generation and propagation of action potentials and the transmission of electric signals across synaptic clefts. Therefore, it can be properly conjectured that neural memories can be stored in conformational states of ion channel proteins. This conjecture reveals the possible molecular basis of neural memory. It also suggests that hysteresis models may become an integral part of neural memory models.

The book consists of four chapters. The first two chapters deal with the Preisach-type models of hysteresis. These models are constructed as assemblies of the simplest hysteresis elements, i.e., rectangular loops with various switching-up and switching-down values. The sparse parallel connectivity of these loops results in the emergence of distributed memory selectively extracted from time varying inputs. The diversity of rectangular loops is crucial for the formation of selective and distributed memory. These selectively extracted memories are not immutable, but they continuously evolve over time by being modified, distorted or suppressed into oblivion by subsequent input variations. This memory feature of the Preisach-type hysteresis models is due to the erasure property of these models. It is also shown that engrams (i.e., memory traces) of distributed memories of Preisach-type hysteresis models can be clearly identified by using a special diagram technique. These engrams reveal that selectively extracted memories are not stored in particular rectangular loops. Instead, all rectangular loops are involved in the collective storage of extracted input data. The necessary and sufficient conditions for the applicability of the Preisach-type models of hysteresis are studied along with their identification. The latter is done by using the measured first-order reversal curves (FORC) in the case of the classical Preisach model and second-order reversal curves (SORC) in the case of far-reaching generalizations of this model. These curves are also instrumental in the numerical implementation of these models. Finally, it is demonstrated that the Preisach models of hysteresis can be useful for the analysis of certain problems of nonlinear diffusion with finite speed of propagation of zero front. This is illustrated for the case of nonlinear diffusion in type-II superconductors with sharp resistive transitions. It turns out that somewhat similar nonlinear diffusion problems are encountered in neural science and they are discussed in Chapter 3.

The third chapter deals with hysteresis and neural memory. This chapter begins with a brief review of the structure of neurons. Hence, only very basic and selected facts are presented for the case of pyramidal neurons. These neurons are abundant in the cerebral cortex and the hippocampus which are the brain parts involved in neural memory formation and cognition. In the second section of this chapter, the basic facts related to ion channels and synapses are discussed. A novel part of this discussion is related to the random nature of ion currents through single protein channels observed in patch-clamp technique measurements. The classical kinetic theory was developed to account for this randomness. This theory is based on the underlying Markovian assumption concerning the random nature of ion channel currents. This assumption is not fully justified and is regarded as questionable. It is suggested in the book to abandon the Markovian assumption and treat stochastic binary channel currents as being produced by random switching of rectangular hysteresis loops. Mathematically, the hysteresis based random switching between open and closed channel conformations can be treated as exit problems for stochastic processes. These problems are among the well-studied problems of random process theory. Another approach to random switchings of rectangular loops is based on the theory of Markov processes on graphs. This theory, as well as the theory of exit problems, are discussed in detail in the fourth chapter of the book.

The next section of the third chapter deals with the discussion of generation and propagation of action potentials. These potentials are generated and propagated due to the collective action of sodium and potassium ion channels. It is demonstrated that the collective deterministic action of these channels exhibit hysteresis. This demonstration is accomplished by using the inverse problem approach to the nonlinear deterministic Hodgkin-Huxley diffusion equation. The analysis is presented for the case of non-myelinated axons, as well as myelinated axons with Ranvier nodes.

The fourth and most important section of the third chapter (and the book) deals with hysteresis and neural memory. It is often emphasized that brains are similar to computers. The whole research area of neural networks has been developed to explore these similarities. However, as far as memory is concerned, brains are strikingly different from computers. In computers, binary storage is employed, while this is not the case for brain memory storage. Furthermore, identical storage elements are used in computers, while ubiquitous biological diversity is probably utilized for distributed storage in brains. In computers, binary data are assigned to be stored in addressable memory locations. However, in the case of brains, data are not assigned for storage but rather extracted from incoming analog sensory inputs. This extraction is selective. This means that only most distinct features are extracted from incoming sensory data for storage. The selectively extracted data stored in brains are not immutable. Instead, the stored data continuously evolve over time by being updated and modified.

It turns out that memory of Preisach hysteresis models may imitate important properties observed in neural memory. These properties are:

- Selective nature of neural memories extracted from sensory inputs,
- Distributed nature of neural memories and their engrams (i.e., memory traces),
- Neural memory formation as an emerging property of sparse connectivity,
- Neural memory stability with respect to protein turnover,
- Neural memory storage plasticity,
- Neural memory recalls and their effect on storage.

Some words of caution are in order here. Hysteresis models of neural memory (as any model) are products of mind, while actual neural memory is a product of the evolution process. The scientific process of modelling is driven by observations, intuition and logical reasoning. Whereas, the slow and convoluted evolution process is driven by random mutations and survivalistic selection. For this reason, hysteresis models of neural memory may only imitate certain important properties of actual neural memory but they may never fully reflect or account for its immense complexity.

The final section of the third chapter is not related to neural memory. The purpose of this section is to suggest that unique features of Preisach hysteresis models may be explored for future developments of novel data storage devices, as well as hardware-based global optimizers. The Preisach approach may lead to the implementation of such global optimizers by employing classical means without resorting to quantum computing.

The last and fourth chapter of the book is the most sophisticated from the mathematical point of view. This chapter deals with hysteresis driven by random processes which model noise in actual physical systems. The chapter begins with the brief review of the basic facts related to stochastic processes. It is emphasized that these processes can be mathematically studied on two equivalent levels: 1) on the level of random realizations which are described by nonlinear stochastic ordinary differential equations, and 2) on the level of transition probability densities described by deterministic linear partial differential equations. Then, the simple case of hysteresis driven by discrete time i.i.d. (independent and identically distributed) processes is discussed and analytical formulas are derived for expected values of the output processes.

The next two sections of the chapter deal with hysteresis driven by continuous-time stochastic processes. Two different approaches are explored for the analysis of output processes. The first approach is based on the mathematical machinery of exit problems for stochastic processes. This approach is quite transparent from the physical point of view. However, its analytical and computational implementation may be quite cumbersome. For this reason, another and entirely different approach is developed which is based on the theory of stochastic processes on graphs. This theory has recently been developed to study random perturbations of Hamiltonian dynamical systems. It is demonstrated that this theory is naturally suitable for the analysis of random output processes of hysteretic systems driven by noise. As a by-product of this demonstration, analytical expressions for the stationary characteristics of these output processes are developed. It is stressed that the presented techniques can be directly used in the study of random currents of ion channels as well as the phenomena of fading memory. The developed mathematical tools are applied in the book to the calculation of the spectral density of random outputs of hysteretic systems driven by stationary stochastic processes. This problem is of considerable mathematical difficulty because hysteretic transformations of input stochastic processes are highly nonlinear in nature. Nevertheless, the mathematical machinery of stochastic processes on graphs makes this problem tractable.

The last section of the fourth chapter deals with functional (path) integration models of hysteresis. Stochastic processes are used here in the definition of such models, and it is demonstrated that in some typical cases these models are reduced to the classical Preisach model. This reduction attests to the generality of the classical Preisach model of hysteresis.

In writing this book, special efforts have been made to produce a book that will be accessible and appealing to a broad audience. To achieve this goal, a special emphasis has been placed on the clarity of exposition of various concepts and facts related to hysteresis and neural memory. It is for readers to judge to what extent these efforts have been successful. It is believed that this book may be of interest to neuroscientists, biologists, bioengineers, electrical engineers, applied mathematicians and physicists interested in neural memory and its molecular basis.

In conclusion, the authors would like to acknowledge the help of Siddharth Tyagi and Vaishnavi Murthy in the preparation of the book manuscript. Their help is greatly appreciated. Our thanks to Steven Patt from World Scientific Publishing Company for his assistance and patience.

I. D. Mayergoyz and C. E. Korman

Contents

Chapter 1

Classical Preisach Model

1.1 What is Hysteresis?

The phenomenon of hysteresis is ubiquitous, and it is encountered in many different areas of science, technology and social life. The most known example of this phenomenon is magnetic hysteresis. This hysteresis is utilized in the design of magnetic data storage devices as well as in applications of permanent magnets. Other examples of hysteresis include mechanical hysteresis, superconducting hysteresis, optical hysteresis, electron-beam hysteresis, adsorption hysteresis, economic hysteresis, etc. The phenomenon of hysteresis is also encountered in biology and neuroscience. In the area of neuroscience, hysteresis of ion channels is probably most important as far as the understanding of neural memory formation is concerned. This topic will be extensively discussed in the third chapter of this book.

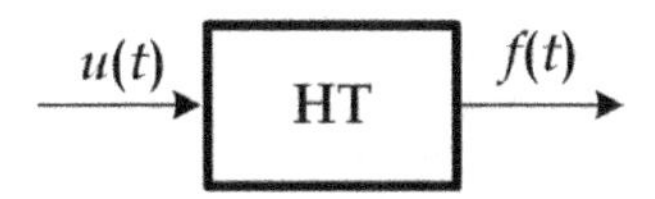

Fig. 1.1

So, what is hysteresis? To make the discussion very general and applicable to hysteresis phenomena of different origins, we shall adopt the language of system theory. Namely, we consider a transducer (a device) that converts an input $u(t)$ into an output $f(t)$ (see Fig. 1.1). This transducer is called a hysteresis transducer (HT) if its input-output relationship exhibits hysteresis. The most known and simplest manifestation of hysteresis is a hysteresis loop (see Fig. 1.2). Such a loop is formed for periodic (back and forth) variations of input between two extremum values. For symmetric loops, these extremum values are minimum value $-u_m$ and maximum value u_m. A hysteresis loop has two branches: an ascending branch corresponding to monotonic increase of input from $-u_m$ to u_m and a descending branch corresponding to monotonic decrease of input from u_m to $-u_m$. On Fig. 1.2, the tracing of these branches are marked by upward and downward arrows. Figure 1.2 presents only one symmetric loop. However, quite often there exists a family of minor symmetric hysteresis loops confined within the major symmetric loop (see Fig. 1.5). There are also minor nonsymmetric loops which appear for periodic input variations between two values u_1 and u_2 when $u_1 > u_2$ and $u_1 \neq -u_2$ (see Figs. 1.11 and 1.12).

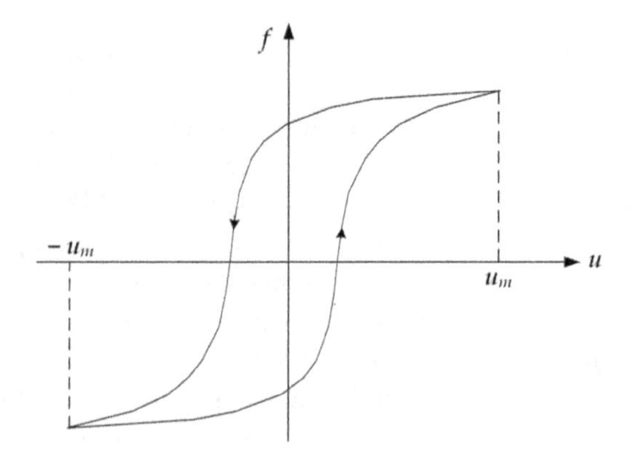

Fig. 1.2

The term "hysteresis" was introduced by the physicist J. A. Ewing. This word is of Greek origin with the meaning of "lagging behind". Indeed, when a symmetric hysteresis loop is traced, variations of output $f(t)$ lag behind the variations of input $u(t)$. Namely, when a descending branch is traced, input $u(t)$ reaches zero while the output $f(t)$ is still positive. Furthermore, output $f(t)$ reaches zero when input $u(t)$ is already negative. Similar lagging behind variations of output $f(t)$ are observed in tracing the ascending branch of a symmetrical hysteresis loop.

Although loops are the most known manifestation of hysteresis, they do not fully reflect the essence of hysteresis phenomenon. The essence of this phenomenon is history dependent branching. In other words, hysteresis can be defined as a multibranch input-output relation for which transition from one branch to another occur after each input extremum. Such a multibranch nonlinearity is shown in Fig. 1.3. It is apparent that the formation

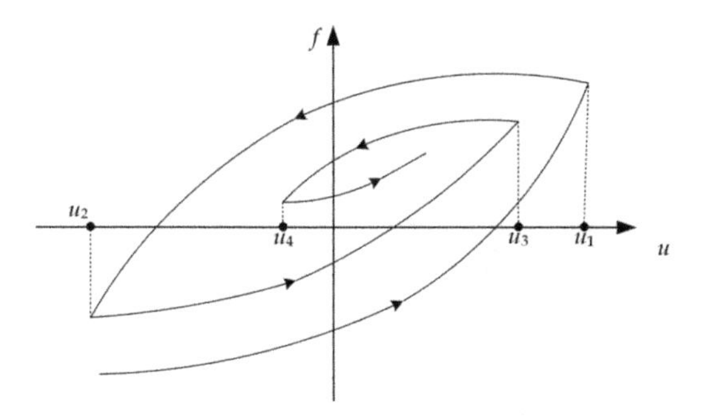

Fig. 1.3

of hysteresis loops is a particular case of history-dependent branching. This case is realized for periodic variations of inputs, while branching occurs for arbitrary input variations.

In summary, hysteresis can be viewed as an input-output nonlinearity with memory of past history which reveals itself through branching. This branching has a relatively simple structure in the case of **rate-independent hysteresis**. The term "rate-independent" means that branches of hysteresis are controlled only by the past extremum values of input, while the speed and particular manner of monotonic input variations between input extremum points has no influence on branching. The above statement is illustrated by Figs. 1.4a, 1.4b and 1.4c. Here, Figs. 1.4a and 1.4b represent two different inputs $u^{(1)}(t)$ and $u^{(2)}(t)$ that successively assume the same extremum values u_1, u_2, u_3 and u_4 but vary in time differently between these values. Then, for rate-independent hysteresis these two inputs will result in the same branching (see Fig. 1.4c) provided that the initial state of hysteresis is the same. This implies that rate-independent hysteresis is endowed with discrete memory structure which consists of past-extremum values of input.

The given definition of rate-independent hysteresis is consistent with many experimental facts. For instance, it is known in the area of magnetic hysteresis that shapes of major and minor symmetrical loops can be specified without referring to how fast magnetic field H varies between two extremum values $-H_{m_k}$ and H_{m_k} (see Fig. 1.5). This indicates that time effects are negligible, and the presented definition of rate-independent hysteresis is an adequate one. It is worthwhile to keep in mind that for very fast input variations, the time effects may become important and the given definition of rate-independent hysteresis may fail.

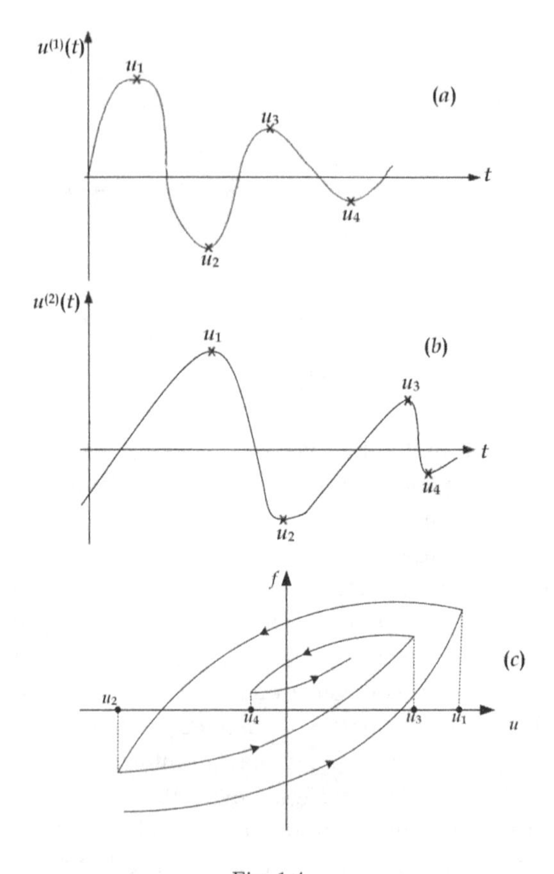

Fig. 1.4

It turns out that all rate-independent hysteresis nonlinearities fall into two general categories: (a) hysteresis nonlinearities with *local* memories, and (b) hysteresis nonlinearities with *nonlocal* memories. The hysteresis nonlinearity with local memory have the following property: the value of output $f(t_0)$ at any instant of time t_0 and the values of input $u(t)$ at all subsequent instants of time $t \geq t_0$ uniquely define the value of output $f(t)$ for all $t \geq t_0$. In other words, in hysteresis with local memory the past exerts its influence upon the future through the current value of output. This is not true in the case of hysteresis with nonlocal memories. For such hysteresis, future values of output $f(t)$, $(t \geq t_0)$, depend not only on the current value of output $f(t_0)$ but on past extremum values of inputs as well. By analogy with the theory of random processes, hysteresis with local

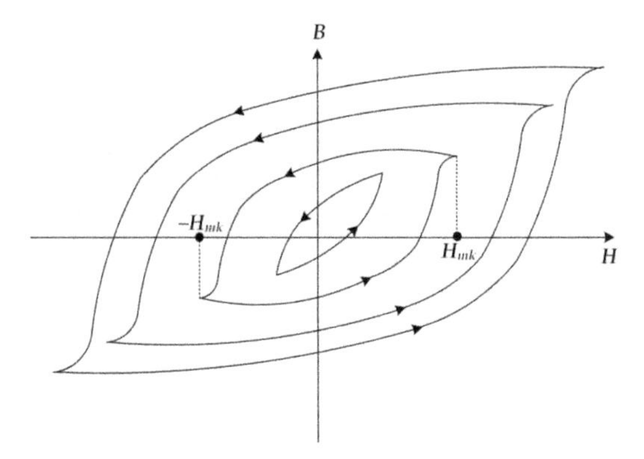

Fig. 1.5

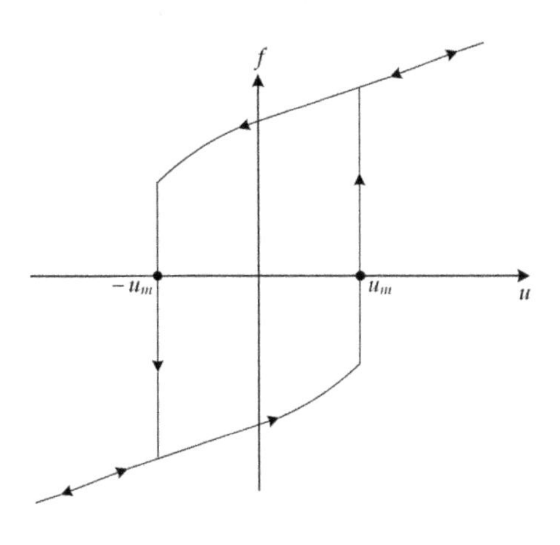

Fig. 1.6

memories can be called Markovian hysteresis, while hysteresis with nonlocal memory can be defined as non-Markovian hysteresis.

Typical examples of hysteresis nonlinearities with local memories are shown in Figs. 1.6, 1.7 and 1.8. Figure 1.6 presents the simplest hysteresis with local memory. This hysteresis is specified by only one loop formed by ascending and descending branches. These branches are only partially reversible (their vertical sections are not reversible). This type of hysteresis is characteristic, for instance, for Stoner-Wohlfarth magnetic particles [1]. For this type of hysteresis, branching occurs if extremum values exceed u_m or $-u_m$.

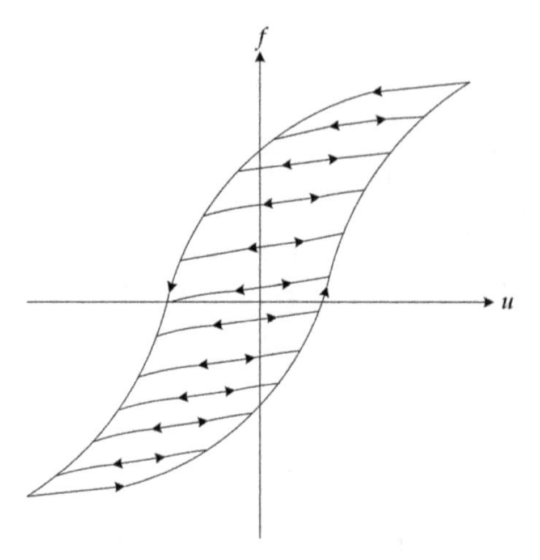

Fig. 1.7

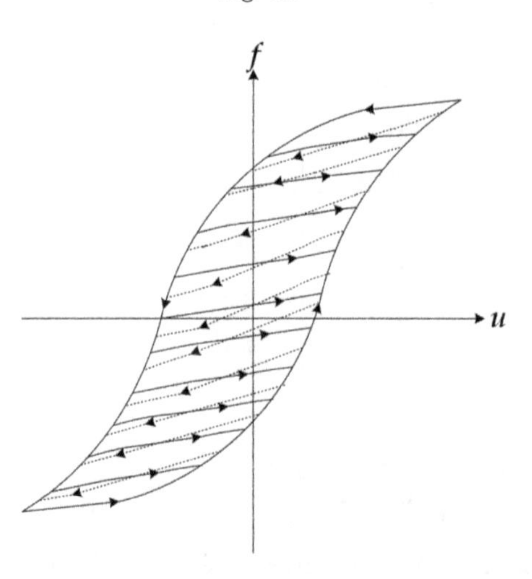

Fig. 1.8

A more complicated type of hysteresis with local memory is illustrated by Fig. 1.7. Here, there is a set of inner curves within the major hysteresis loop and only one curve passes through each point. These curves are fully reversible and can be traced in both directions corresponding to a monotonically increasing and decreasing input, respectively. For this type of hysteresis, branching may only occur when ascending or descending branches of the major loop are reached.

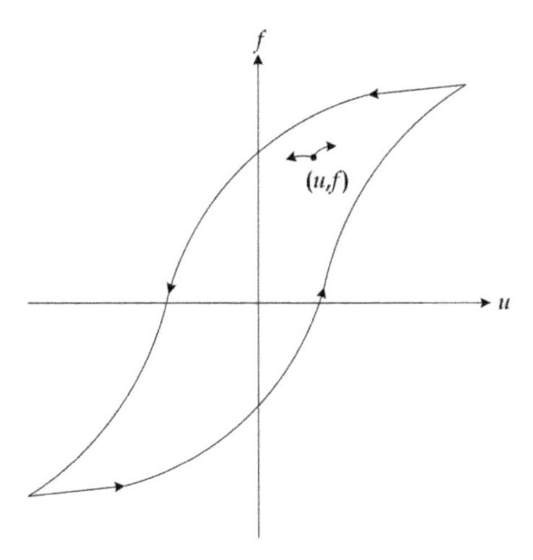

Fig. 1.9

A furthermore complicated type of hysteresis with two sets of inner curves (the ascending and descending curves) is shown in Fig. 1.8. This type of hysteresis was probably first described by Madelung [2] in the beginning of the last century, and afterwards it was independently rediscovered by many authors time and again (see, for instance, [3] and [4]. For this type of hysteresis, only one curve from each set passes through each point within the major hysteresis loop. If the input $u(t)$ is monotonically increased, one of the ascending curves is followed. However, if the input is monotonically decreased, one of the descending curves is traced. For this reason, branching may occur for any input extremum.

It is clear from the above examples that hysteresis with local memory has the following feature: every reachable point on the $u - f$ plane corresponds to a uniquely defined state, and the future time evolution of output is uniquely defined by this state for both monotonically increasing and decreasing inputs. In other words, at any point on the $u - f$ plane there are only one or two curves that may represent the future evolution of output (see Fig. 1.9). This is not true for hysteresis with nonlocal memory. In the latter case, at any reachable point (u, f) there are infinitely many (continuum set of) curves that may represent the future evolution of hysteresis output (see Fig. 1.10). The choice of each of these curves is determined by a particular past input history, namely, by a particular sequence of past input extrema.

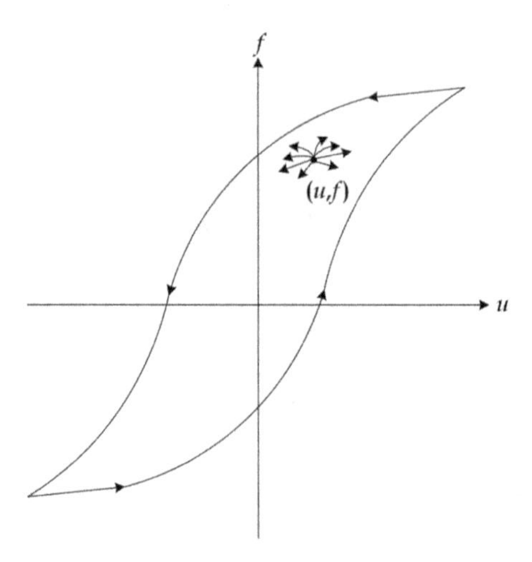

Fig. 1.10

Mathematical models of hysteresis with local memory have been extensively studied by using differential and algebraic equations. These models achieved some level of sophistication that is reflected, for instance, in publications [5]–[8]. However, the notion of hysteresis with local memory is not consistent with experimental facts. For instance, it is reported in [9] that crossing and even partially coincident minor loops have been experimentally observed. Such loops are schematically shown in Figs. 1.11 and 1.12, respectively. The existence of crossing minor loops attached to a major loop is more or less obvious, while the existence of partially coincident minor loops is a subtler effect. The existence of crossing and partially coincident minor loops clearly suggests that the states of hysteresis are not uniquely specified by instantaneous values of output and input. This means that such a hysteresis does not have a local memory.

This book is solely concerned with mathematical (Preisach-type) models of hysteresis with nonlocal memories. The question can be posed: why are these models needed? The answer is that a hysteresis transducer is usually a part of a system. For this reason, transducer's input is not known beforehand because it is determined by the interaction of the transducer with the rest of the system. This means that it is impossible to specify in advance the hysteresis branches which will be followed in a particular regime of the system. This is the main difficulty as far as self-consistent mathematical descriptions of systems with nonlocal memory hysteresis is

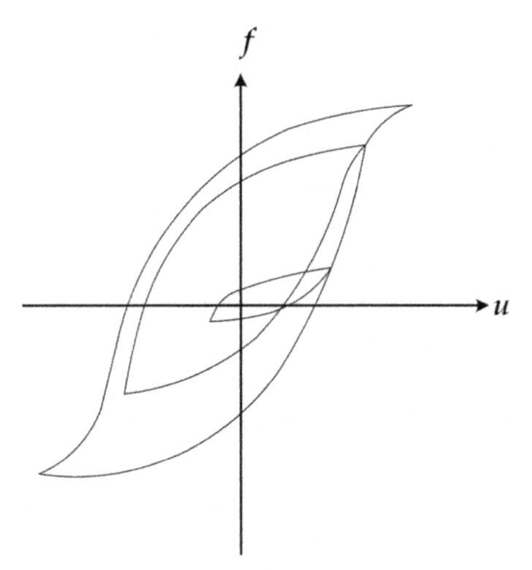

Fig. 1.11

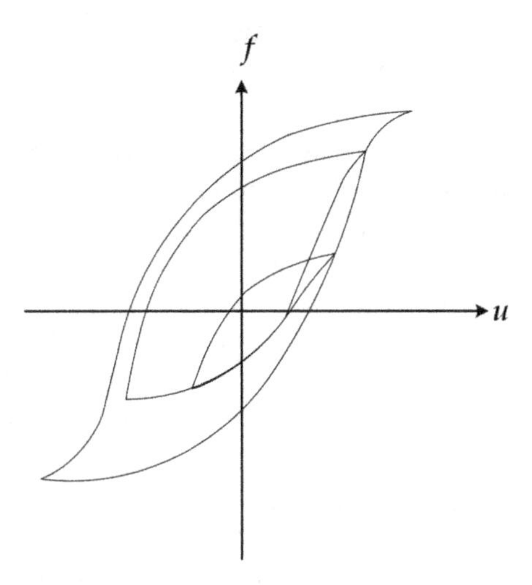

Fig. 1.12

concerned. To overcome this difficulty, mathematical models of hysteresis with nonlocal memories are needed. These models represent mathematical tools which themselves (due to their structure) are able to detect and store input extrema and choose appropriate hysteresis branches in accordance with the stored memories of past input extrema. Such models coupled together with mathematical descriptions of the rest of systems can provide complete mathematical descriptions of systems with nonlocal memory hysteresis.

This book deals exclusively with the mathematical models of hysteresis which are purely phenomenological in nature. Essentially, these models are mathematical tools which describe and generalize experimental facts. They provide no insights into the physical origin of hysteresis. In many applications related to physics, chemistry and biology, the origin of hysteresis can be traced back to the multiplicity of local energy minima of specific systems. These local energy minima represent metastable states which may persist for a long time. These persisting metastable states are responsible for the origin of hysteresis.

In neuroscience, proteins of ion channels have many metastable (conformational) states which manifest themselves in hysteretic behavior of these channels. For this reason, it can be conjectured that metastable states of channel proteins may be related to the formation of neural memory. As far as the authors are aware, the papers of B. G. Cragg and H. N. V. Temperley "Memory: The Analogy with Ferromagnetic Hysteresis" [10] and A. Kathalsky and E. Nuemann "Hysteresis and Molecular Memory Record" [11] are among the very first publications which suggested the possible relations between neural memory and hysteresis. However, these papers did not deal with Preisach-type models of hysteresis with nonlocal (non-Markovian) memories. At the time of publication of the above-mentioned papers, these hysteresis models were not sufficiently developed. The purpose of this book is to demonstrate that by using the Preisach-type models of hysteresis the connection between the neural memory and hysteresis can be further elaborated to account for many observed and unique properties of neural memory. The possible relation between neural memory and Preisach hysteresis models was first pointed out by the first author in his paper [12] (see also [13]–[15]), which was subsequently reviewed by Sir John Maddox in Nature [16]. The interesting point of this relation is that the sparse connectivity of simple hysteresis elements in the Presiach model results in distributed memory storage, whose "engrams" (i.e. memory traces) can be clearly identified.

1.2 Definition of the Classical Preisach Model of Hysteresis

This model has a long and instructive history that can be best characterized by the following eloquent statement of J. Larmor in his preface to the book of H. Poincare [17]: " ... *scientific progress, considered historically, is not a strictly logical process, and does not proceed by syllogisms. New ideas emerge dimly into intuition, come into consciousness from nobody knows where, and become the material on which the mind operates, forging them gradually into consistent doctrine, which can be welded on to existing domains of knowledge.*"

This is exactly what has happened with the Preisach model of hysteresis. The origin of this model can be traced back to the paper of F. Preisach "On the Magnetic Aftereffect" [18] published in 1935, where the idea of the hysteresis model is briefly outlined. Its English translation has recently appeared in [19]. This paper dealt exclusively with magnetic hysteresis. For this reason, the Preisach model was long regarded as a physical model. It was primarily known in the area of magnetics, where it was the focus of considerable research for many years [20]–[27]. The first author of this book initially heard about the Preisach paper during his conversation with Professor K. M. Polivanov about 45 years ago.

Somewhat in parallel, the Preisach model was independently discovered and then extensively studied for adsorption hysteresis by D. H. Everett and his collaborators [28]–[31]. This clearly indicated the generality of the Preisach model, and that its applications were not limited to specific areas, such as magnetics and adsorption.

The next step in the development of the Preisach model was made in the late 1970s and the beginning of 1980s. At that time, it was realized in the work of M. Krasnoselskii, A. Pokrovskii and the first author of this book, that the Preisach model contained a new mathematical idea and can be stated without referring to any physical phenomena. As a result, this model was separated from its physical connotation and represented in purely mathematical terms that are similar to the spectral decomposition of operators [32]. In this way, a new mathematical tool has evolved that can now be used for the mathematical description of hysteresis of various physical nature. For instance, this model is widely used in the description and analysis of hysteresis of naturally consolidated rocks, nonlinear elasticity and plasticity, shape memory alloys and piezoelectric materials. In those areas, this model is often referred to as "Preisach-Mayergoyz (PM) space".

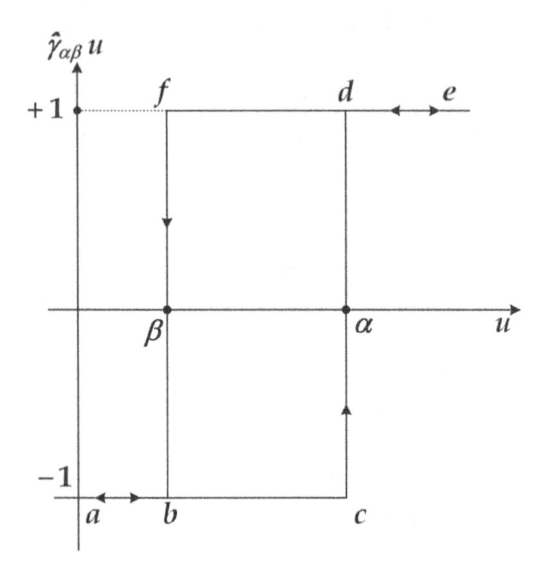

Fig. 1.13

We next proceed to the purely mathematical definition of the Preisach model. To do this, let us consider an infinite set of simplest hysteresis operators $\hat{\gamma}_{\alpha\beta}$. Each of these operators can be represented by a rectangular loop on the input-output diagram (see Fig. 1.13).

Numbers α and β correspond to "up" and "down" switching values of input, respectively. It will be assumed in the sequel that $\alpha \geq \beta$ which is quite natural from the physical point of view. Outputs of the above elementary hysteresis operators may assume only two values, +1 and −1. In other words, these operators can be interpreted as two-position relays with "up" and 'down" positions, respectively,

$$\hat{\gamma}_{\alpha\beta}u(t) = +1 , \tag{1.1}$$

or,

$$\hat{\gamma}_{\alpha\beta}u(t) = -1 . \tag{1.2}$$

As the input, $u(t)$, is monotonically increased, the ascending branch *abcde* is followed. When the input is monotonically decreased, the descending branch *edfba* is traced. It is clear that the operators $\hat{\gamma}_{\alpha\beta}$ represent hysteresis nonlinearities with local memories (see Section 1.1).

Along with the set of operators $\hat{\gamma}_{\alpha\beta}$, consider an arbitrary weight function $\mu(\alpha, \beta)$ that is often referred to as the Preisach function. Then, the

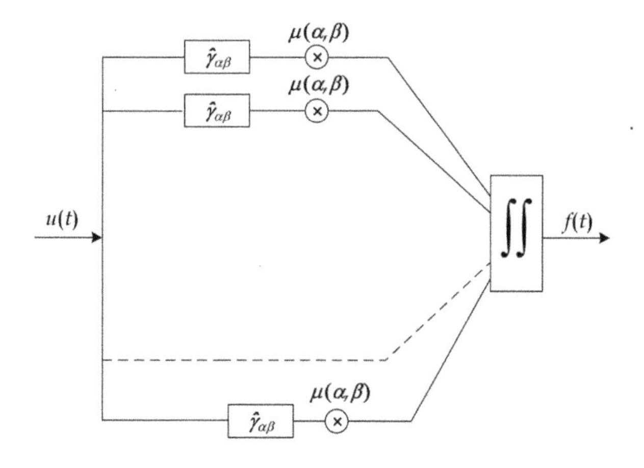

Fig. 1.14

Preisach model can be written as follows:

$$f(t) = \hat{\Gamma}u(t) = \iint\limits_{\alpha \geq \beta} \mu(\alpha, \beta)\hat{\gamma}_{\alpha\beta}u(t)d\alpha d\beta \ . \tag{1.3}$$

Here $\hat{\Gamma}$ is used for the concise notation of the Preisach hysteresis operator that is defined by the integral in (1.3).

It is apparent that the Preisach model (1.3) can be interpreted as a continuous analog of a system of parallely connected two-position relays. This interpretation is illustrated by the block diagram shown in Fig. 1.14. According to this diagram, the same input $u(t)$ is applied to each of two-position relays. Their individual outputs are multiplied by $\mu(\alpha, \beta)$ and then integrated over all appropriate values of α and β. As a result, the output, $f(t)$, is obtained. Discrete approximation to the above block-diagram can be used as device realizations of the Preisach model (1.3).

It is clear from the above discussion that the Preisach model is constructed as a superposition of simplest hysteresis operators $\hat{\gamma}_{\alpha,\beta}$. These operators can be construed as the main building blocks for the model (1.3). The idea that a complicated operator can be represented as a superposition of simplest operators is not entirely new and was exploited before in mathematics, particularly in functional analysis [32]. For instance, according to the spectral decomposition theory for self-adjoint (Hermitian) operators, any self-adjoint operator can be represented as a superposition of projection operators that are, in a way, the simplest self-adjoint operators. The above analogy shows that the Preisach model (1.3) can be interpreted from

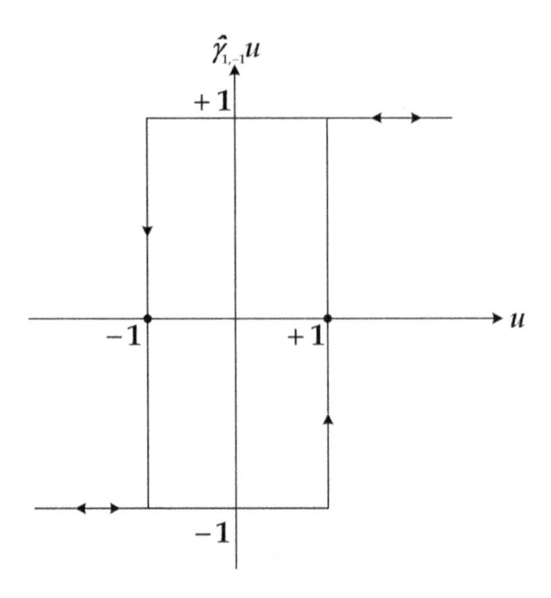

Fig. 1.15

the mathematical point of view as a spectral decomposition of complicated hysteresis operator $\hat{\Gamma}$ into the simplest hysteresis operators $\hat{\gamma}_{\alpha,\beta}$. There is also an interesting parallel between the Preisach model and wavelet transforms which are currently very popular in the area of signal processing. Indeed, all rectangular loop operators $\hat{\gamma}_{\alpha,\beta}$ can be obtained by translating and dilating the rectangular loop operator, $\hat{\gamma}_{1,-1}$, (see Fig. 1.15), that can be regarded as the "mother loop operator." Thus, the Preisach model can be viewed as a "wavelet operator transform."

The Preisach hysteresis nonlinearity (1.3) is constructed as a superposition of elementary hysteresis nonlinearities $\hat{\gamma}_{\alpha,\beta}$ with local memories. Nevertheless, it usually has a nonlocal memory. (This fact will be established in the next section.) It is remarkable that this new qualitative property of nonlocal memory emerges as a collective property of a system of a large number of simple (and qualitatively similar), sparsely interconnected components. This suggests that the emergence of nonlocal memory can be viewed as a connectivity effect.

Having defined the Preisach model, it is appropriate to describe the directions along which the further discussion will proceed. The subsequent discussion in this chapter will be centered around the following five questions.

(1) **How does the Preisach model work? In other words, how does this model detect local input extrema, store them and choose the appropriate branches of hysteresis nonlinearity according to the stored history?**
The answer to this question will reveal the mechanism of memory formation in the Preisach model. It will require the development of a special diagram technique that will constitute the mathematical foundation for the subsequent analysis of the Preisach model. In particular, this diagram technique will reveal the distributed nature of the Preisach model's memory, whose engrams (i.e., memory traces) can be clearly identified.

(2) **What experimental data are needed for the determination of the Preisach function, $\mu(\alpha, \beta)$, for a given hysteresis transducer (device)?**
This is the so-called identification problem. The solution to this problem is very important as far as the practical applications of the Preisach model are concerned.

(3) **What are the necessary and sufficient conditions for the representation of actual hysteresis nonlinearities by the Preisach model?**
The significance of this problem is that its solution will clearly establish the limits on applicability of the Preisach model.

(4) **How can the Preisach model be implemented numerically?**
This is an important question because it seems at first that the numerical evaluation of two-dimensional integrals is required for the numerical implementation of the Preisach model. However, it will be shown that the evaluation of the above integrals can be completely avoided.

(5) **How can the Preisach model be useful for the computation of hysteresis energy dissipation?**
It is well known that the hysteresis energy dissipation can be easily evaluated for the case of periodic (cyclic) input variations. However, the problem of computing hysteresis energy losses for arbitrary (not necessarily periodic) input variations has remained unsolved. It will be shown in this chapter (see Section 1.5) that the Preisach model can bring about the solution of this problem. This can be useful for the computation of entropy production and, in this way, may facilitate the development of irreversible thermodynamics of hysteretic media.

There is another problem which has not been mentioned above

but has been extensively studied by mathematicians M. Krasnoselskii, A. Pokrovskii, A. Visintin and M. Brokate, and their colleagues. This problem is related to the fact that hysteresis nonlinearities are naturally defined on the set of continuous and piecewise monotonic inputs. However, the above set of functions does not form a complete function space. This constitutes the main difficulty as far as the rigorous mathematical treatment of differential (or integral) equations with hysteresis nonlinearities is concerned. Thus, the problem of continuous extension of hysteresis operators from the above set of piecewise monotonic inputs to some complete function spaces presents itself. The essence of this problem is in the finding of such complete function spaces. The solution to this problem is important because these function spaces form the natural "environment" for the rigorous mathematical study of equations with hysteresis nonlinearities. Nevertheless, this problem is by and large of purely mathematical nature. It is not directly related to applications, and for this reason will not be discussed in the book. The reader interested in the discussion of this problem is referred to the book of Krasnoselskii and Pokrovskii [33] as well as to more recent publications [34]–[38].

It is apparent from the above discussion that the Preisach model has been defined without any reference to a particular physical origin of hysteresis. This clearly reveals the phenomenological nature of the model and its mathematical generality. This suggests that it can be used for the description of hysteresis of any physical nature, including hysteresis in neural systems.

1.3 Diagram Technique and the Basic Properties of the Preisach Model

The mathematical analysis of the Preisach model is considerably facilitated by its geometric interpretation. This interpretation is based on the following simple fact. There is the one-to-one correspondence between operators $\hat{\gamma}_{\alpha,\beta}$ and points (α, β) of the half-plane $\alpha \geq \beta$ (see Fig. 1.16). In other words, each point of the half-plane $\alpha \geq \beta$ can be identified with only one particular $\hat{\gamma}$-operator whose "up" and "down" switching values are respectively equal to α and β coordinates of the point. It is clear that this identification is possible because both $\hat{\gamma}_{\alpha,\beta}$ operators and the points of the half-plane $\alpha \geq \beta$ are uniquely defined by pairs of numbers, α and β.

Consider a right triangle T (see Fig. 1.16). Its hypotenuse is a part of the line $\alpha = \beta$, while the vertex of its right angle has the coordinates α_0

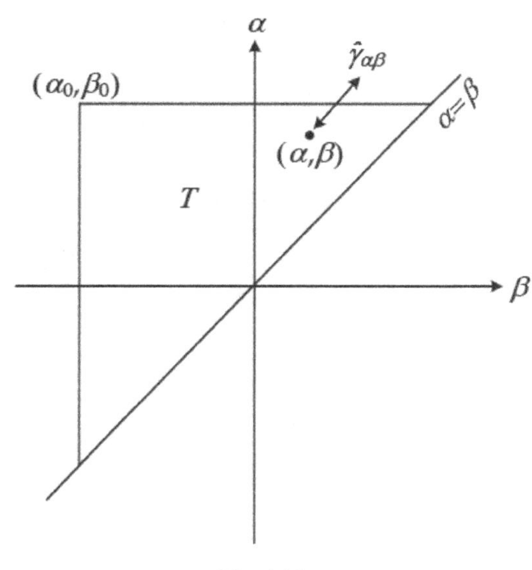

Fig. 1.16

and β_0 with $\beta_0 = -\alpha_0$. In the sequel, this triangle will be called the limiting triangle and the case when $\mu(\alpha, \beta)$ is a finite function with a support within T will be discussed. This means that, it will be assumed that the function $\mu(\alpha, \beta)$ is equal to zero outside the triangle T. This case covers the important class of hysteresis nonlinearities with closed major loops. At the same time, the above case will not essentially limit the generality of our future discussions.

To start the discussion, we first assume that the input $u(t)$ at some instant of time t_0 has the value that is less than β_0. Then, the outputs of all $\hat{\gamma}$-operators which correspond to the points of the triangle T are equal to -1. In other words, all $\hat{\gamma}$-operators are in the "down" position. This corresponds to the state of "negative saturation" of the hysteresis nonlinearity represented by the model (1.3).

Now, we assume that the input is monotonically increased until it reaches at time t_1 some maximum value u_1. As the input is being increased, all $\hat{\gamma}$-operators with "up" switching values α less than the current input value $u(t)$ are being turned into the "up" position. This means that their outputs become equal to $+1$. Geometrically, it leads to the subdivision of the triangle T into two sets: $S^+(t)$ consisting of points (α, β) for which the corresponding $\hat{\gamma}$-operators are in the "up" position, and $S^-(t)$ consisting of points (α, β) such that the corresponding $\hat{\gamma}$-operators are still

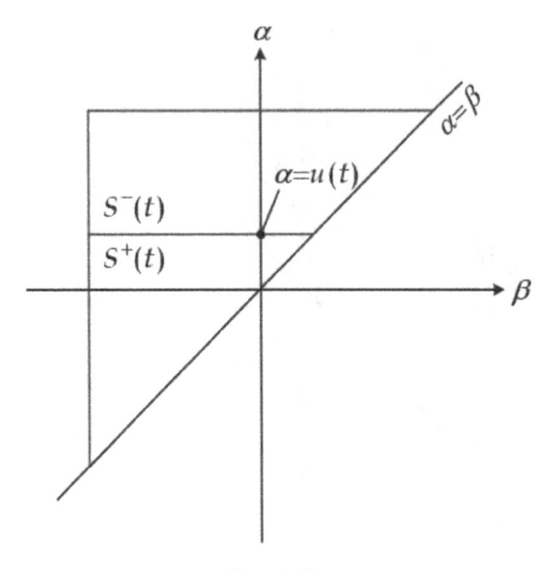

Fig. 1.17

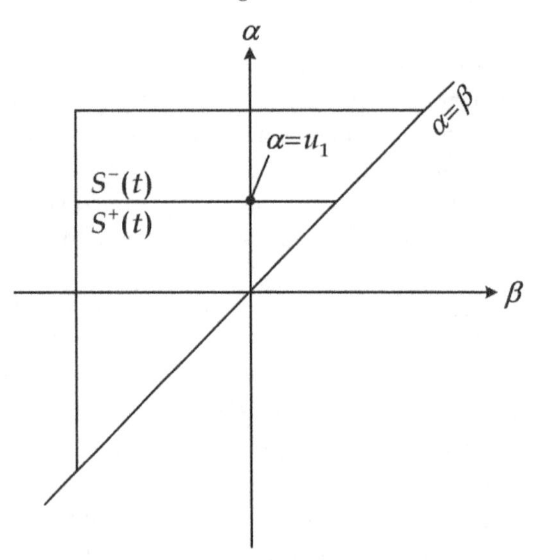

Fig. 1.18

in the "down" position. This subdivision is made by the line $\alpha = u(t)$ (see Fig. 1.17) that moves upwards as the input is being increased. This upward motion is terminated when the input reaches the maximum value u_1. The subdivision of the triangle T into $S^+(t)$ and $S^-(t)$ is shown in Fig. 1.18.

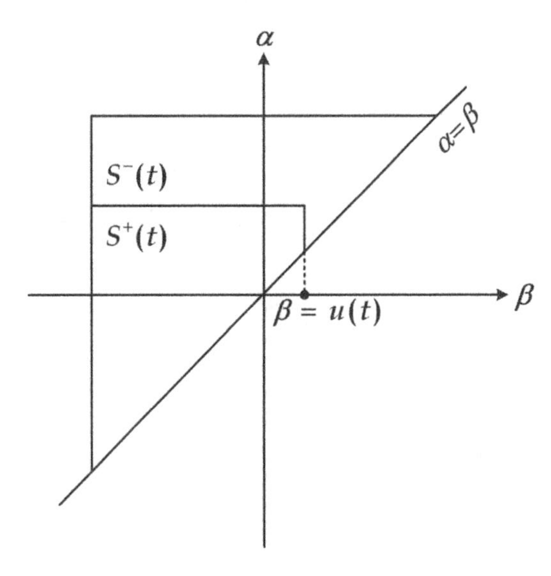

Fig. 1.19

Next, we assume that the input is monotonically decreased until it reaches at time t_2 some minimum value u_2. As the input is being decreased, all $\hat{\gamma}$-operators with "down" switching values β above the current input value, $u(t)$, are being turned back into the "down" position. This changes the previous subdivision of T into positive and negative sets. Indeed, the interface $L(t)$ between $S^+(t)$ and $S^-(t)$ has now two links, the horizontal and vertical ones. The vertical link moves from right to left and its motion is specified by the equation $\beta = u(t)$. This is illustrated by Fig. 1.19. The above motion of the vertical link is terminated when the input reaches its minimum value u_2. The subdivision of the triangle T for this particular instant of time is shown in Fig. 1.20. The vertex of the interface $L(t)$ at the above instant of time has the coordinates $\alpha = u_1$ and $\beta = u_2$.

Now, we assume that the input is increased again until it reaches at time t_3 some maximum value u_3 that is less than u_1. Geometrically, this increase results in the formation of a new horizontal link of $L(t)$ which moves upwards. This upward motion is terminated when the maximum u_3 is reached. This is shown in Fig. 1.21.

Next, we assume that the input is decreased again until it reaches at time t_4 some minimum value u_4 that is above u_2. Geometrically, this input

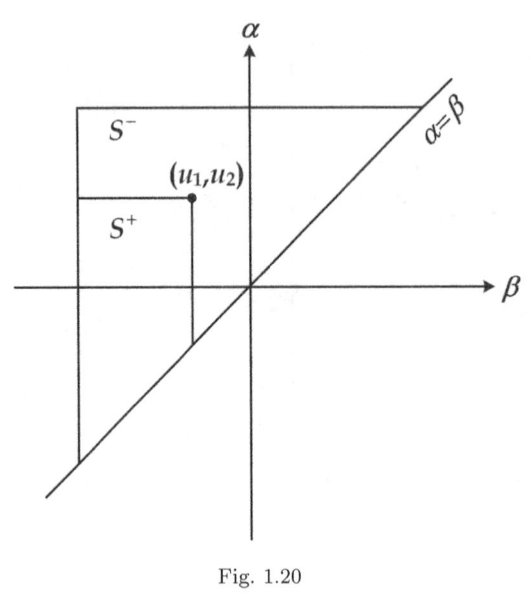

Fig. 1.20

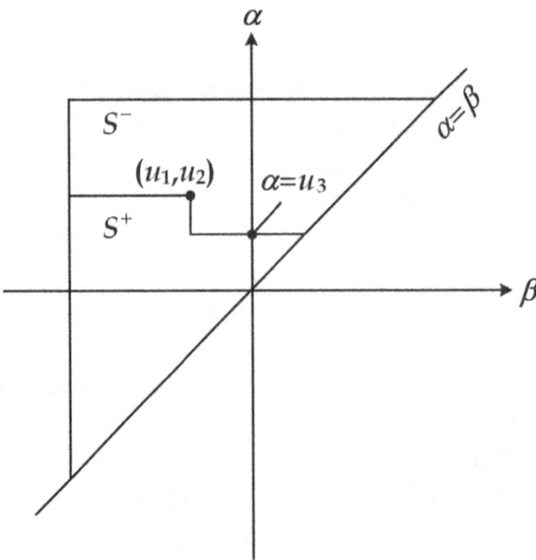

Fig. 1.21

variation results in the formation of a new vertical link that moves from right to left. This motion is terminated as the input reaches its minimum value u_4. As a result, a new vertex of $L(t)$ is formed that has the coordinates $\alpha = u_3$ and $\beta = u_4$. This is illustrated by Fig. 1.22.

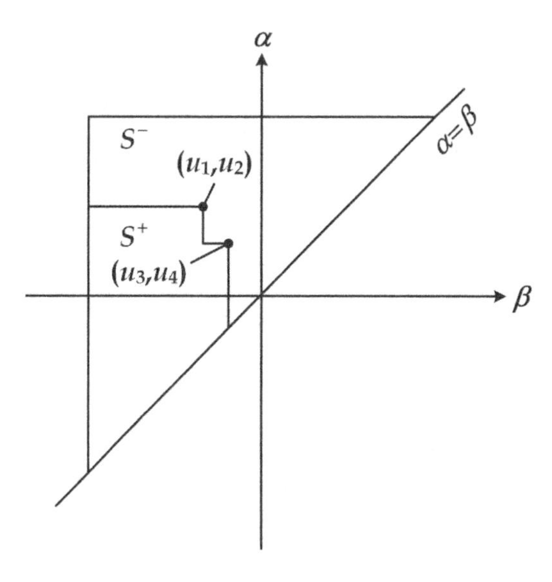

Fig. 1.22

By generalizing the previous analysis, the following conclusion can be reached. At any instant of time, the triangle T is subdivided into two sets: $S^+(t)$ consisting of points (α, β) for which the corresponding $\hat{\gamma}$-operators are in the "up" position, and $S^-(t)$ consisting of points for which the corresponding $\hat{\gamma}$-operators are in the "down" position. The interface $L(t)$ between $S^+(t)$ and $S^-(t)$ is a staircase line whose vertices have α and β coordinates coinciding respectively with local maxima and minima of input at past instants of time. The final link of $L(t)$ is attached to the line $\alpha = \beta$ and it moves when the input is changed. This link is a horizontal one and it moves upwards as the input is increased (see Fig. 1.23). The final link is a vertical one and it moves from right to left as the input is decreased (see Fig. 1.24).

Thus, at any instant of time the integral in formula (1.3) can be subdivided into two integrals, over $S^+(t)$ and $S^-(t)$, respectively:

$$f(t) = \hat{\Gamma}u(t) = \iint\limits_{S^+(t)} \mu(\alpha, \beta)\hat{\gamma}_{\alpha,\beta}u(t)d\alpha d\beta + \iint\limits_{S^-(t)} \mu(\alpha, \beta)\hat{\gamma}_{\alpha,\beta}u(t)d\alpha d\beta. \tag{1.4}$$

Since,

$$\hat{\gamma}_{\alpha,\beta}u(t) = +1, \quad \text{if } (\alpha, \beta) \in S^+(t) \tag{1.5}$$

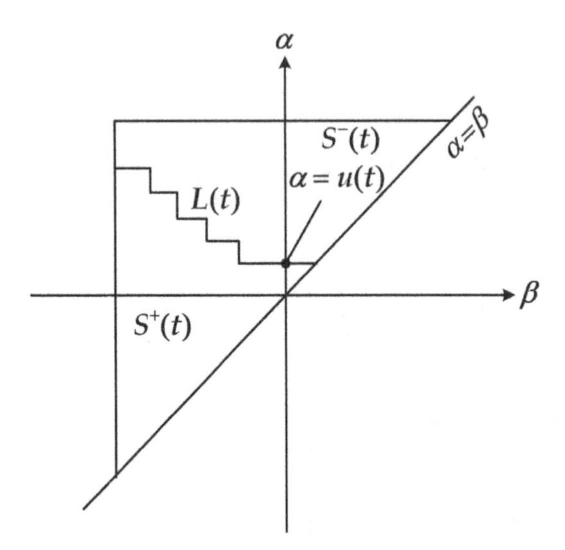

Fig. 1.23

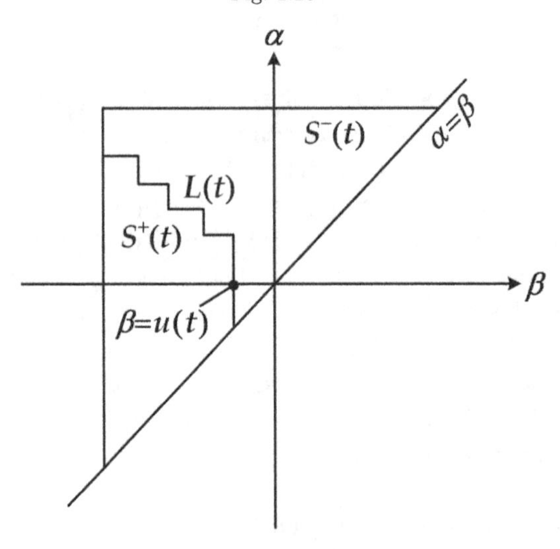

Fig. 1.24

and

$$\hat{\gamma}_{\alpha,\beta} u(t) = -1, \quad \text{if } (\alpha, \beta) \in S^-(t), \tag{1.6}$$

from formula (1.4) we find

$$f(t) = \iint_{S^+(t)} \mu(\alpha, \beta) d\alpha d\beta - \iint_{S^-(t)} \mu(\alpha, \beta) d\alpha d\beta. \tag{1.7}$$

From the above expression, it follows that an instantaneous value of output depends on a particular subdivision of the limiting triangle T into positive and negative sets $S^+(t)$ and $S^-(t)$. This subdivision is determined by a particular shape of the interface $L(t)$. This shape, in turn, depends on the past extremum values of input because these extremum values are the coordinates of the vertices of $L(t)$. Consequently, the past extremum values of input shape the staircase interface, $L(t)$, and in this way they leave their mark upon the future.

To make the above point perfectly clear, consider two inputs $u_1(t)$ and $u_2(t)$ with two different past histories for $t < t'$. This means that they had different local extrema for $t < t'$. It is next assumed that these inputs coincide for $t \geq t'$. Then according to formula (1.7), the outputs $f_1(t)$ and $f_2(t)$ corresponding to the above inputs are given by the formulas:

$$f_1(t) = \iint\limits_{S_1^+(t)} \mu(\alpha,\beta)d\alpha d\beta - \iint\limits_{S_1^-(t)} \mu(\alpha,\beta)d\alpha d\beta \tag{1.8}$$

$$f_2(t) = \iint\limits_{S_2^+(t)} \mu(\alpha,\beta)d\alpha d\beta - \iint\limits_{S_2^-(t)} \mu(\alpha,\beta)d\alpha d\beta \ , \tag{1.9}$$

where $S_1^+(t)$ and $S_1^-(t)$, $S_2^+(t)$ and $S_2^-(t)$ are positive and negative sets of two subdivisions of T associated with $u_1(t)$ and $u_2(t)$, respectively.

The above two subdivisions are different because they correspond to two different input histories. Thus, from formulas (1.8) and (1.9) we conclude that

$$f_1(t) \neq f_2(t) \text{ for } t > t'. \tag{1.10}$$

It is clear that the inequality (1.10) holds even if the outputs $f_1(t')$ and $f_2(t')$ are somehow the same at t'. This means that the Preisach model (1.3) describes, in general, hysteresis nonlinearities with nonlocal (non-Markovian) memories.

The above discussion reveals the mechanism of memory formation in the Preisach model. The memory is formed as a result of two different rules for the modification of the interface $L(t)$. Indeed, for a monotonically increasing input, we have a horizontal final link of $L(t)$ moving upwards, while for a monotonically decreasing input, we have a vertical final link of $L(t)$ moving from right to left. These two different rules result in the formation of the staircase interface, $L(t)$, whose vertices have coordinates equal to past input extrema.

It is apparent from the previous analysis that the Preisach model can be defined in purely geometric terms, without any reference to the analytical definition (1.3). Indeed, the formula (1.7), along with the above two rules for the modification of $L(t)$, can be interpreted as an independent definition of the Preisach model. This definition is fully equivalent to the previous one. However, the geometric definition may be convenient for further generalization of the Preisach model. For instance, new and more general rules for the subdivision of T into positive and negative sets, $S^+(t)$ and $S^-(t)$, may be introduced. In these rules, the links of $L(t)$ may not necessarily be the segments of straight lines parallel to coordinate axes. Furthermore, different functions $\mu^+(\alpha, \beta)$ and $\mu^-(\alpha, \beta)$ may be defined on the positive and negative sets, respectively. All these modifications may result in some meaningful generalizations of the Preisach model. However, the above possibilities have not been examined enough in the existing literature.

Having described the geometric interpretation of the Preisach model, we are now well equipped for the discussion of the main properties of this model. We begin with the simplest property which expresses the fact that the output value, f^+, in the state of positive saturation is equal to the minus output value, $-f^-$, in the state of negative saturation. In the state of positive saturation, the input $u(t)$ is more than α_0 and all the $\hat{\gamma}$-operators are in the "up" position. Hence, according to formula (1.7), we find:

$$f^+ = \iint_T \mu(\alpha, \beta) d\alpha d\beta. \tag{1.11}$$

Similarly, in the state of negative saturation the input $u(t)$ is less than β_0 and all $\hat{\gamma}$-operators are in the "down" position. As a result, we obtain

$$f^- = -\iint_T \mu(\alpha, \beta) d\alpha d\beta. \tag{1.12}$$

From formulas (1.11) and (1.12), we have

$$f^+ = -f^-. \tag{1.13}$$

It is important to keep in mind that the saturation values f^+ and f^- remain constant for any value of input $u(t)$ above α_0 and below β_0, respectively. In other words, after ascending and descending branches merge together, they become flat. Partly for this reason, it is often said that the Preisach model does not describe reversible components of hysteresis nonlinearities. These components are regarded as being responsible for finite slopes of ascending and descending branches after they merge together. The inability of the Preisach model to describe the reversible components of hysteresis nonlinearities has long been viewed as a deficiency of the model. It will be shown later in the book that this deficiency along with some others can be removed by the appropriate generalization of the Preisach model.

We next proceed to the more interesting property which further elucidates the mechanism of memory formation in the Preisach model. It turns out that this model does not accumulate all past extremum values of input. Some of them can be erased by subsequent input variations. To make this property clear, consider a particular past history that is characterized by a finite decreasing sequence $\{u_1,\ u_3,\ u_5,\ u_7\}$ of local input maxima and an increasing sequence $\{u_2,\ u_4,\ u_6,\ u_8\}$ of local input minima. A typical $\alpha-\beta$ diagram for this kind of history is shown in Fig. 1.25. Now, we assume that the input $u(t)$ is monotonically increased until it reaches some maximum u_9 that is above u_3. This monotonic increase of input $u(t)$ results in the formation of a horizontal final link of $L(t)$ that moves upwards until the maximum value u_9 is reached. This results in a modified $\alpha - \beta$ diagram shown in Fig. 1.26. It is evident that all vertices whose α-coordinates were below u_9 have been erased. It is also clear that the erasure of vertices is equivalent to the erasing of the memory associated with these vertices. Namely, the past input maxima and minima that were respectively equal to α-and β-coordinates of the erased vertices have been erased. We have illustrated how the erasure of vertices occurs for monotonically increasing inputs. However, it is obvious that the erasure of vertices may occur in a similar manner for monotonically decreasing inputs as well. Thus, we can formulate the following property of the Preisach model.

ERASURE PROPERTY *Each local input maximum erases the vertices of $L(t)$ whose α-coordinates are below this maximum, and each local minimum erases the vertices whose β-coordinates are above this minimum.*

The erasure property is asserted above in purely geometric terms. This makes this property quite transparent. However, the same property can also be described in analytical terms. The analytical formulation complements the geometric one because it is directly phrased in terms of time input variations.

Consider a particular input variation shown in Fig. 1.27 for the time interval $t_0 \leq t \leq t'$. We assume that at the initial instant of time t_0 the input value $u(t_0)$ was below β_0. This means that the initial state is the state of negative saturation. Consequently, the whole history (i.e., memory) has been written by the input variations after time t_0. We would like to specify

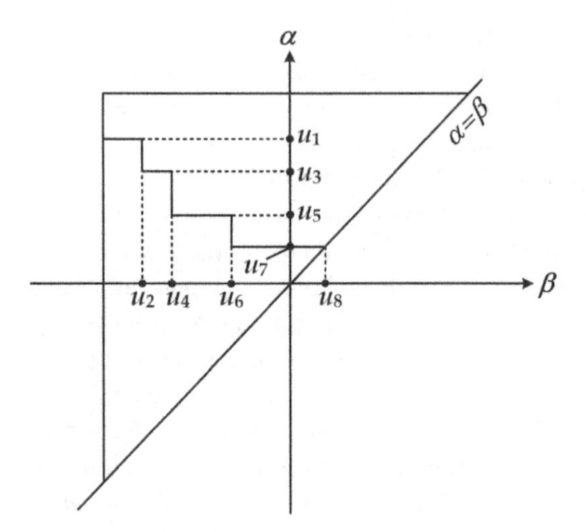

Fig. 1.25

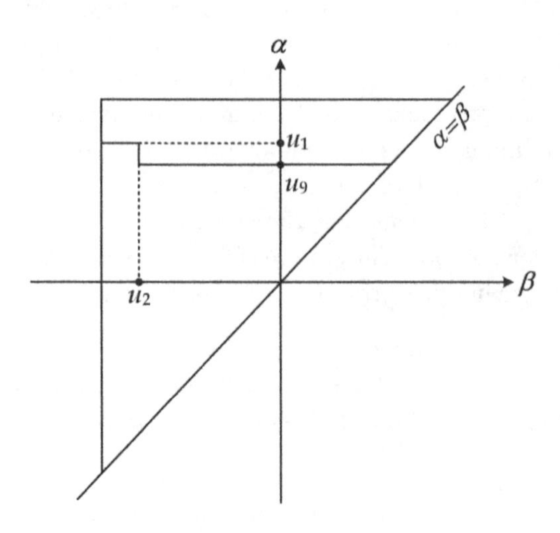

Fig. 1.26

explicitly local input extrema that will be stored by the Preisach model at time $t^{'}$. Consider the global maximum of the input at the time interval $[t_0, t^{'}]$. We will use the notations M_1 for this maximum and t_1^+ for the instant of time the maximum was reached:

$$M_1 = u(t_1^+) = \max_{[t_0, t^{'}]} u(t). \tag{1.14}$$

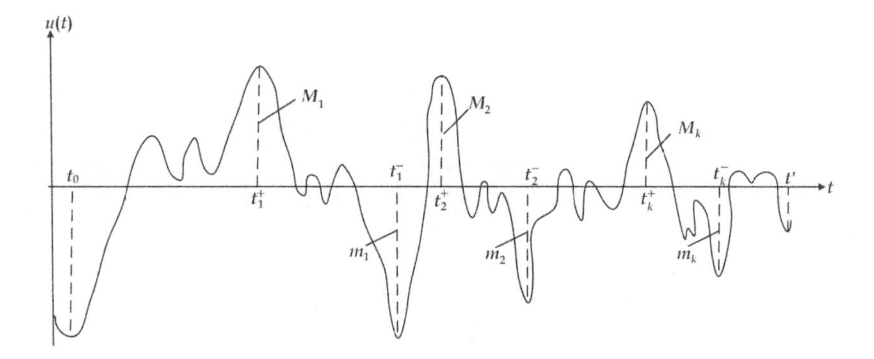

Fig. 1.27

It is clear that all previous input extrema were erased by this maximum. Now, consider the global minimum of the input at the interval $[t_1^+, t']$. We will use the notation m_1 for this minimum and t_1^- for the time it was reached:

$$m_1 = u(t_1^-) = \min_{[t_1^+, t']} u(t). \tag{1.15}$$

It is apparent that all intermediate input extrema that occurred between t_1^+ and t_1^- were erased by the minimum m_1.

Next, consider the global maximum of the input at the interval $[t_1^-, t']$. The notations M_2 and t_2^+ are appropriate for this maximum and the time it occurred, respectively:

$$M_2 = u(t_2^+) = \max_{[t_1^-, t']} u(t). \tag{1.16}$$

It is obvious that this maximum erased all intermediate input extrema that occurred between t_1^- and t_2^+. As before, consider the global minimum of input at the time interval $[t_2^+, t']$, and the notations m_2 and t_2^- will be used for this minimum and the time it was achieved:

$$m_2 = u(t_2^-) = \min_{[t_2^+, t']} u(t). \tag{1.17}$$

It is clear that this minimum erased all intermediate input extrema.

Continuing the above line of reasoning, we can inductively introduce the global maxima M_k and global minima m_k:

$$M_k = u(t_k^+) = \max_{[t_{k-1}^-, t']} u(t) \tag{1.18}$$

and

$$m_k = u(t_k^-) = \min_{[t_k^+, t']} u(t). \tag{1.19}$$

Only these input extrema were accumulated by the Preisach model, while all intermediate input extrema were erased. It is natural to say that M_k and m_k $(k = 1, 2, \dots)$ form a sequence of alternating dominant maxima and minima.

It is evident from the above analysis that α- and β-coordinates of vertices of the interface $L(t')$ are equal to M_k and m_k, respectively. It is also clear that the sequence of alternating dominant extrema is modified with time. This means that new dominant extrema can be introduced by the time varying input, while the previous ones can be erased. In other words, M_k and m_k are functions of t' as it is clearly suggested by their definitions (1.18) and (1.19).

Now, the erasure property can be stated in the following form.

ERASURE PROPERTY *Only the sequence of alternating dominant input extrema are stored by the Preisach model. All other input extrema are erased.*

It is worth noting that the erasure property is in some sense natural and consistent with experimental facts. Indeed, experiments in the area of magnetics show the existence of major hysteresis loops whose shapes do not depend on how these loops were traced. In other words, the major hysteresis loops are well-defined. It means that any past history is erased by input oscillations of sufficiently large magnitude. This is in complete agreement with the erasure property.

Consider another characteristic property of the Preisach model that is valid for periodic input variations. Let $u_1(t)$ and $u_2(t)$ be two inputs that may have different past histories (different alternating series of dominant extrema). However, starting from some instant of time t_0, these inputs vary back and forth between the same two consecutive extremum values, u_+ and u_-. It can be shown that these periodic input variations result in minor hysteresis loops. Let Figs. 1.28 and 1.29 represent $\alpha - \beta$ diagrams for the inputs $u_1(t)$ and $u_2(t)$, respectively. As the inputs vary back and forth between u_+ and u_-, the final links of staircase interfaces $L_1(t)$ and $L_2(t)$, move within the identical triangles T_1 and T_2. This results in periodic shape variations for $L_1(t)$ and $L_2(t)$ which in turn produce periodic variations of the outputs, $f_1(t)$ and $f_2(t)$. This means that some minor hysteresis loops are traced in the $f - u$ diagram for both inputs (see Fig. 1.30). The positions

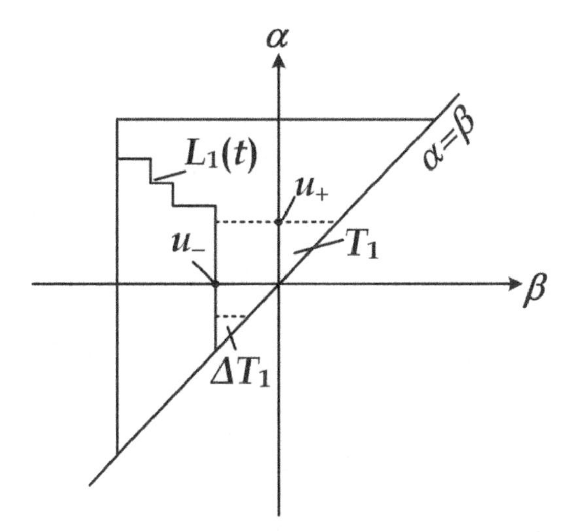

Fig. 1.28

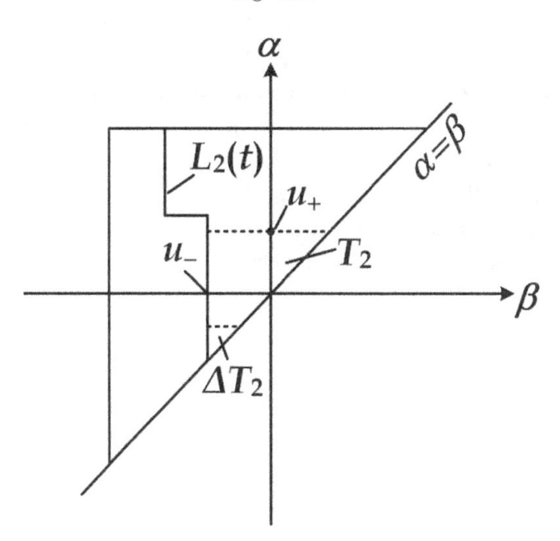

Fig. 1.29

of these two loops with respect to the f-axis are different. This is because the above two inputs have different past histories that lead to different shapes for staircase interfaces, $L_1(t)$ and $L_2(t)$. As a result, the values of outputs for the same values of inputs are different. This is easily seen from the formula (1.7). However, it can be proved that the above two hysteresis

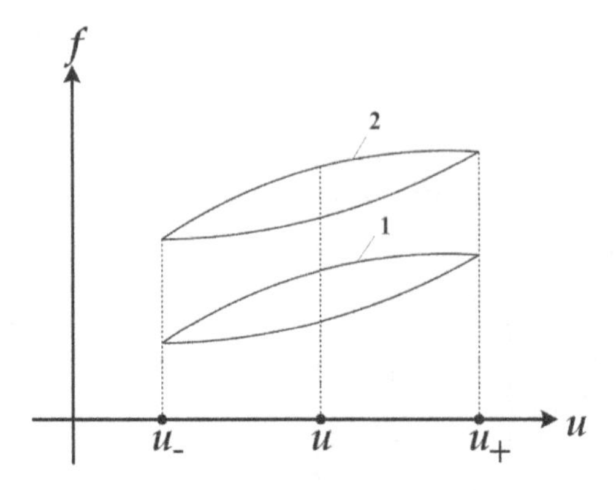

Fig. 1.30

loops are congruent. It means that the coincidence of these loops can be achieved by the appropriate translation of these loops along the f-axis

The proof of the congruency of the above loops is equivalent to showing that any equal increments of inputs $u_1(t)$ and $u_2(t)$ result in equal increments of outputs $f_1(t)$ and $f_2(t)$. To this end, let us assume that both inputs after achieving the same minimum value u_- are increased by the same amount: $\Delta u_1 = \Delta u_2 = \Delta u$. As a result of these increases, the identical triangles ΔT_1 and ΔT_2 are added to the positive sets $S_1^+(t)$ and $S_2^+(t)$ and subtracted from the negative sets $S_1^-(t)$ and $S_2^-(t)$ (see Figs. 1.28 and 1.29). Now, using the formula (1.7), we find that the corresponding output increments are given by formulas

$$\Delta f_1 = 2 \iint_{\Delta T_1} \mu(\alpha, \beta) d\alpha d\beta \tag{1.20}$$

$$\Delta f_2 = 2 \iint_{\Delta T_2} \mu(\alpha, \beta) d\alpha d\beta. \tag{1.21}$$

Since $\Delta T_1 = \Delta T_2$ we conclude

$$\Delta f_1 = \Delta f_2. \tag{1.22}$$

The equality (1.22) has been proved for the case when inputs $u_1(t)$ and $u_2(t)$ are monotonically increased by the same amount after achieving the same minimum value u_-. Thus, this equality means the congruency for the ascending branches of the above minor loops. By literally repeating the previous reasoning, we can prove that the same equality (1.22) holds when the inputs $u_1(t)$ and $u_2(t)$ are monotonically decreased by the same amount Δu after achieving the maximum value u^+. This means that the descending branches of the above minor loops are congruent as well. Thus, we have established the following property of the Preisach model.

CONGRUENCY PROPERTY *All minor hysteresis loops corresponding to back-and-forth variations of inputs between the same two consecutive extremum values are congruent.*

We conclude this section with a remark on the possible applications of the Preisach model beyond the area of hysteresis modelling. It is clear from the previous discussion that the Preisach model has the ability to detect, extract and store the alternating series of dominant extrema of input. In this sense, the Preisach model is endowed with memory. For this reason, the Preisach model might have an appeal as a mathematical model of memory with some interesting properties, and its (discrete) device realization (see Fig. 1.14) might be utilized as an unusual storage device. We will discuss below only a few peculiarities of this memory.

First, the mechanism of memory formation in the Preisach model is quite simple and results from the parallel connection of qualitatively similar but quantitatively different elements (two-position cells) $\hat{\gamma}_{\alpha\beta}$. Since this model employs very simple elements and has little structure, its memory formation can be interpreted as a connectivity effect.

Second, storage of information is not localized. Indeed, the model (1.3) stores the information (extremum values of input) not in particular separate cells (as in the case of computer storage devices), but some ensembles of the cells $\hat{\gamma}_{\alpha\beta}$ participate in storage of each bit of information. As a result, if some of the cells are destroyed, the stored information might still be preserved.

The fact that the Preisach-model based storage does not require identical storage elements suggests that this type of storage may find applications in future computer systems. Indeed, relentless process of miniaturization has resulted in the transition of digital electronic devices from microscale to nanoscale. It is well known that nanoscale devices will be very susceptible to random dopant fluctuations [39] that occur due to random nature of ion implantation and diffusion. These random dopant fluctuations lead to fabrication deviations that are strongly pronounced at the nanoscale and which appreciably affect the characteristics of digital semiconductor devices. This makes the production of almost identical storage elements very expensive and probably unattainable. This nonidentical property of digital devices is detrimental to the existing principles of computer storage, whereas this nonidentical nature of storage elements is beneficial to Preisach storage. It is actually at the very foundation of this storage. It is also apparent that the stored information must be represented as sequences of alternating dominant maxima and minima to be suitable for Preisach storage without any erasure, i.e. without any information loss. Such representation requires special formatting of the data subject to storage. This matter will be further discussed in Chapter 3.

Finally, it is clear that in the Preisach model very simple (parallel) connectivity of rectangular loop elements $\hat{\gamma}_{\alpha\beta}$ results in nonlocal distributed memory storage. It is also evident that the staircase interface $L(t)$ may be regarded as an **"engram"** (i.e. memory trace) of this distributed storage. This point will be discussed in detail in Chapter 3, which deals with Preisach models of neural memory.

1.4 Identification Problem, FORCs and Representation Theorem

Now, we proceed to the discussion of the identification problem for the Preisach model. The essence of this problem is the determination of the weight function $\mu(\alpha, \beta)$. The set of first-order reversal curves (FORCs) will be used for this purpose. These curves can be defined as follows. First, the input $u(t)$ should be decreased to a value that is less than β_0. This brings a hysteresis nonlinearly to the state of negative saturation. Next, the input is monotonically increased until it reaches some value α'. The corresponding $\alpha - \beta$ diagram is shown in Fig. 1.31. As the input is increased, an ascending branch of a major loop is followed (see Fig. 1.32). This branch will also be called the limiting ascending branch because there is no branch below it. The notation $f_{\alpha'}$ will be used for the output value on this branch that corresponds to the input value $u = \alpha'$. A first-order reversal curve is formed as the above monotonic increase of the input is followed by a subsequent monotonic decrease. The term "first-order" is used to emphasize the fact that each of these curves is formed after the first reversal of input. The notation $f_{\alpha'\beta'}$ will be used for the output value on the reversal curve attached to the limiting ascending branch at the point $f_{\alpha'}$. This output value corresponds to the input value $u = \beta'$ (see Fig. 1.32). The above monotonic decrease of input modifies the previous $\alpha - \beta$ diagram shown in Fig. 1.31. A new $\alpha - \beta$ diagram for the instant of time when the input reaches the value β' is illustrated by Fig. 1.33.

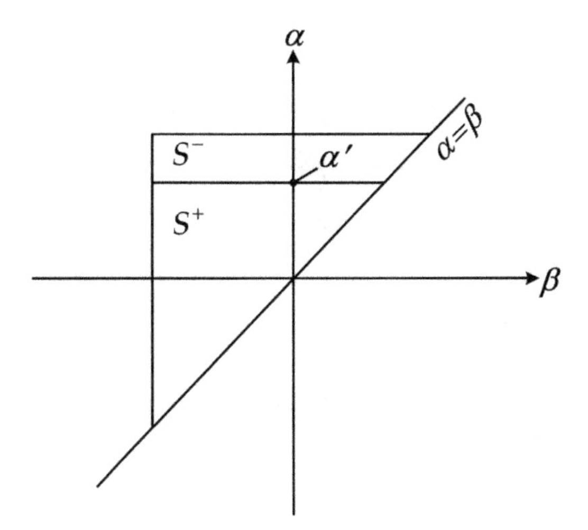

Fig. 1.31

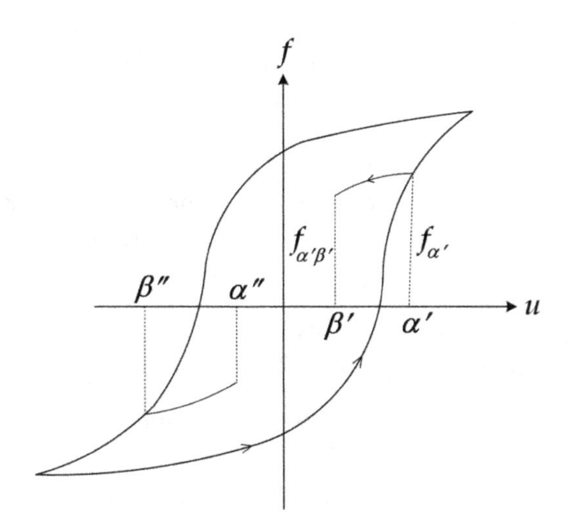

Fig. 1.32

Now, we define the function:

$$F\left(\alpha',\beta'\right) = \frac{1}{2}\left(f_{\alpha'} - f_{\alpha'\beta'}\right). \tag{1.23}$$

This function is equal to one-half of the output increments along the first-order reversal curves. The next step is to express this function in terms of

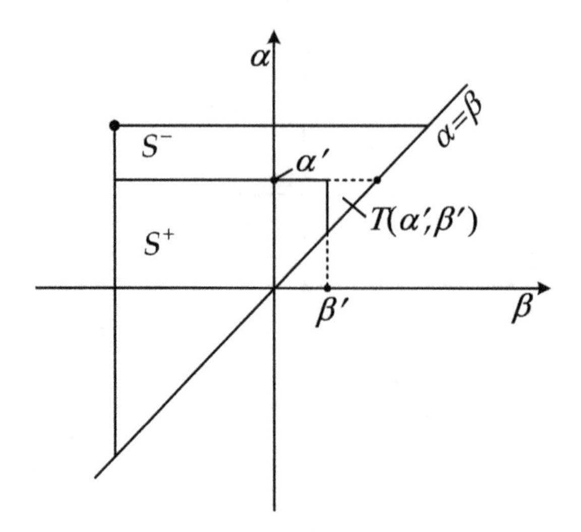

Fig. 1.33

the Preisach function $\mu(\alpha,\beta)$. To this end, we compare the $\alpha-\beta$ diagrams shown in Figs. 1.31 and 1.33. It is clear from these diagrams that the triangle $T(\alpha',\beta')$ is added to the negative set S^- and subtracted from the positive set S^+ as a result of the monotonic input decrease from the value $u=\alpha'$ to the value $u=\beta'$. Using the above fact and the formula (1.7), we find that the Preisach model will match the output increments along the first-order reversal curves if the function $\mu(\alpha,\beta)$ satisfies the equation

$$f_{\alpha'} - f_{\alpha'\beta'} = 2 \iint_{T(\alpha',\beta')} \mu(\alpha,\beta)\,d\alpha\,d\beta. \tag{1.24}$$

By comparing formulas (1.23) and (1.24), we obtain

$$F(\alpha',\beta') = \iint_{T(\alpha',\beta')} \mu(\alpha,\beta)\,d\alpha\,d\beta. \tag{1.25}$$

The integral over the triangle $T(\alpha',\beta')$ can be written as the following double integral:

$$F(\alpha',\beta') = \int_{\beta'}^{\alpha'} \left(\int_{\beta}^{\alpha'} \mu(\alpha,\beta)\,d\alpha \right) d\beta. \tag{1.26}$$

By differentiating the last expression twice (first with respect to β' and then with respect to α'), we find:

$$\mu(\alpha',\beta') = -\frac{\partial^2 F(\alpha',\beta')}{\partial\alpha'\,\partial\beta'}. \tag{1.27}$$

Invoking (1.23), the expression (1.27) can be written in another equivalent form:

$$\mu(\alpha', \beta') = \frac{1}{2} \frac{\partial^2 f_{\alpha' \beta'}}{\partial \alpha' \partial \beta'}. \tag{1.28}$$

The formula (1.28) allows for a simple geometric interpretation of the function $\mu(\alpha', \beta')$. Indeed, for the first derivative of $f_{\alpha' \beta'}$ with respect to β' we have

$$\frac{\partial f_{\alpha' \beta'}}{\partial \beta'} = \tan \theta(\alpha', \beta'), \tag{1.29}$$

where $\theta(\alpha', \beta')$ is the angle between the axis u and the tangent to the first-order reversal curve $f_{\alpha' \beta'}$ at the point $u = \beta'$.

From (1.28) and (1.29), we find

$$\mu(\alpha', \beta') = \frac{1}{2} \frac{\partial \tan \theta(\alpha', \beta')}{\partial \alpha'}. \tag{1.30}$$

From (1.30), we conclude that the Preisach function $\mu(\alpha', \beta')$ is positive if $\tan \theta(\alpha', \beta')$ is a monotonically increasing function of α' for any fixed β'. The last condition is satisfied if all first-order reversal curves are monotonically increasing functions of β', and they do not intersect inside the major loop but merge together at the point where the descending and ascending branches of the major loop meet one another (see Fig. 1.34). To secure the above merge of first-order reversal curves, $\tan \theta(\alpha', \beta')$ should increase as a function of α' for any fixed β' in order to compensate for larger values $f_{\alpha' \beta'}$. It is worthwhile noting that the function $\mu(\alpha', \beta')$ is often treated as a distribution function with some statistical connotation. For this reason, this function is tacitly assumed to be positive. In our treatment, the last property is directly related to experimental facts.

For positive $\mu(\alpha, \beta)$, $F(\alpha', \beta')$ is a monotonically increasing function of α' for any fixed β' and a monotonically decreasing function of β' for any fixed α'. This follows directly from (1.25).

If the Preisach function is determined from formula (1.28) (or formula (1.27)), then the expression (1.24) is satisfied. This means that the Preisach model matches the output increments along the first-order reversal curves. We next show that this also implies that the first-order reversal curves themselves are matched. To this end, consider the particular case when $\beta' = \beta_0$. For this case, we have

$$f_{\alpha' \beta_0} = f^-. \tag{1.31}$$

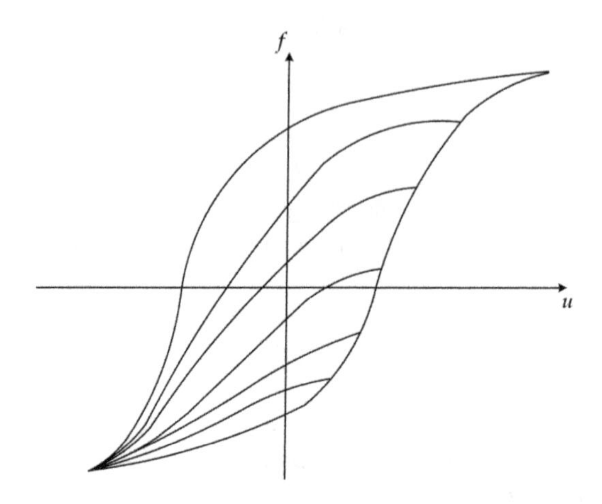

Fig. 1.34

From formulas (1.24) and (1.31), we obtain:

$$f^- - f_{\alpha'} = -2 \iint_{T(\alpha',\beta_0)} \mu(\alpha,\beta)d\alpha d\beta. \tag{1.32}$$

Thus, the Preisach model matches the output increment, $f^- - f_{\alpha'}$, along the limiting ascending branch.

For $\alpha' = \alpha_0$, we have

$$f_{\alpha_0} = f^+. \tag{1.33}$$

From formulas (1.32) and (1.33), we find

$$f^- - f^+ = -2 \iint_T \mu(\alpha,\beta)d\alpha d\beta, \tag{1.34}$$

where $T = T(\alpha_0, \beta_0)$ is the limiting triangle.

Since major hysteresis loops are usually symmetric, the following equality holds:

$$f^+ = -f^- \, . \tag{1.35}$$

From formulas (1.34) and (1.35) we derive:

$$f^- = -\iint_T \mu(\alpha,\beta)d\alpha d\beta \, . \tag{1.36}$$

This means that the Preisach model matches the output value in the state of negative saturation. From the last fact and formula (1.32), we conclude

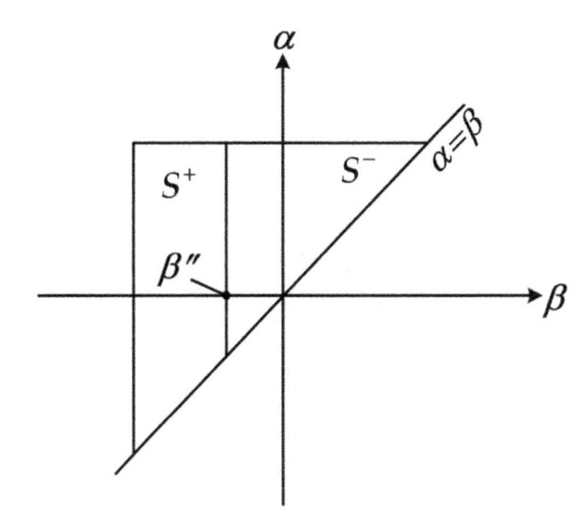

Fig. 1.35

that the model matches the limiting ascending branch. Since the limiting ascending branch and the output increments along first-order reversal curves are matched, we conclude that the first-order reversal curves themselves are matched.

The Preisach function, $\mu(\alpha, \beta)$, has been found by using the first-order reversal curves. These curves are attached to the limiting ascending branch, and each of them is formed when a monotonic increase along this branch is followed by a subsequent input decrease. For this reason, these curves can be called first-order *decreasing* reversal curves. However, by almost literally repeating the previous reasoning, a similar expression for $\mu(\alpha, \beta)$ can be found by using the first-order *increasing* reversal curves. These curves are attached to the descending branch of the major loop. Each of these first-order increasing reversal curves is formed when a monotonic decrease along the limiting descending branch is followed by a subsequent input increase. The notation $f_{\beta''}$ will be used for the output value on the limiting descending branch. This value is achieved when the input is monotonically decreased from some value above α_0 to the value $u = \beta''$. The corresponding $\alpha - \beta$ diagram is shown in Fig. 1.35. The notation $f_{\beta''\alpha''}$ will be used for the output value on the first-order increasing reversal curve that is attached to the limiting descending branch at the point $f_{\beta''}$. This output value corresponds to $u = \alpha''$ (see Fig. 1.32). The corresponding $\alpha - \beta$ diagram is shown in Fig. 1.36.

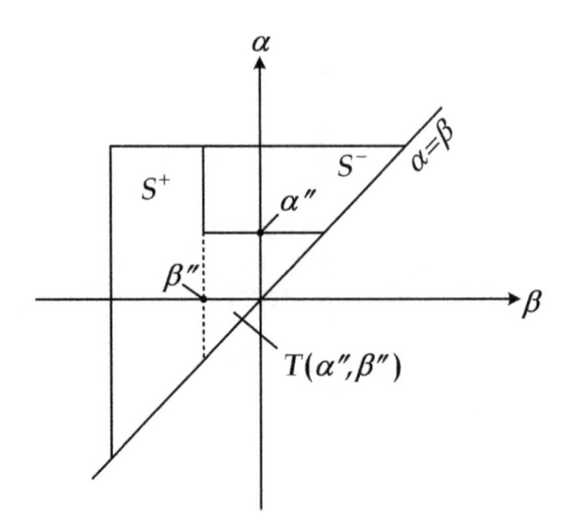

Fig. 1.36

By using the function

$$F(\alpha'', \beta'') = \iint_{T(\alpha'', \beta'')} \mu(\alpha, \beta) d\alpha d\beta, \tag{1.37}$$

from Figs. 1.35 and 1.36 and the formula (1.7), we obtain

$$F(\alpha'', \beta'') = \frac{1}{2}(f_{\beta''\alpha''} - f_{\beta''}). \tag{1.38}$$

From equality (1.37), as before we find

$$\mu(\alpha'', \beta'') = -\frac{\partial^2 F(\alpha'', \beta'')}{\partial \alpha'' \partial \beta''} . \tag{1.39}$$

It is clear on symmetry grounds that first-order decreasing and increasing reversal curves are congruent. In mathematical terms, this means that if

$$\beta'' = -\alpha' \text{ and } \alpha'' = -\beta' , \tag{1.40}$$

then

$$f_{\beta''} = -f_{\alpha'} \text{ and } f_{\beta''\alpha''} = -f_{\alpha'\beta'} . \tag{1.41}$$

From (1.23), (1.38) and (1.41) we find that if (1.40) holds, then

$$F(\alpha'', \beta'') = F(\alpha', \beta') . \tag{1.42}$$

By substituting (1.40) into (1.42), we obtain

$$F(-\beta', -\alpha') = F(\alpha', \beta') . \tag{1.43}$$

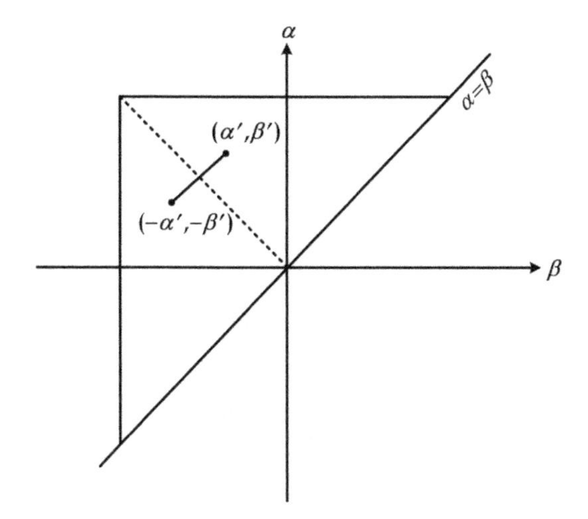

Fig. 1.37

Next, substituting (1.42) and (1.40) into (1.39), we derive

$$\mu(-\beta', -\alpha') = -\frac{\partial^2 F(\alpha', \beta')}{\partial\beta' \partial\alpha'} . \tag{1.44}$$

By comparing (1.44) and (1.27), we find

$$\mu(-\beta', -\alpha') = \mu(\alpha', \beta') . \tag{1.45}$$

The formulas (1.43) and (1.45) express the mirror symmetry of functions $F(\alpha, \beta)$ and $\mu(\alpha, \beta)$ with respect to the line $\alpha = -\beta$ (see Fig. 1.37). This symmetry is a consequence of the congruency of the first-order decreasing and increasing reversal curves.

If the line $\alpha = -\beta$ is the interface between the positive and negative sets, $S^+(t)$ and $S^-(t)$, then, according to the above symmetry and formula (1.7), we find that the output is equal to zero:

$$f(t) = 0 . \tag{1.46}$$

For this reason, the state corresponding to the above interface is called in magnetics "the demagnetized state." However, this state cannot be exactly achieved. This is because an interface $L(t)$ is always a staircase line whose links are parallel to α and β axes. As a result, an actual staircase interface can only approximate the line $\alpha = -\beta$. Such an approximation can be achieved, for instance, if the input $u(t)$ is an oscillating function whose amplitude is slowly decreased to zero starting from some value above α_0 (see Fig. 1.38). The corresponding staircase interface is shown in Fig. 1.39.

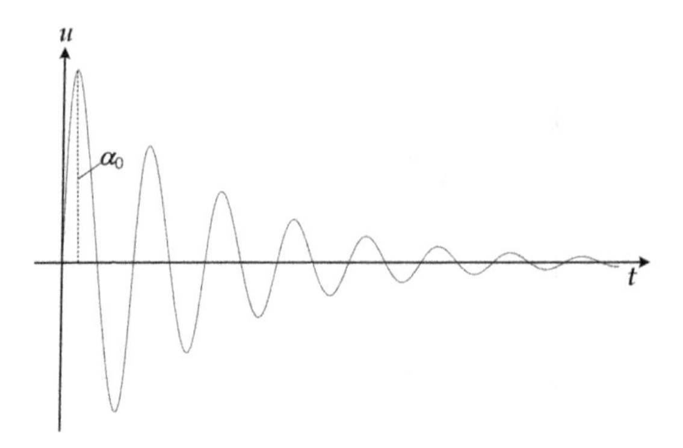

Fig. 1.38

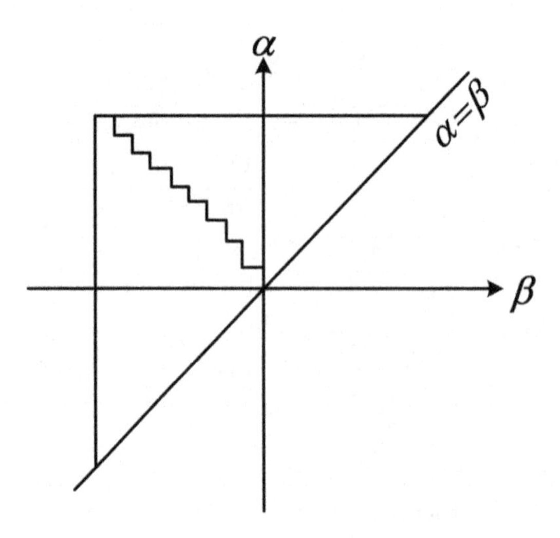

Fig. 1.39

We next proceed to the formulation and the proof of the fundamental theorem which gives the necessary and sufficient conditions for the representation of actual hysteresis nonlinearities by the Preisach model.

REPRESENTATION THEOREM *The erasure property and the congruency property constitute the necessary and sufficient conditions for the representation of an actual hysteresis nonlinearity by the Preisach model for piece-wise monotonic inputs.*

PROOF. **Necessity:** Let a hysteresis transducer be representable by the Preisach model. Then, this transducer should have the same properties as the model. In particular, it should have the erasure and congruency properties.

Sufficiency: Consider a hysteresis transducer that has both the erasure property and the congruency property. It can be recalled that the erasure property means that the future values of output do not depend on all past extremum values of input but only on those that form a sequence of alternating dominant input extrema. The congruency property, on the other hand, suggests that all minor hysteresis loops formed as a result of back-and-forth input variations between the same two consecutive input extrema are congruent. We intend to prove that the above properties imply that the hysteresis transducer can be represented by the Preisach model.

The proof is constructive. First, it is assumed that the weight function, $\mu(\alpha, \beta)$, is found for the given transducer by matching its first-order reversal curves. This can be accomplished by using the formula (1.27). This formula is equivalent to (1.24), which means that the integrals of $\mu(\alpha, \beta)$ over triangles $T(\alpha^{'}, \beta^{'})$ are equal to one-half of output increments, $(1/2)\Delta f = (1/2)(f_{\alpha'} - f_{\alpha'\beta'})$ along the first-order reversal curves. Next, it will be proved that if the above weight function is substituted in (1.3), then the Preisach model and the given transducer will have the same input-output relationships. This statement is true for the first-order reversal curves due to the very way the weight function, $\mu(\alpha, \beta)$, is determined. The induction argument will be next used to prove that the same statement holds for higher-order reversal curves as well. Let us assume that the above statement is true for reversal curves with number $1, 2, \ldots, k$. Then, for the induction inference, we need to prove that this statement holds for a reversal curve number $k + 1$.

Let a be a point at which the reversal curve number $k + 1$ starts (see Fig. 1.40). The point a corresponds to some input value $u = \alpha^{'}$. According to the induction assumption, the output values of the transducer and the Preisach model coincide at this point. Thus, it remains to be proved that the output increments along the reversal curve number $k + 1$ are the same for the actual transducer and for the Preisach model.

Consider an arbitrary input value $u = \beta^{'} < \alpha^{'}$. The output increment for the transducer will be equal to the increment of f along some curve ab (see Fig. 1.40). Let Figs. 1.41 and 1.42 represent $\alpha - \beta$ diagrams for the Preisach model at the time instants when $u = \alpha^{'}$ and $u = \beta^{'}$, respectively. From these diagrams we find that the input decrease from $\alpha^{'}$ to $\beta^{'}$ results

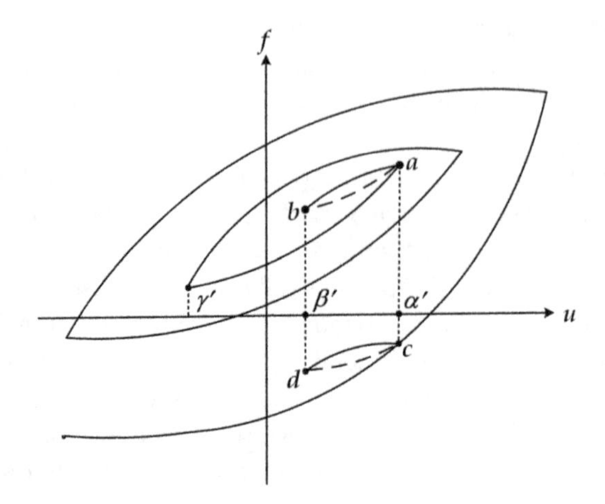

Fig. 1.40

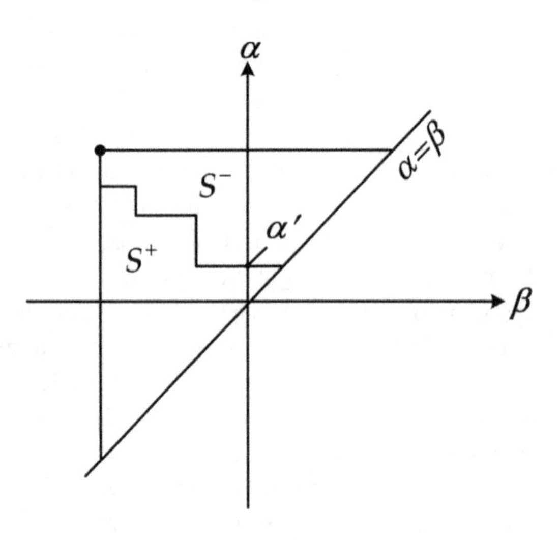

Fig. 1.41

in adding the triangle $T(\alpha^{'}, \beta^{'})$ to the negative set S^{-} and subtracting the same triangle from the positive set S^{+}. Using the above fact and the formula (1.7), we find that for the Preisach model the output increment along the reversal curve number $k+1$ is given by

$$\Delta f = 2 \iint\limits_{T(\alpha^{'}, \beta^{'})} \mu(\alpha, \beta) d\alpha d\beta. \tag{1.47}$$

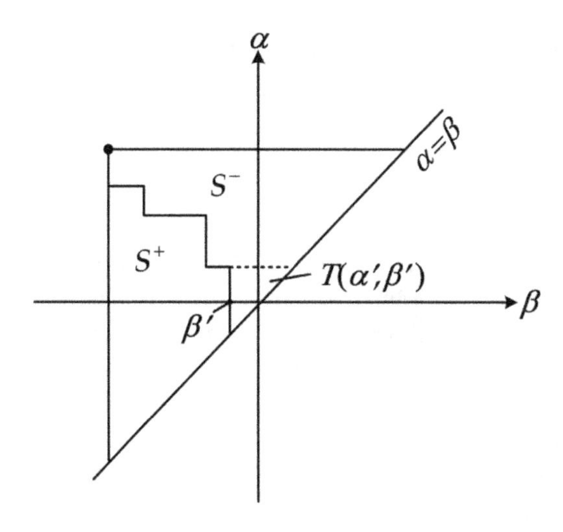

Fig. 1.42

However, according to the way the function, $\mu(\alpha, \beta)$ is defined, the right-hand side of (1.47) is equal to the increment of the transducer output along the first-order reversal curve *cd* (see Fig. 1.40). Thus, it remains to be shown that the output increments along the curves *ab* and *cd* are the same. It is here that the erasure and congruency properties will be used. The proof proceeds as follows. If starting from the point *b* we monotonically increased the input value from β' back to α', then, according to the erasure property, we would arrive at the same point *a* by moving along some curve *ba* (see Fig. 1.40). Indeed, the erasure property implies that as soon as the input exceeds the value α', the history associated with back-and-forth input variations between α' and β' should be erased and the subsequent output variation should follow the reversal curve number k. But, this would be possible if only for $u = \alpha'$ we arrived back at the point a. Similarly, if starting from the point d on the first-order reversal curve we monotonically increase the input value from β' to α', then, according to the same erasure property, we should arrive at the point c moving along some curve *dc* (see Fig. 1.40). Now, by invoking the congruency property, we conclude that the hysteresis loops *bab* and *dcd* are congruent. This is true because both loops result from back and forth input variations between the same two consecutive input extrema, α' and β'. From the congruency of the above loops, we find that the output increments along the curves *ab* and *cd* are the same. Consequently, the output values of the transducer and the Preisach model coincide along the reversal curve number $k+1$. The last fact has been proved for any $\beta' \geq \gamma'$ (see Fig. 1.40). However, according to the erasure property, the reversal curve number $k+1$ should coincide with the reversal curve number $k-1$ for $\beta' < \gamma'$. Thus, the case $\beta' < \gamma'$ falls in the domain of the induction assumption.

In the above discussion, we have considered the reversal curve number $k+1$ corresponding to the monotonically decreasing input. However, the case when the reversal curve number $k+1$ is formed as a result of monotonically increasing input can be treated similarly. The only difference in the proof will be that the first-order *increasing* reversal curves must be employed instead of the first-order *decreasing* reversal curves used in the above reasoning. This completes the proof of the theorem.

It is easy to see that the essence of the given proof is in the reduction of higher-order reversal curves to the first-order reversal curves. This reduction rests on both the erasure property and congruency property.

The proven theorem is important because it clearly establishes the limits of applicability of the Preisach model. These limits are formulated in purely phenomenological terms, without any reference to the actual physical nature of hysteresis. This reveals the physical universality of the Preisach model. The theorem also explicitly indicates the factors which affect the accuracy of the Preisach model. Indeed, deviations from the conditions of the representation theorem may serve as the measure of model accuracy.

The above theorem allows for a simple explanation of so-called statistical instability of the Preisach model. This instability has been a very popular topic in the "magnetics" literature. It usually means that weight functions, $\mu(\alpha, \beta)$, determined from different experimental data are not identical. Since these functions have been construed in magnetics as "particle distributions" (with some statistical connotation), the dependence of $\mu(\alpha, \beta)$ on a particular experimental way of its determination has been termed as "statistical instability." The origin of this "statistical instability" can be easily understood from the following discussion.

The formula (1.27) for $\mu(\alpha, \beta)$ has been derived from the expression (1.25). This means that the weight function, $\mu(\alpha, \beta)$, can be always determined if the integrals of $\mu(\alpha, \beta)$ over the triangles $T(\alpha', \beta')$ are somehow experimentally found. It has been proposed before (see formula (1.24)) to find these integrals by matching the first-order reversal curves. However, this is not the only way it can be done. Indeed, according to the formula (1.47), the same integrals can be found by matching the output increments along any particular reversal curves. But, we will end up with the same values for these integrals if and only if higher-order reversal curves and the first-order reversal curves are congruent. According to the proof of the representation theorem, this congruency takes place if and only if the erasure and congruency properties are valid for hysteresis transducers. If these properties are not valid, then, by matching different reversal curves, we will end up with different values for the integrals over the triangles $T(\alpha', \beta')$ and, consequently, with different values of $\mu(\alpha, \beta)$. This is exactly what had happened when the "statistical instability" was discovered (see [25]). Thus, from the phenomenological point of view, the origin of "statistical instability" comes from the fact that the erasure and congruency properties may not be exactly satisfied for actual hysteresis nonlinearities. Under these circumstances, the Preisach model cannot serve as an absolutely accurate representation for actual hysteresis nonlinearities, but it can still be used as an approximation. The quality of this approximation will depend on the extent to which the erasure and congruency properties are satisfied.

It has been mentioned before that the weight function, $\mu(\alpha, \beta)$, can be found by matching output increments along any reversal curves. Thus, the question arises: "*Which reversal curves should be used for the above purpose*?" If the erasure and congruency properties are valid, then it really does not matter which reversal curves are used for the determination of $\mu(\alpha, \beta)$. All of them will theoretically lead to the same result. However, from the practical point of view, the first-order reversal curves have some clear advantages. First, it is easier to measure these curves than higher-order reversal curves. Second, measurements of these curves start from a well-defined state, namely, the state of negative (or positive) saturation. In these states all the past history was erased. This is not the case for some experimental techniques described in the literature. For instance, it has been suggested in the literature to use a demagnetized state as a starting state in the experimental determination of $\mu(\alpha, \beta)$. But, as it was pointed out before, the demagnetized state is not well defined for the Preisach model. This state depends on a particular way it has been prepared. As a result, some errors and discrepancies may be introduced if the demagnetized state is used as the initial state for the experimental determination of $\mu(\alpha, \beta)$.

It is often asserted in the literature that the Preisach model describes reversal curves with zero initial slopes. This statement is based on the following reasoning. Let $f_{\alpha'\beta'}$ be a reversal curve which is traced for a monotonically decreasing input. This curve starts at the point $f_{\alpha'}$ which corresponds to the local input maximum $u = \alpha'$. The difference $f_{\alpha'\beta'} - f_{\alpha'}$ is then given by (1.24) and the slope of this reversal curve at the point

$\beta = \beta'$ can be found from (1.29). By using formulas (1.24), (1.25), (1.26), and (1.29), it is easy to derive the following expression for the initial slope

$$\lim_{\beta' \to \alpha'} \tan\theta(\alpha', \beta') = 2 \lim_{\beta' \to \alpha'} \int_{\beta'}^{\alpha'} \mu(\alpha, \beta') d\alpha. \tag{1.48}$$

In the literature, the function $\mu(\alpha, \beta)$ is often construed as a distribution function for particles with rectangular hysteresis loops and, for this reason, it is tacitly assumed to be bounded. This assumption and the last formula result in zero initial slopes for the reversal curves $f_{\alpha' \beta'}$. This property is sometimes regarded as an intrinsic property of the Preisach model. However, this is not true. Indeed, if the phenomenological approach is adopted, then there is no need to interpret μ as a distribution for particles and the assumption that μ is bounded can be removed. The freedom of choice of function $\mu(\alpha, \beta)$ should be used in order to match as many experimental facts as possible. It is easy to show that experimentally observed nonzero initial slopes of reversal curves $f_{\alpha' \beta'}$ can be matched by the Preisach model if we allow for delta-type (Dirac function) singularities of $\mu(\alpha, \beta)$ along the line $\alpha = \beta$. It is easy to see that these singularities lead to an additional (and fully reversible) term in the Preisach model consisting of degenerate (zero width) rectangular loop (or step) operators $\hat{\gamma}_{\alpha\alpha}$:

$$f(t) = \iint_{\alpha \geq \beta} \mu(\alpha, \beta) \hat{\gamma}_{\alpha,\beta} u(t) d\alpha d\beta + \int_{-\infty}^{\infty} k(\alpha) \hat{\gamma}_{\alpha,\alpha} u(t) d\alpha, \tag{1.49}$$

where function $\mu(\alpha, \beta)$ is now free of singularities.
This form of the Preisach model leads to the following modification of formulas (1.24)–(1.26):

$$f_{\alpha' \beta'} - f_{\alpha'} = -2 \int_{\beta'}^{\alpha'} \left(\int_{\beta}^{\alpha'} \mu(\alpha, \beta) d\alpha \right) d\beta - 2 \int_{\beta'}^{\alpha'} k(\alpha) d\alpha. \tag{1.50}$$

From the last formula, we derive:

$$\tan\theta(\alpha', \beta') = \frac{\partial f_{\alpha' \beta'}}{\partial \beta'} = 2 \int_{\beta'}^{\alpha'} \mu(\alpha, \beta') d\alpha + 2k(\beta'), \tag{1.51}$$

and

$$\lim_{\beta' \to \alpha'} \tan\theta(\alpha', \beta') = 2k(\alpha'). \tag{1.52}$$

Thus, the actual nonzero initial slopes of the first-order reversal curves can be matched by the appropriate choice of function $k(\alpha)$.

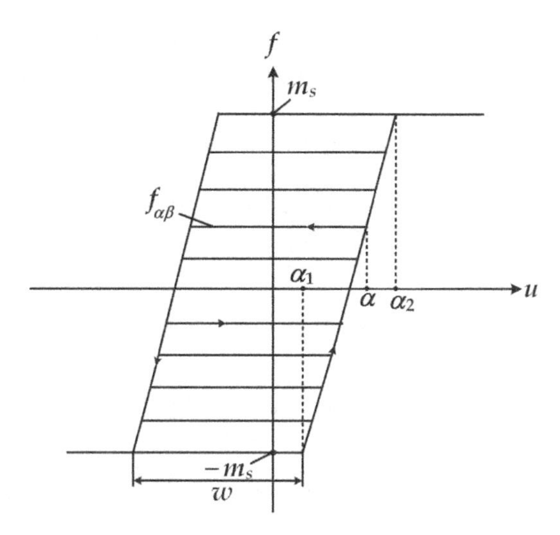

Fig. 1.43

Next consider a simple example that illustrates the application of the formula (1.28) in the case of a hysteresis nonlinearity with a local memory shown in Fig. 1.43. This hysteresis nonlinearity has a set of inner curves that are parallel to u-axis. The above hysteresis nonlinearity is completely characterized by the following parameters: m_s, α_1, α_2, w. It is our intention to find the Preisach representation (1.3) for this nonlinearity. To this end, we have to find the weight function $\mu(\alpha, \beta)$. This requires the specification of first-order transition curves $f_{\alpha\beta}$ and the subsequent application of the formula (1.28). It is clear from Fig. 1.43 that for any α such that $\alpha_1 < \alpha < \infty$ the corresponding first-order reversal curve $f_{\alpha\beta}$ consists of two parts: (a) a particular inner curve and (b) a part of the limiting descending branch if $\alpha_1 - w \leq \beta \leq \alpha_2 - w$ and $\beta + w \leq \alpha < \infty$. It is apparent that $f_{\alpha\beta}$ varies only along the second part.

From the above remark, we find

$$f_{\alpha\beta} = -m_s + \frac{2m_s}{\alpha_2 - \alpha_1}(\beta - \alpha_1 + w) \tag{1.53}$$

if

$$\alpha_1 - w \leq \beta \leq \alpha_2 - w \text{ and } \beta + w \leq \alpha < \infty \tag{1.54}$$

and

$$f_{\alpha\beta} = \text{ constant} \tag{1.55}$$

for all other possible values of β.

It is worthwhile to keep in mind that, depending on a particular value of β, the constant in (1.55) may assume one of the following two values: $-m_s$ or $-m_s + ((2m_s)/(\alpha_2 - \alpha_1))(\alpha - \alpha_1)$.

From formulas (1.53), (1.54) and (1.55), we derive:

$$\frac{\partial f_{\alpha\beta}}{\partial \beta} = \frac{2m_s}{\alpha_2 - \alpha_1}, \quad \text{if } (\alpha, \beta) \in \Omega \,, \tag{1.56}$$

if

$$\alpha_1 - w \leq \beta \leq \alpha_2 - w \text{ and } \beta + w \leq \alpha < \infty \tag{1.57}$$

and

$$\frac{\partial f_{\alpha\beta}}{\partial \beta} = 0 \tag{1.58}$$

for all other values of α and β. The last three formulas can be written in the following equivalent form

$$\frac{\partial f_{\alpha\beta}}{\partial \beta} = \frac{2m_s}{\alpha_2 - \alpha_1}, \quad \text{if } (\alpha, \beta) \in \Omega \,, \tag{1.59}$$

and

$$\frac{\partial f_{\alpha\beta}}{\partial \beta} = 0, \quad \text{if } (\alpha, \beta) \notin \Omega \,, \tag{1.60}$$

where Ω is the region defined by the inequalities (1.57) (see also Fig. 1.44).

From formulas (1.59) and (1.60), we obtain

$$\frac{\partial^2 f_{\alpha\beta}}{\partial \alpha \partial \beta} = \frac{2m_s}{\alpha_2 - \alpha_1} \delta(\alpha - \beta - w) \,, \tag{1.61}$$

if

$$\alpha_1 \leq \alpha \leq \alpha_2 \tag{1.62}$$

and $\partial^2 f_{\alpha\beta}/\partial\alpha\partial\beta$ is zero otherwise. From expressions (1.28), (1.61) and (1.62) we find that

$$\mu(\alpha, \beta) = \frac{m_s}{\alpha_2 - \alpha_1} \delta(\alpha - \beta - w) \tag{1.63}$$

for

$$\alpha_1 \leq \alpha \leq \alpha_2 \tag{1.64}$$

and $\mu(\alpha, \beta)$ is equal to zero otherwise.

Thus, the weight function $\mu(\alpha, \beta)$ has the support on the line $\alpha - \beta - w = 0$. This support is the bold segment (see Fig. 1.44) of the above line.

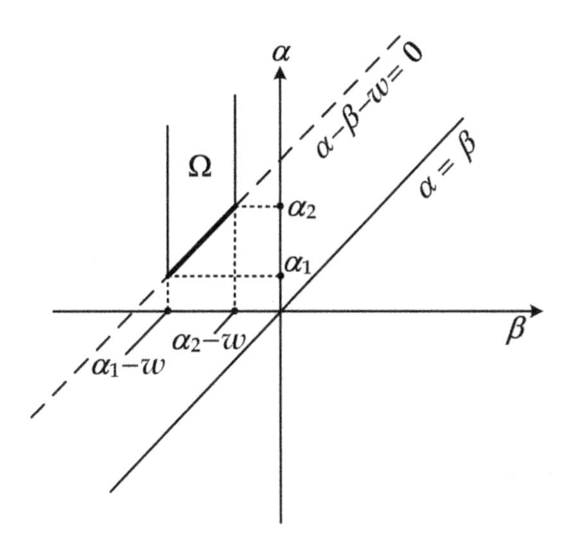

Fig. 1.44

By using formulas (1.63) and (1.64) in (1.3), after simple transformations we obtain

$$f(t) = \frac{m_s}{\alpha_2 - \alpha_1} \int_{\alpha_1}^{\alpha_2} \hat{\gamma}_{\alpha,\alpha-w} u(t) d\alpha \ . \tag{1.65}$$

This is the Preisach representation of the hysteresis nonlinearity shown in Fig. 1.43. It is left to the reader as a useful exercise to verify that formula (1.65) indeed describes all branches of this hysteresis nonlinearity.

The hysteresis nonlinearity shown in Fig. 1.43 is usually called hysteresis "play-operator" or "backlash" operator. Superpositions (parallel-connections) of such operators result in Prandtl-Ishlinskii model of hysteresis [33] which is extensively used in the study (and compensations) of hysteresis of piezoelectric actuators. It is clear from formula (1.65) that the Prandtl-Ishlinskii model can be always reduced to the Preisach model. It is also clear that the Preisach representation of the Prandtl-Ishlinskii model is very attractive due to the most elementary nature of rectangular loop operators $\hat{\gamma}_{\alpha\beta}$.

It is not accidental that in the Preisach representation of a play-operator the function $\mu(\alpha, \beta)$ has a "line-support" (see Fig. 1.44). This is related to the fact that the play-operators have a local memory. In general, it can be proved that if a hysteresis nonlinearity with a local memory can be represented by the Preisach model, the weight function $\mu(\alpha, \beta)$ has a

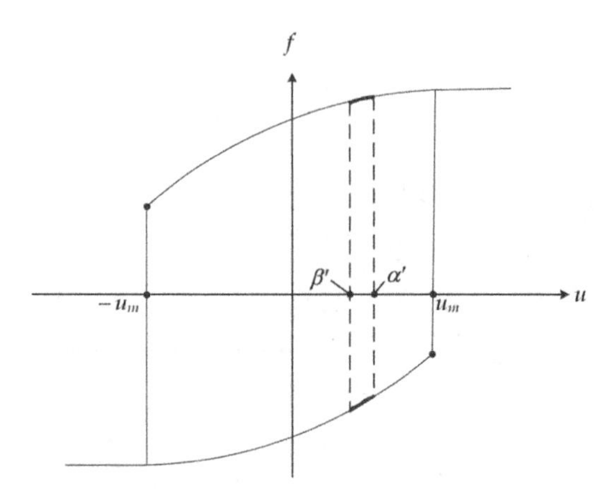

Fig. 1.45

support along some particular curve and this curve may intersect all possible staircase interfaces $L(t)$ only once.

It was emphasized before that the Preisach model can describe (and usually does describe) hysteresis with nonlocal memories. These nonlinearities are much more complex than those with local memories. However, it would be a mistake to think that any hysteresis nonlinearity with local memory can be represented by the Preisach model. In fact, there are very simple hysteresis nonlinearities with local memories that cannot be described by the model. For instance, this is true for the hysteresis nonlinearity shown in Fig. 1.45. Indeed, let the input vary back and forth between two consecutive extremum values α' and β', $-u_m < \beta' < \alpha' < u_m$. Then, depending on the past history, the bold reversible parts of descending and ascending branches will be traced back and forth. These parts can be construed as degenerate minor loops. Since these parts are not congruent, the congruency property of the representation theorem is not satisfied. Consequently, the hysteresis nonlinearity shown in Fig. 1.45 cannot be represented by the Preisach model. However, this hysteresis nonlinearity is typical for single Stoner-Wohlfarth magnetic particles. It is known from the theory of these particles that the reversible parts of their hysteresis loops result from uniform rotations of magnetization within these particles, that is from reversible processes. Incongruence of the above parts is the reason why the Preisach model cannot describe the hysteresis loops of single Stoner-Wohlfarth particles. For this reason, it is often asserted that the Preisach model does not fully account for reversible processes. It will be shown in the next chapter that this deficiency of the Preisach model can be removed by its appropriate generalization.

Next, we consider how the Preisach model can be numerically implemented. It is apparent that this can be done by using formula (1.7) for the computation of the output, $f(t)$, and the formula (1.28) for the determination of the weight function, $\mu(\alpha, \beta)$. Although the above approach is straightforward, it encounters two main difficulties. First, it requires the numerical evaluation of double integrals in (1.7). This is a time-consuming procedure. Second, the determination of the weight function by employing the formula (1.28) requires differentiations of experimentally obtained data. These differentiations may strongly amplify errors (noise) inherently present in any experimental data. It turns out that another approach can be developed for the numerical implementation of the Preisach model. This approach completely circumvents the above two difficulties. It is based on the explicit formula for the integrals in (1.7). This formula directly involves (without any differentiation) the experimental data used for the identification of $\mu(\alpha, \beta)$. Moreover, the above formula will be a valuable tool for the theoretical investigation of the Preisach model as well.

The starting point for the derivation of the explicit formula for $f(t)$ is the expression (1.7). It is worthwhile to remind here that the positive $(S^+(t))$ and negative $(S^-(t))$ sets in (1.7) are separated by the staircase interface $L(t)$. This interface has vertices whose α and β coordinates are equal to M_k and m_k, respectively (see Fig. 1.46). As discussed before, numbers M_k and m_k form the sequence of dominant input extrema.

By adding and subtracting the integral of $\mu(\alpha, \beta)$ over $S^+(t)$, the expression (1.7) can be represented in the form:

$$f(t) = -\iint_T \mu(\alpha, \beta) d\alpha d\beta + 2 \iint_{S^+(t)} \mu(\alpha, \beta) d\alpha d\beta, \tag{1.66}$$

where, as before, T is the limiting triangle.

According to formula (1.25), we find

$$\iint_T \mu(\alpha, \beta) d\alpha d\beta = F(\alpha_0, \beta_0) . \tag{1.67}$$

The positive set, $S^+(t)$, can be subdivided into n trapezoids Q_k (see Fig. 1.46). As a result, we have

$$\iint_{S^+(t)} \mu(\alpha, \beta) d\alpha d\beta = \sum_{k=1}^{n(t)} \iint_{Q_k(t)} \mu(\alpha, \beta) d\alpha d\beta . \tag{1.68}$$

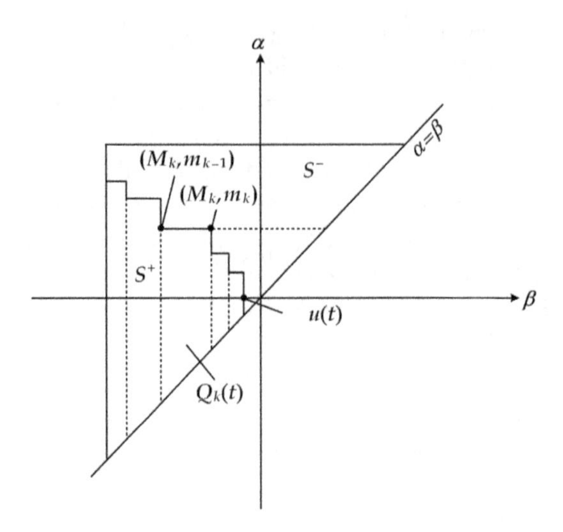

Fig. 1.46

It is clear that the number of these trapezoids and their shapes may change with time. For this reason, n and Q_k are written in formula (1.68) as functions of time.

Each trapezoid Q_k can be represented as a difference of two triangles, $T(M_k, m_{k-1})$ and $T(M_k, m_k)$. Thus, we obtain

$$\iint\limits_{Q_k(t)} \mu(\alpha,\beta)d\alpha d\beta = \iint\limits_{T(M_k,m_{k-1})} \mu(\alpha,\beta)d\alpha d\beta - \iint\limits_{T(M_k,m_k)} \mu(\alpha,\beta)d\alpha d\beta, \tag{1.69}$$

where, for the case $k = 1$, m_0 in (1.69) is naturally equal to β_0.

According to formula (1.25), we find:

$$\iint\limits_{T(M_k,m_{k-1})} \mu(\alpha,\beta)d\alpha d\beta = F\big(M_k, m_{k-1}\big) \tag{1.70}$$

and

$$\iint\limits_{T(M_k,m_k)} \mu(\alpha,\beta)d\alpha d\beta = F\big(M_k, m_k\big)\ . \tag{1.71}$$

From formulas (1.69), (1.70) and (1.71), we derive

$$\iint\limits_{Q_k(t)} \mu(\alpha,\beta)d\alpha d\beta = F\big(M_k, m_{k-1}\big) - F\big(M_k, m_k\big)\ . \tag{1.72}$$

From formulas (1.66), (1.67), (1.68) and (1.72), we obtain

$$f(t) = -F(\alpha_0, \beta_0) + 2\sum_{k=1}^{n(t)} \Big[F(M_k, m_{k-1}) - F(M_k, m_k)\Big] . \tag{1.73}$$

It is clear from Fig. 1.46 that m_n is equal to the current value of input

$$m_n = u(t) . \tag{1.74}$$

Consequently, the expression (1.73) can be written as

$$\begin{aligned} f(t) = -F(\alpha_0, \beta_0) + 2 \sum_{k=1}^{n(t)-1} \Big[F(M_k, m_{k-1}) - F(M_k, m_k)\Big] \\ + 2\Big[F(M_n, m_{n-1}) - F(M_n, u(t))\Big] . \end{aligned} \tag{1.75}$$

The last expression has been derived for monotonically decreasing input, that is, when the final link of interface $L(t)$ is a vertical one. If the input $u(t)$ is being monotonically increased, then the final link of $L(t)$ is a horizontal one and the $\alpha - \beta$ diagram shown in Fig. 1.46 should be slightly modified. The appropriate diagram is shown in Fig. 1.47. This diagram can be considered as a particular case of the previous one. This case is realized when

$$m_n(t) = M_n(t) = u(t) . \tag{1.76}$$

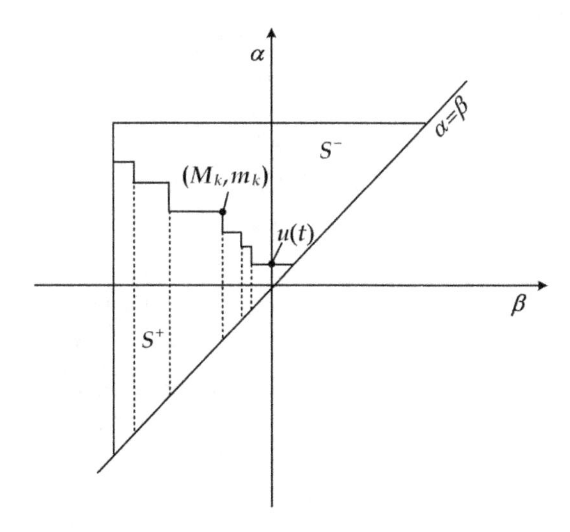

Fig. 1.47

According to the definition (1.25) of $F(\alpha, \beta)$, we find

$$F(M_n, m_n) = F\big(u(t), u(t)\big) = 0\ . \tag{1.77}$$

From formulas (1.73), (1.76) and (1.77), we derive the following expression for $f(t)$ in the case of monotonically increasing input:

$$\begin{aligned} f(t) = -F(\alpha_0, \beta_0) + 2 \sum_{k=1}^{n(t)-1} \Big[F(M_k, m_{k-1}) - F(M_k, m_k)\Big] \\ + 2\Big[F\big(u(t), m_{n-1}\big)\Big]\ . \end{aligned} \tag{1.78}$$

The function $F(\alpha, \beta)$ is related to experimentally measured first-order reversal curves by the formula (1.23). Using this formula, expressions (1.75) and (1.78) can be written in terms of the above experimental data as follows:

$$f(t) = -f^+ + \sum_{k=1}^{n-1} \Big[f_{M_k m_k} - f_{M_k m_{k-1}}\Big] + f_{M_n u(t)} - f_{M_n m_{n-1}}\ , \tag{1.79}$$

$$f(t) = -f^+ + \sum_{k=1}^{n-1} \Big[f_{M_k m_k} - f_{M_k m_{k-1}}\Big] + f_{-m_{n-1}} - f_{-m_{n-1}, -u(t)}\ . \tag{1.80}$$

Here, f^+ is, as before, the positive saturation value of output, and the last term in (1.78) has been transformed by using the formulas (1.23) and (1.43). Thus, we have derived the explicit expressions (1.79) and (1.80) for $f(t)$ in terms of experimentally measured data. These expressions constitute the basis for the numerical implementation of the Preisach model.

As was pointed out before, the derived formulas (1.79) and (1.80) (or (1.75)) and (1.78) are useful not only for the numerical implementation of the Preisach model but for its theoretical investigation as well. For instance, by using (1.79) and (1.80), the following proposition can easily be proven.

PROPOSITION *Any $f - u$ path of hysteresis transducer representable by the Preisach model is piecewise congruent to first-order transition curves.*

PROOF Suppose that the input $u(t)$ is being monotonically decreased from its previous maximum value $u = M_n$ until it reaches the value $u = m_{n-1}$. Then, the formula (1.79) is valid. In this formula, all terms except $f_{M_n u(t)}$ do not vary. Consequently, the $f - u$ path traced during the above input variation is congruent to the first-order reversal curve $f_{M_n u}$ which is attached to the limiting ascending branch at the point f_{M_n}. As the input reaches the value m_{n-1}, the cancellation of the last two terms in (1.79) occurs. If the input is being further decreased remaining between $u = m_{n-1}$ and $u = m_{n-2}$, then the formula (1.79) is modified as follows:

$$f(t) = -f^+ + \sum_{k=1}^{n-2} \left[f_{M_k m_k} - f_{M_k m_{k-1}} \right] + f_{M_{n-1} u(t)} - f_{M_{n-1} m_{n-2}} \,. \quad (1.81)$$

From this formula, as before, we conclude that the $f - u$ path traced during the above input variation is congruent to the first-order transition curve $f_{M_{n-1}u}$ that is attached to the limiting ascending branch at the point $f = f_{M_{n-1}}$. By continuing the same line of reasoning, we find that if the input is being monotonically decreased between $u = m_k$ and $u = m_{k-1}$, then the corresponding $f - u$ path is congruent to the first-order reversal curve $f_{M_k u}$. For the case when the input is monotonically increased, the formula (1.80) is valid. From this formula, we find that if the input is monotonically increased between the values $u = M_k$ and $u = M_{k-1}$, then the time varying part of the output is described by the term $f_{-m_{k-1}, -u(t)}$. Thus, the corresponding $f - u$ path is congruent to the first-order reversal curve $f_{-m_{k-1}, -u}$ that is attached to the limiting descending branch at the point $f = f_{-m_{k-1}}$. This completes the proof.

It is clear from the presented discussion, that the first-order reversal curves (FORCs) play the central role in the theory of the classical Preisach model. Indeed, these curves are used for the identification of this model, in the proof of the Representation Theorem and in the algebraic expressions for the output of the Preisach model. Furthermore, measurements of the first-order reversal curve start from well-defined state of negative (or positive) saturation when all the past history is erased. For this reason, these curves are not "contaminated" by past variations of input. This property as well as the simplicity of measurements of first-order reversal curves make them very attractive for general characterization of hysteretic materials; the characterizations that may not be directly related to the Preisach model. These curves were first introduced by the first author of the book more than thirty years ago [12], [13]. Since then, they have become a standard tool for the characterization of hysteresis in various areas of science and technology. One example is their use in geology. Currently, the first-order reversal curves are even used for the extraction of various microscopic properties of hysteretic materials. Quite often, this is done without rigorous justification, which has led to some critical discussion of this matter (see, for instance, [40]). It must be remarked that FORCs represent the simplest class of reversal curves. In the next chapter, the second order reversal curves are introduced and they are extensively used in the theory and identification of generalized Preisach models which are far reaching extensions of the classical Preisach model.

1.5 Hysteresis Energy Losses

A hysteresis phenomenon is associated with some energy dissipation which is often referred to as hysteresis energy loss. The problem of determining hysteresis energy losses is a classical one. It has been attracting considerable attention because the hysteresis energy loss is an important component of "core losses" occurring in almost all electromagnetic power devices as well as in many high frequency microwave devices. For this reason, the means for accurate predictions of hysteresis losses and their reduction are important for optimal design of various equipment. The solution to the above problem has long been known for the particular case of periodic (cyclic) input variations. In magnetics, this solution is most often associated with the name of C. P. Steinmetz [41]. This solution implies that a hysteresis energy loss per cycle is equal to an area enclosed by a loop resulting from periodic input variations (see Fig. 1.48). However, energy dissipation occurs for arbitrary (not necessary periodic) variations of input. The problem of computing hysteresis energy losses for arbitrary input variations has remained unsolved. A solution to this problem would be of both theoretical and practical importance. From the theoretical point of view, the solution to the above problem will allow for the calculation of internal entropy production that is a key point in the development of irreversible thermodynamics of hysteretic media. In magnetics, it may also allow one to separate a dissipated energy from an energy stored in magnetic field. This eventually may lead to expressions for electromagnetic forces in hysteretic media. From the practical viewpoint, the solution to the above problem may bring new experimental techniques for the measurement of hysteresis energy losses occurring for arbitrary input variations.

It should not be surprising that the expression for hysteresis energy losses has been found only for the case of periodic input variations. The reason behind this fact is that the hysteresis energy losses occurring for periodic input variations can be easily evaluated by using only the energy conservation principle; no knowledge of actual mechanisms of hysteresis or its model is required. The situation is much more complicated when arbitrary input variations are considered. Here, the energy conservation principle alone is not sufficient, and an adequate model of hysteresis should

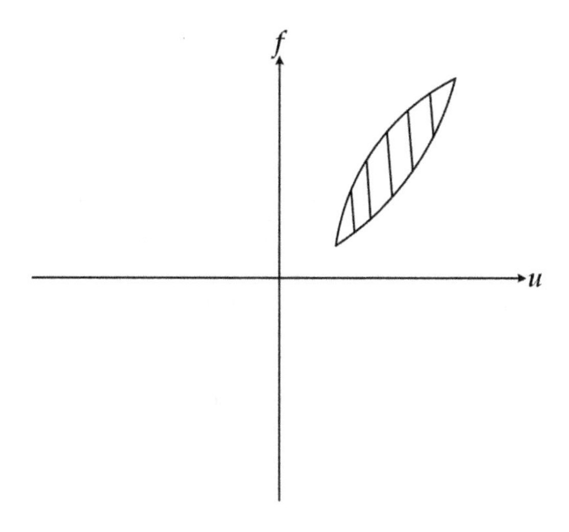

Fig. 1.48

be employed in order to arrive at the solution to the problem. It turns out that the Preisach hysteresis model is very well suited for this purpose.

In this section, the Preisach model will be used for the derivation of general expressions for hysteresis energy losses. These expressions will be given in terms of the weight function, $\mu(\alpha, \beta)$, as well as in terms of experimentally measured first-order transition curves. Furthermore, a formula that relates the hysteresis energy losses occurring for arbitrary input variations to the losses occurring for certain periodic input variations will be derived. This formula may result in simple techniques for the measurement of hysteresis losses occurring for arbitrary input variations. The application of the mentioned results to the irreversible thermodynamics of hysteretic media will be discussed as well.

We begin by defining the input, $u(t)$, and the output, $f(t)$, as work variables. This means that the infinitesimal energy supplied to the transducer (media) in the form of work is given by the formula

$$\delta W = u \, df \, . \tag{1.82}$$

In magnetics, u is the magnetic field H, f is the magnetization M, and the formula (1.82) becomes the classical expression for the work done in magnetizing a unit volume of magnetic media:

$$\delta W = H \, dM \, . \tag{1.83}$$

Similarly, in mechanics, u is the force F, f is the specific length L, and from formula (1.82) we find the standard relation

$$\delta W = F\, dL \; . \tag{1.84}$$

Now, we proceed to the derivation of expressions for hysteresis energy losses. We first consider the case when a hysteresis nonlinearity is represented by a rectangular loop shown in Fig. 1.49. If a periodic variation of input is such that the whole loop is traced, then the hysteresis energy loss for one cycle, Q_{cycle}, is equal to the area enclosed by the loop

$$Q_{\text{cycle}} = 2(\alpha - \beta) \; . \tag{1.85}$$

It is clear that the horizontal links of the loop are fully reversible and, for this reason, no energy losses occur as these links are traced. Thus, it can be concluded that only "switching-up" and "switching-down" result in energy losses. It can be assumed (on the physical grounds) that there is symmetry between these switchings. In other words, these switchings are identical as far as energy losses are concerned. Consequently, the same energy loss occurs for each of these switchings. As a result, we conclude that the energy loss per switching, q, is given by

$$q = (\alpha - \beta) \; . \tag{1.86}$$

The product $\mu(\alpha, \beta)\hat{\gamma}_{\alpha,\beta}$ can be construed as a rectangular hysteresis loop with output values equal to $\pm\mu(\alpha, \beta)$. For this reason, switchings of such loops will result in energy losses equal to $\mu(\alpha, \beta)(\alpha - \beta)$. In the Preisach model, any input variation is associated with switchings of specific rectangular loops $\mu(\alpha, \beta)\hat{\gamma}_{\alpha,\beta}$. These switchings represent irreversible processes occurring during input variations. Consequently, it is natural to equate the hysteresis energy loss occurring for some input variation to the sum of energy losses resulting from the switching of rectangular loops during this input variation. Since in the Preisach model we are dealing with continuous ensembles of rectangular loops, the above summation should be replaced by integration. Thus, if Ω denotes the region of points on $\alpha - \beta$ diagram for which rectangular loops were switched during some input variation, then the hysteresis energy loss, Q, for this input variation is given by

$$Q = \iint\limits_{\Omega} \mu(\alpha, \beta)(\alpha - \beta) d\alpha d\beta \; . \tag{1.87}$$

This is the fundamental formula for hysteresis energy losses, and all subsequent discussion will follow from this expression. It is clear from the

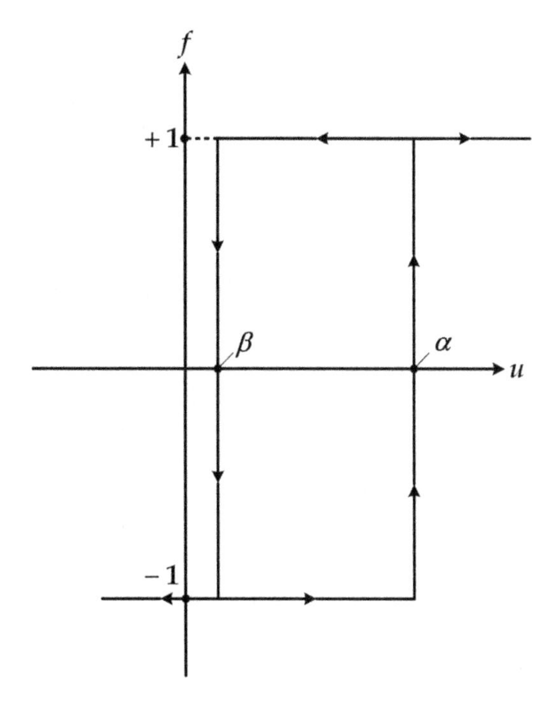

Fig. 1.49

above reasoning that the derivation of the formula (1.87) rests on the following two facts: (a) for rectangular hysteresis loops, hysteretic losses can be evaluated for arbitrary input variations, (b) the Preisach model represents complicated hysteresis nonlinearities as superpositions of rectangular loops. The above two facts make the Preisach model a very convenient tool for the solution of the problem at hand. However, it has to be kept in mind that the formula (1.87) cannot be applied to any hysteresis nonlinearity. It has certain limits of applicability that are the same as for the Preisach model itself.

A typical shape of the region Ω is shown in Fig. 1.50. It is clear from this figure that Ω can be always subdivided into a triangle and some trapezoids. The trapezoids, in turn, can be represented as differences of triangles. Thus, if the integral in (1.87) can be evaluated for any triangular region, then it will be easy to determine this integral for any possible shape of Ω. For this reason, it makes sense to compute the values of the above integrals over various triangles. By using these values, hysteresis losses can be easily found for any input variations. In the case when Ω is a triangle, the integral (1.87)

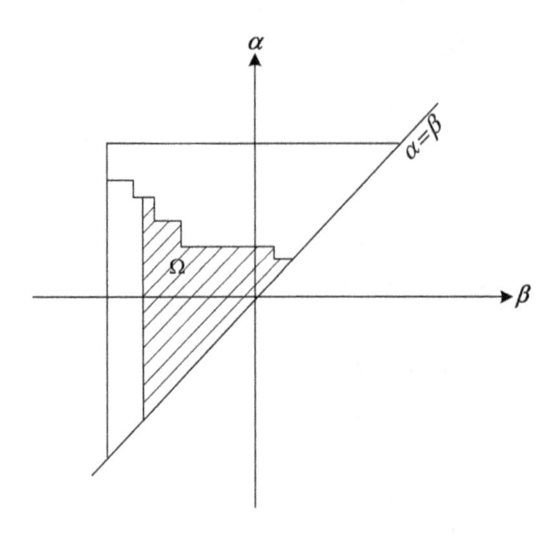

Fig. 1.50

can be evaluated in terms of first-order reversal curves. The derivation proceeds as follows.

Consider the function $(\alpha-\beta)F(\alpha,\beta)$. By differentiating this function, we find

$$\frac{\partial^2}{\partial\alpha\partial\beta}\left[(\alpha-\beta)F(\alpha,\beta)\right]=\frac{\partial F(\alpha,\beta)}{\partial\beta}-\frac{\partial F(\alpha,\beta)}{\partial\alpha}+(\alpha-\beta)\frac{\partial^2 F(\alpha,\beta)}{\partial\alpha\partial\beta}\,. \quad (1.88)$$

By using formulas (1.27) and (1.88), we derive

$$\mu(\alpha,\beta)(\alpha-\beta)=\frac{\partial F(\alpha,\beta)}{\partial\beta}-\frac{\partial F(\alpha,\beta)}{\partial\alpha}-\frac{\partial^2}{\partial\alpha\partial\beta}\left[(\alpha-\beta)F(\alpha,\beta)\right]\,. \quad (1.89)$$

Let $T(u_+,u_-)$ be a triangle (see Fig. 1.51) swept during the monotonic increase of input from u_- to u_+. According to (1.87) the above input variation results in the hysteretic loss $Q(u_-,u_+)$ that is given by

$$Q(u_-,u_+)=\iint\limits_{T(u_+,u_-)}\mu(\alpha,\beta)(\alpha-\beta)d\alpha d\beta\,. \quad (1.90)$$

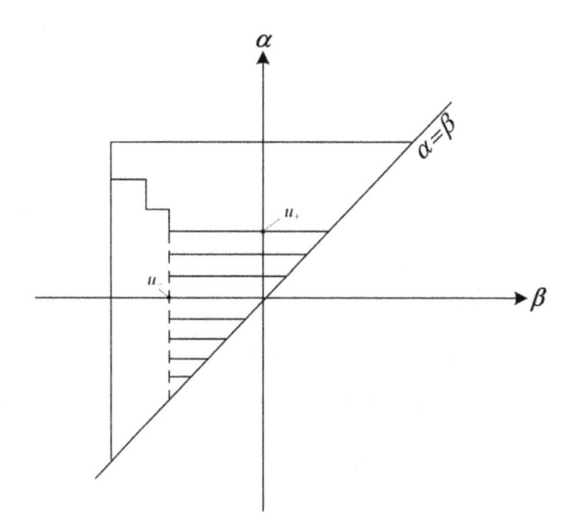

Fig. 1.51

Substituting the expression (1.89) into (1.90), we find:

$$Q(u_-,u_+) = \iint_{T(u_+,u_-)} \frac{\partial F(\alpha,\beta)}{\partial \beta} d\alpha d\beta - \iint_{T(u_+,u_-)} \frac{\partial F(\alpha,\beta)}{\partial \alpha} d\alpha d\beta - \iint_{T(u_+,u_-)} \frac{\partial^2}{\partial\alpha\partial\beta}\big[(\alpha-\beta)F(\alpha,\beta)\big] d\alpha d\beta \,. \tag{1.91}$$

The first integral in formula (1.91) can be evaluated as follows:

$$\begin{aligned}\iint_{T(u_+,u_-)} \frac{\partial F(\alpha,\beta)}{\partial \beta} d\alpha d\beta &= \int_{u_-}^{u_+} \left(\int_{u_-}^{\alpha} \frac{\partial F(\alpha,\beta)}{\partial \beta} d\beta \right) d\alpha \\ &= \int_{u_-}^{u_+} F(\alpha,\alpha) d\alpha - \int_{u_-}^{u_+} F(\alpha,u_-) d\alpha \\ &= -\int_{u_-}^{u_+} F(\alpha,u_-) d\alpha,\end{aligned} \tag{1.92}$$

since $F(\alpha,\alpha) = 0$.

Similarly, for the second integral in (1.91) we obtain

$$\iint_{T(u_+,u_-)} \frac{\partial F(\alpha,\beta)}{\partial \alpha} d\alpha d\beta = \int_{u_-}^{u_+} F(u_+,\beta) d\beta \,. \tag{1.93}$$

Finally, for the third integral in formula (1.91)), we derive

$$\iint_{T(u_+,u_-)} \frac{\partial^2}{\partial\alpha\partial\beta}\big[(\alpha-\beta)F(\alpha,\beta)\big]d\alpha d\beta$$

$$= \int_{u_-}^{u_+}\left(\int_{\beta}^{u_+} \frac{\partial^2}{\partial\alpha\partial\beta}\big[(\alpha-\beta)F(\alpha,\beta)\big]d\alpha\right)d\beta \qquad (1.94)$$

$$= \int_{u_-}^{u_+} \frac{\partial}{\partial\beta}\big[(u_+-\beta)F(u_+,\beta)\big]d\beta$$

$$= -(u_+-u_-)F(u_+,u_-)\,.$$

Substituting formulas (1.92), (1.93) and (1.94) into equation (1.91), we find

$$Q(u_-,u_+) = (u_+-u_-)F(u_+,u_-) - \int_{u_-}^{u_+} F(\alpha,u_-)d\alpha - \int_{u_-}^{u_+} F(u_+,\beta)d\beta\,. \qquad (1.95)$$

The last formula has two main advantages over expression (1.90). First, its application requires the evaluation of one-dimensional integrals. Second, this formula expresses the losses directly in terms of experimentally measured first-order reversal curves.

By using the expression (1.95), the hysteresis energy losses can be evaluated for arbitrary input variations. Consider some input variation for which the region Ω has the shape shown in Fig. 1.50. Then, the corresponding energy losses are given by (1.87) that can be written as follows:

$$Q = Q(M_n,m_n) + \sum_{i=1}^{k}\big[Q(M_{n-i},m_{n-i}) - Q(M_{n-i},m_{n-i-1})\big]\,, \qquad (1.96)$$

where it is assumed that

$$m_{n-k-1} = u(t)\,, \qquad (1.97)$$

and each term in equation (1.96) can be evaluated by employing the formula (1.95).

Next, we discuss some interesting qualitative properties of energy losses occurring in hysteresis transducers described by the Preisach model. Consider a cyclic variation of input between two consecutive extremum values u_- to u_+. During the monotonic increase of input from u_- to u_+, the final horizontal link of $L(t)$ sweeps the triangle $T(u_+,u_-)$ (see Fig. 1.51). Consequently, the losses occurring during this monotonic increase are given by (1.90). On the other hand, during the monotonic decrease of input from u_+ to u_-, the final vertical link of $L(t)$ sweeps the same triangle, and the corresponding losses $Q(u_+, u_-)$ will be given by the same integral in (1.90). Thus,

$$Q(u_+, u_-) = Q(u_-, u_+) , \tag{1.98}$$

and we obtain the following result.

For any loop, the hysteretic losses occurring along ascending and descending branches are the same.

The above result can be used to find the formula which relates hysteretic losses occurring for arbitrary input variations to certain cyclic hysteretic losses. Suppose that the input $u(t)$ is monotonically increased from some minimum value u_- and it reaches successively the values u_1 and u_2 with $u_2 > u_1$ (see Fig. 1.52). We are concerned with the hysteretic losses $Q(u_1, u_2)$ during the monotonic input increase between u_1 and u_2. For this input increase we have (see Fig. 1.53)

$$\Omega = T(u_2, u_-) - T(u_1, u_-) . \tag{1.99}$$

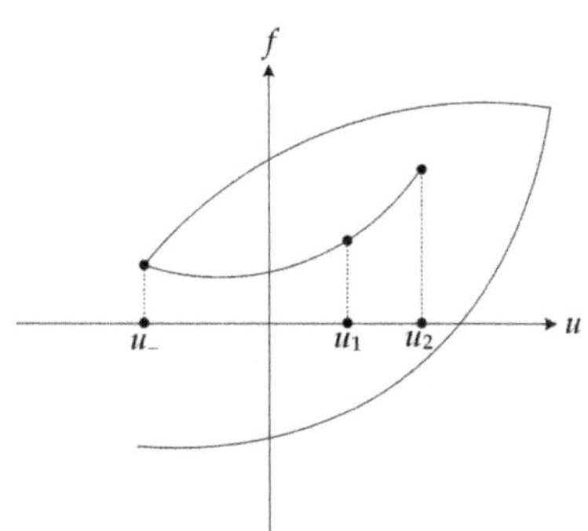

Fig. 1.52

Fig. 1.53

Consequently,

$$Q(u_1, u_2) = Q(u_-, u_2) - Q(u_-, u_1) . \tag{1.100}$$

Using the formula (1.98), the losses $Q(u_-, u_2)$ and $Q(u_-, u_1)$ can be expressed in terms of cyclic losses

$$Q(u_-, u_1) = \frac{1}{2}\bar{Q}(u_-, u_1), \qquad Q(u_-, u_2) = \frac{1}{2}\bar{Q}(u_-, u_2), \tag{1.101}$$

where $\bar{Q}(u_-, u_1)$ is the hysteretic loss per cycle when the input is periodically varied between u_- and u_1; the notation $\bar{Q}(u_-, u_2)$ has a similar meaning.

By substituting formulas (1.101) into (1.100), we obtain

$$Q(u_1, u_2) = \frac{1}{2}\left[\bar{Q}(u_-, u_2) - \bar{Q}(u_-, u_1)\right] . \qquad (1.102)$$

The last formula expresses the loss occurring during the monotonic increase of input. By literally repeating the same line of reasoning, a similar formula can be derived for the case of monotonic input decrease between u_1 and u_2 ($u_1 > u_2$):

$$Q(u_1, u_2) = \frac{1}{2}\left[\bar{Q}(u_+, u_2) - \bar{Q}(u_+, u_1)\right], \qquad (1.103)$$

where u_+ is the last input maximum.

The formulas (1.102) and (1.103) may be useful from the practical point of view, because it is much easier to measure cyclic losses than those occurring for nonperiodic input variations.

It is instructive to show that the derived expressions for hysteresis energy losses are consistent with the classical result: *hysteresis energy losses occurring for a cyclic input variation are equal to the area enclosed by the loop resulting from this cyclic input variation.*

Consider a cyclic input variation between u_- and u_+. According to formulas (1.98) and (1.95), we find that the hysteretic loss per cycle for the above input variation is given by the expression

$$\begin{aligned}\bar{Q}(u_+, u_+) &= 2Q(u_+, u_+)\\ &= 2\left[(u_+ - u_-)F(u_+, u_-) - \int_{u_-}^{u_+} F(u_+, \beta)d\beta - \int_{u_-}^{u_+} F(\alpha, u_-)d\alpha\right] .\end{aligned} \qquad (1.104)$$

On the other hand, the area enclosed by the corresponding loop is given by the formula

$$W = \oint_{u_- u_+ u_-} u \, df . \qquad (1.105)$$

Since

$$\oint_{u_- u_+ u_-} u \, df + \oint_{u_- u_+ u_-} f \, du = \oint_{u_- u_+ u_-} d(uf) = 0 , \qquad (1.106)$$

we find

$$W = - \oint_{u_- u_+ u_-} f \, du = - \oint_{u_- u_+} f \, du - \oint_{u_+ u_-} f \, du . \qquad (1.107)$$

To evaluate the last two integrals, we shall use the formulas (1.75) and (1.78). In the case of monotonic input increase, the formula (1.78) is appropriate. This formula can be written in the form

$$f(t) = C + 2\, F\big(u(t), u_-\big)\ , \tag{1.108}$$

where u_- is used instead of m_{n-1} and the constant C is given by the formula

$$C = -F(\alpha_0, \beta_0) + 2\sum_{k=1}^{n-1}\Big[\, F(M_k, m_{k-1}) - F(M_k, m_k)\,\Big]\ . \tag{1.109}$$

From formula (1.108), we find

$$\int\limits_{u_- u_+} f\, du \;=\; C\,(u_+ - u_-) + 2\int_{u_-}^{u_+} F(u, u_-)du\ . \tag{1.110}$$

In the case of monotonic input decrease from u_+ to u_-, the formula (1.75) is appropriate. This formula can be rearranged as follows

$$f(t) = C + 2\,\Big[F\big(u_+, u_-\big) - F\big(u_+, u(t)\big)\Big]\ , \tag{1.111}$$

where u_+ is used instead of M_n, and the constant C is the same history-dependent constant as in equation (1.108).

From formula (1.111), we obtain

$$\int\limits_{u_+ u_-} f\, du = C(u_- - u_+) + 2(u_- - u_+)F\big(u_+, u_-\big) - 2\int_{u_+}^{u_-} F\big(u_+, u\big)du\ . \tag{1.112}$$

Using formulas (1.107), (1.110) and (1.112), we derive

$$W = 2\left[(u_+ - u_-)F(u_+, u_-) - \int_{u_-}^{u_+} F(u_+, u)du - \int_{u_-}^{u_+} F(u, u_-)du\right]\ . \tag{1.113}$$

It is apparent that the expressions (1.104) and (1.113) are identical. This proves that the expressions for hysteresis energy losses derived above are consistent with the classical result (1.105).

We next discuss the applications of the above results to the irreversible thermodynamics of hysteretic media. It is clear that any hysteresis phenomenon is accompanied with energy dissipation. This means that hysteretic processes are irreversible and consequently, they fall in the domain of irreversible thermodynamics. Irreversible thermodynamics is the far-reaching extension of classical thermodynamics which describes reversible processes. For this reason, it is appropriate to begin with the brief review of the formal structure of classical thermodynamics.

Classical thermodynamics is based upon three main principles. The first principle of classical thermodynamics is the law of energy conservation. According to this principle, there exists a function of state, called the internal energy, U, of a closed system. This state function is such that its infinitesimally small change dU may occur as a result of energy exchange with the surroundings in the form of heat $đQ$, as well as a result of energy $đW$ added to the system (or spent by the system) in the form of work. Mathematically, the first principle is expressed by

$$dU = đQ + đW \,, \tag{1.114}$$

where a stroke is put across the symbol d in (1.114) to emphasize that the quantities $đQ$ and $đW$ are path-dependent infinitesimals, which are sometimes called imperfect differentials. In other words, the above quantities depend on particular path traced by the system during its transition from one equilibrium state to another.

The second principle of classical thermodynamics postulates the existence of another state function, called the entropy S. This principle also relates $đQ$ to the differential of entropy dS for reversible processes by the formula

$$dS = \frac{đQ}{T} \,, \tag{1.115}$$

where T is the absolute temperature.

For irreversible processes, the above equality is replaced by the inequality

$$dS > \frac{đQ}{T} \,. \tag{1.116}$$

The formulas (1.114) and (1.115) are often combined into one formula:

$$dS = \frac{1}{T}(dU - đW) \tag{1.117}$$

that constitutes the mathematical foundation of classical thermodynamics. The factor $1/T$ in equations (1.115) and (1.117) can be mathematically interpreted as an integrating factor for the imperfect differential $đQ$.

The first and second principles of classical thermodynamics are complemented by the Nernst-Plank postulate which is sometimes called the third principle of thermodynamics. According to this principle, the entropy of any system vanishes at zero temperature. This principle provides some useful information concerning the asymptotic behavior of entropy. However, the bulk of phenomenological thermodynamics does not require this principle. For this reason, the above postulate cannot be compared in its importance with the first and second principles of classical thermodynamics.

Classical thermodynamics has by and large been extended in two main directions. The first extension is based on the introduction of new variables describing the composition of the system. This approach has been very successful in applications of thermodynamics to chemical reactions. It has led to the development of chemical thermodynamics. The second extension is based on the generalization of the second principle of classical thermodynamics; it has led to the development of thermodynamic theory of irreversible processes that is often called irreversible thermodynamics. This theory has been mainly developed by I. Prigogine and his collaborators.

As mentioned above, the basic difference between classical and irreversible thermodynamics lies in the way in which the second principle is stated. In irreversible thermodynamics, the second principle is formulated as follows.

(1) The change in entropy dS can be split into two parts:

$$dS = đ_e S + đ_i S , \tag{1.118}$$

where $đ_e S$ is due to the flow of entropy into the system from its surroundings, while $đ_i S$ is the generation of entropy by irreversible processes within the system. The term $đ_i S$ is often called internal entropy production.

(2) The internal entropy production $đ_i S$ is never negative. It is zero if only the system undergoes a reversible process and positive if it undergoes an irreversible process. Thus,

$$đ_i S \geq 0 . \tag{1.119}$$

(3) For closed systems, the term $đ_e S$ is related to the energy $đ_e Q$ received in the form of heat by the formula that is similar to (1.115):

$$đ_e S = \frac{đ_e Q}{T} , \tag{1.120}$$

where T is the absolute temperature that is assumed to be definable (at least locally) for nonequilibrium situations.

It is also assumed in irreversible thermodynamics that the formula (1.117) holds with dS meaning the total change in entropy. From equations (1.118) and (1.120), we find

$$T\,dS = đ_e Q + T\,đ_i S . \tag{1.121}$$

The last expression allows one to relate the entropy production to the dissipated energy within the system. Indeed, from formulas (1.117) and (1.120) we find

$$dU = đW + đ_e Q + T đ_i S \,. \tag{1.122}$$

The first two terms in (1.122) have the same meaning as in (1.114) while the last term can be interpreted as the energy supplied to the system as a result of dissipating (irreversible) processes. This interpretation is especially clear for adiabatically isolated ($đ_e Q = 0$) systems that undergo cyclic changes $\oint đW = 0$. The increase in internal energy during one cycle ($\oint đU$) of such systems is only due to dissipating processes within the system ($\oint T đ_i S$). From formula (1.122) and the foregoing discussion, we find that the entropy production can be related to the dissipated energy $đ_i Q$ by the formula:

$$đ_i S = \frac{đ_i Q}{T} \,. \tag{1.123}$$

It is apparent that the novel part of the above formulation of the second principle is the introduction of internal entropy production $đ_i S$. However, this new quantity is useful only if it can be evaluated (in a mathematical form) for different irreversible processes. This is the central problem of irreversible thermodynamics and it has been emphasized in many books on this subject. For instance, in the book [42] (p. 90) by I. Prigogine we find: "*The main feature of the thermodynamics of irreversible processes consists of the evaluation of the entropy productions...* ." Similarly, in [43] (p. 21) we read: "*In thermodynamics of irreversible process, however, one of the important objectives is to relate the quantity $đ_i S$, the entropy production, to the various irreversible phenomena which may occur inside the system.*" Finally, in [44] (p. 69) it is noted: "*A central problem of irreversible thermodynamics, in fact, is the development of formulas for the entropy production $đ_i S$ in specific cases.*"

The above problem has been resolved for various irreversible processes which are caused by *macroscopic non-uniformities* of the system. Examples of such processes include heat flows due to temperature gradients, diffusion due to density gradients, electric current flows due to electric potential gradients, and so forth. For the above processes, the so-called entropy balance equation (1.118) is written in local (differential) form in which the entropy production, $đ_i S$, is replaced by the entropy source. The entropy source is then found as a sum of several terms each being product of a flux characterizing a particular irreversible process and a quantity, called thermodynamic force, which is related to a particular macroscopic nonuniformity of the system (temperature gradient, for instance). In this way, many useful results have been established. The celebrated L. Onsager reciprocity principle [45]–[46] for phenomenological coefficients is the most known example of these results. However, the above developments cannot cover hysteresis phenomena. This is because hysteresis is not necessarily caused by macroscopic nonuniformities and therefore cannot be linked to gradients of some physical quantities. As a result, different approaches should be developed for the calculation of entropy production in the case of irreversible hysteretic processes. It is logical to expect that mathematical models of hysteresis may help to solve the above problem. It is shown below that by using the Preisach model and the expressions for hysteresis energy losses derived on the basis of this model, the entropy production for hysteresis processes can indeed be found.

Consider the input $u(t)$ which is monotonically increased from its previous local minimum value u_-. If the current input value, $u(t)$, is lower than M_n, then by using (1.95), for the dissipated energy we find

$$Q(u_-, u) = (u - u_-)F(u, u_-) - \int_{u_-}^{u} F(u, \beta)d\beta - \int_{u_-}^{u} F(\alpha, u_-)d\alpha \ . \quad (1.124)$$

Employing formula (1.124), it is easy to conclude, that the energy dissipation, $đ_i Q$, that occurs as a result of the input increase from u to $u + du$, is given by

$$đ_i Q = \frac{\partial Q(u_-, u)}{\partial u} du \ . \quad (1.125)$$

From relations (1.123) and (1.125), we derive:

$$đ_i S = \frac{1}{T} \frac{\partial Q(u_-, u)}{\partial u} du \ . \quad (1.126)$$

By differentiating in formula (1.124) with respect to u and substituting the result into (1.126), after simple transformations we obtain:

$$đ_i S = \frac{du}{T} \int_{u_-}^{u} \frac{\partial}{\partial u} \Big[F(u, u_-) - F(u, \beta) \Big] d\beta \ . \quad (1.127)$$

If the input is monotonically decreased from its previous local maximum value, then the internal entropy production occurring as a result of the input decrease from u to $u - du$ is given by

$$đ_i S = \frac{du}{T} \int_{u}^{u_+} \frac{\partial}{\partial u} \Big[F(u_+, u) - F(\alpha, u) \Big] d\alpha \ . \quad (1.128)$$

The derivation of the last formula is similar to that of relation (1.127). It has been tacitly assumed in the previous derivation that the monotonic input variations are such that no previous history is wiped out. However, by using (1.96), it is easy to extend the last two relations to the most general case. The details of this extension are left to the reader.

References

[1] E. C. Stoner and E. P. Wohlfarth, "A mechanism of magnetic hysteresis in heterogeneous alloys," Philosophical Transactions of the Royal Society of London, Series A, Mathematical and Physical Sciences, Vol. 240, pp. 599-642, 1948.

[2] E. Madelung, "Über Magnetisierung durch schnellverlaufende Ströme und die Wirkungsweise des Rutherford-Marconischen Magnetdetektors," Annaleu der Physik., Vol. 17, p. 861, 1905.

[3] D. H. Everett and F. W. Smith, "A general approach to hysteresis. Part 2: Development of the domain theory," pp. 187-197, Vol. 50, 1954.

[4] R. I. Potter and R. J. Schmulian, "Self-consistently computed magnetization patterns in thin magnetic recording media," IEEE Transactions on Magnetics, Vol. MAG-7, pp. 873-880, 1971.

[5] L. Chua and K. Stromsmoe, "Lumped-circuit models for nonlinear inductors exhibiting hysteresis loops," IEEE Transactions on Circuit Theory, Vol. CT-17, pp. 564-574, 1970.

[6] L. Chua and S. Bass, "A Generalized Hysteresis Model," IEEE Transactions on Circuit Theory, Vol. CT-19, pp. 35-48, 1972.

[7] C. D. Boley and M. L. Hodgdon, "Model and simulations of hysteresis in magnetic cores," IEEE Transactions on Magnetics, Vol. 25, Issue: 5, pp. 3922-3924, 1989.

[8] D. D. Jiles and J. B. Thoelke, "Theory of ferromagnetic hysteresis: determination of model parameters from experimental hysteresis loops," Vol. 25, Issue: 5, pp. 3928-3930, 1989.

[9] J. A. Barker, D. E. Schreiber, B. G. Huth and D. H. Everett, "Magnetic hysteresis and minor loops: models and experiments," Proc. Roy. Soc., Vol. 386, Issue 1791, p. 251, 1985.

[10] B. G. Cragg and H. N. Temperley, "Memory: The analogy with ferromagnetic hysteresis," Brain, London 78(2), pp. 304-16, 1955.

[11] A. Katchalsky and E. Neumann, "Hysteresis and Molecular Memory Record," International Journal of Neuroscience, Vol. 3, Issue 4, pp. 175-182, 1972.

[12] I. D. Mayergoyz, "Mathematical Models of Hysteresis," Phys. Rev. Lett., Vol. 56, pp. 1518-1521, 1986.

[13] I. D. Mayergoyz, "Hysteresis models from the mathematical and control theory points of view," Journal of Applied Physics, Vol. 57, pp. 3803-3805, 1985.

[14] I. D. Mayergoyz, "Mathematical Models of Hysteresis", Springer, 1991.

[15] I. Mayergoyz, "Mathematical Models of Hysteresis and Their Applications", Academic Press (an imprint of Elsevier), 2003.

[16] J. Maddox, "Is there inanimate memory?," Nature, Vol. 321, p. 11, 1986.

[17] H. Poincare, "Science and Hypothesis," Dover, New York, 1952.

[18] F. Z. Preisach, Zeitschrift für Physik, Volume 94, Issue 5-6, pp. 277-302, 1935.

[19] Ferenc Preisach, “On the Magnetic Aftereffect,” IEEE Transactions on Magnetics, Vol. 53, No. 3, 0700111, 2017.
[20] L. Neel, Academie des Sciences, Paris, Comptes-Rendus Hebdomaines des Seances, Vol. 246, pp. 2313-2319, 1958.
[21] G. Biorci and D. Pescetti, “Analytical theory of the behaviour of ferromagnetic materials,” Nuovo Cimento, Vol. 7, pp. 829-842, 1958.
[22] G. Biorci and D. Pescetti, “Some consequences of the analytical theory of the ferromagnetic hysteresis,” J. Phys. Radium, Vol. 20 (2-3), pp. 233-236, 1959.
[23] G. Biorci and D. Pescetti, “Some Remarks on Hysteresis,” Journal of Applied Physics, Vol. 37, pp. 425-427, 1966.
[24] W. F. Brown, “Failure of the Local-Field Concept for Hysteresis Calculations,” Journal of Applied Physics, Vol. 33, pp. 1308-1309, 1962.
[25] G. Bate, “Statistical Stability of the Preisach Diagram for Particles of γ-Fe_2O_3,” Journal of Applied Physics, Vol. 33, pp. 2263-2269, 1962.
[26] E. Della Torre, “Measurements of Interaction in an Assembly of γ-Iron Oxide Particles,” Journal of Applied Physics, Vol. 36, pp. 518-522, 1965.
[27] A. Damlamian and A. Visintin, “Une généralisation vectorielle du modèle de Preisach pour l’hystérésis,” C.R. Acad. Sci. Paris, Série I 297, pp. 437-440, 1983.
[28] D. H. Everett and W. I. Whitton, “A general approach to hysteresis,” Transactions of the Faraday Society, Vol. 48, pp. 749-757, 1952.
[29] D. H. Everett, “A general approach to hysteresis. Part 3.—A formal treatment of the independent domain model of hysteresis,” Transactions of the Faraday Society, Vol. 50, pp. 1077-1096, 1954.
[30] D. H. Everett, “A general approach to hysteresis. Part 4. An alternative formulation of the domain model,” Transactions of the Faraday Society, Vol. 51, pp. 1551-1557, 1955.
[31] J. A. Enderby, “The domain model of hysteresis. Part 2.—Interacting domains,” Transactions of the Faraday Society, Vol. 52, pp. 106-120, 1956.
[32] A. Friedman, “Foundation of Modern Analysis,” Dover Publications, New York, 1982.
[33] M. Krasnosel’skii and A. Pokrovskii, “Systems with Hysteresis,” Springer, 1989.
[34] M. Brokate, “Some mathematical properties of the Preisach model for hysteresis,” IEEE Transactions on Magnetics, Vol. 25, pp. 2922-2944, 1989.
[35] M. Brokate and A. Visintin, “Properties of the Preisach model for hysteresis,” J. Reine Angew Math, Vol. 402, pp. 1-40, 1989.
[36] A. Visintin, “On the Preisach Model for Hysteresis,” Nonlinear Anal., Vol. 9, pp. 977-996, 1984.
[37] A. Visintin, “Differential Models of Hysteresis,” Springer, Berlin, 1994.
[38] M. Brokate and J. Sprekels, “Hysteresis and Phase Transitions,” Springer, Berlin, 1996.
[39] I. D. Mayergoyz and P. Andrei, “Statistical analysis of semiconductor devices,” Journal of Applied Physics, Vol. 90 (6), pp. 3019-3029, 2001.

[40] S. Ruta, O. Hovorka, P. W. Huang, K. Wang, G. Ju and R. Chantrell, "First order reversal curves and intrinsic parameter determination for magnetic materials; limitations of hysteron-based approaches in correlated systems," Scientific Reports 7, Nature, 45218, 2017.

[41] C. P. Steinmetz, "On the law of hysteresis," Trans AIEE, Vol. 9, pp. 3-64, 1892.

[42] I. Prigogine, "Introduction to Thermodynamics of Irreversible Processes," North-Holland, Amsterdam, 1963.

[43] S. R. de Groot and P. Mazur, "Non-Equilibrium Thermodynamics," North-Holland, Amsterdam, 1962.

[44] W. G. Vincenti and C. H. Kruger, "Introduction to Physical Gas Dynamics," Wiley, New York, 1965.

[45] L. Onsager, "Reciprocal Relations in Irreversible Processes. I.", Phys. Rev., Vol. 37, pp. 405-426, 1931.

[46] L. Onsager, "Reciprocal Relations in Irreversible Processes. II.," Phys. Rev., Vol. 38, pp. 2265-2279, 1931.

Chapter 2

Generalized Preisach Models

2.1 "Moving" Preisach Model of Hysteresis

The classical Preisach model of hysteresis has been discussed in detail in the previous chapter. It has been repeatedly emphasized that this model has some intrinsic limitations. The most important of them is the following. The classical Preisach model describes hysteresis nonlinearities which exhibit congruency of minor loops formed for the same reversal values of input. However, many experiments show that actual hysteresis nonlinearities may substantially deviate from this property. To remove (or relax) this limitation, essential generalizations of the classical Preisach model are needed, see [1]–[12]. These generalizations are discussed in this chapter.

We begin this chapter with an interesting modification of the classical Preisach model. This modification will reveal that the Preisach model does describe to a certain extent reversible properties of hysteresis nonlinearities. This fact has been overlooked in the existing literature. Apart from the mentioned fact, this modification will be also instrumental in the further generalizations of the classical Preisach model which are discussed in subsequent sections.

The classical Preisach model has been defined as

$$f(t) = \hat{\Gamma}u(t) = \iint_T \mu(\alpha,\beta)\hat{\gamma}_{\alpha,\beta}u(t)d\alpha d\beta, \tag{2.1}$$

where T is the limiting triangle specified by inequalities $\beta_0 \leq \alpha \leq \beta \leq \alpha_0$. This triangle is the support of the function $\mu(\alpha,\beta)$ and it does not depend on input variations.

We next subdivide the triangle T into three sets $S^+_{u(t)}$, $R_{u(t)}$ and $S^-_{u(t)}$

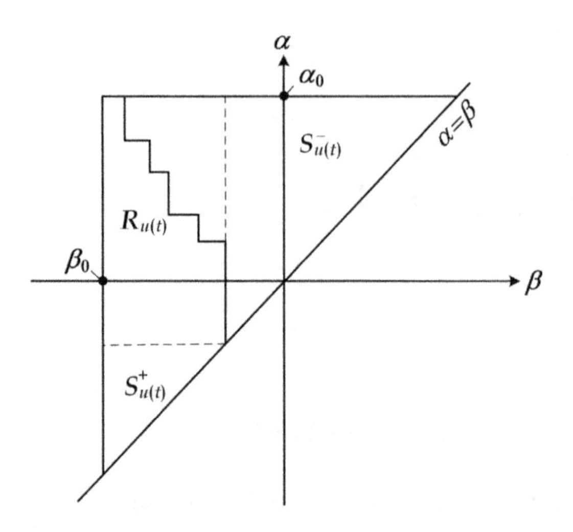

Fig. 2.1

(see Fig. 2.1), that are defined as follows:

$$(\alpha, \beta) \in S^+_{u(t)}, \quad \text{if} \ \ \beta_0 \le \beta \le \alpha \le u(t), \tag{2.2}$$

$$(\alpha, \beta) \in R_{u(t)}, \quad \text{if} \ \ \beta_0 \le \beta \le u(t), \ \ u(t) \le \alpha \le \alpha_0, \tag{2.3}$$

$$(\alpha, \beta) \in S^-_{u(t)}, \quad \text{if} \ \ u(t) \le \beta \le \alpha \le \alpha_0. \tag{2.4}$$

By using the above subdivision, we can represent equation (2.1) in the form

$$f(t) = \iint\limits_{S^+_{u(t)}} \mu(\alpha, \beta)\hat{\gamma}_{\alpha,\beta}u(t)d\alpha d\beta + \iint\limits_{R_{u(t)}} \mu(\alpha, \beta)\hat{\gamma}_{\alpha,\beta}u(t)d\alpha d\beta + \\ + \iint\limits_{S^-_{u(t)}} \mu(\alpha, \beta)\hat{\gamma}_{\alpha,\beta}u(t)d\alpha d\beta \, . \tag{2.5}$$

Since, $u(t) \ge \alpha$ for any $(\alpha, \beta) \in S^+_{u(t)}$, then $\hat{\gamma}_{\alpha,\beta}u(t) = +1$ and

$$\iint\limits_{S^+_{u(t)}} \mu(\alpha, \beta)\hat{\gamma}_{\alpha,\beta}u(t)d\alpha d\beta = \iint\limits_{S^+_{u(t)}} \mu(\alpha, \beta)d\alpha d\beta \, . \tag{2.6}$$

Similarly, $u(t) \le \beta$ for any $(\alpha, \beta) \in S^-_{u(t)}$ and

$$\iint\limits_{S^-_{u(t)}} \mu(\alpha, \beta)\hat{\gamma}_{\alpha,\beta}u(t)d\alpha d\beta = - \iint\limits_{S^-_{u(t)}} \mu(\alpha, \beta)d\alpha d\beta \, . \tag{2.7}$$

By substituting (2.6) and (2.7) in (2.5), we obtain

$$f(t) = \iint\limits_{R_{u(t)}} \mu(\alpha,\beta)\hat{\gamma}_{\alpha,\beta}u(t)d\alpha d\beta \; + \iint\limits_{S^+_{u(t)}} \mu(\alpha,\beta)d\alpha d\beta - \iint\limits_{S^-_{u(t)}} \mu(\alpha,\beta)d\alpha d\beta \, . \tag{2.8}$$

We next find a simple expression for the last two terms in (2.8). Consider a monotonic increase of input from some value below β_0 (state of negative saturation) to some value $u(t)$. Then, the output will change along the ascending branch $f^+_{u(t)}$, and according to (2.8) we find

$$f^+_{u(t)} = - \iint\limits_{R_{u(t)}} \mu(\alpha,\beta)d\alpha d\beta \; + \iint\limits_{S^+_{u(t)}} \mu(\alpha,\beta)d\alpha d\beta - \iint\limits_{S^-_{u(t)}} \mu(\alpha,\beta)d\alpha d\beta \, . \tag{2.9}$$

Similarly, if we consider a monotonic decrease of input from some value above α_0 (state of positive saturation) to the same value $u(t)$, then by using formula (2.8), we obtain

$$f^-_{u(t)} = \iint\limits_{R_{u(t)}} \mu(\alpha,\beta)d\alpha d\beta \; + \iint\limits_{S^+_{u(t)}} \mu(\alpha,\beta)d\alpha d\beta - \iint\limits_{S^-_{u(t)}} \mu(\alpha,\beta)d\alpha d\beta \, . \tag{2.10}$$

By summing up equations (2.9) and (2.10), we get

$$\iint\limits_{S^+_{u(t)}} \mu(\alpha,\beta)d\alpha d\beta - \iint\limits_{S^-_{u(t)}} \mu(\alpha,\beta)d\alpha d\beta = \frac{1}{2}\left(f^+_{u(t)} + f^-_{u(t)}\right). \tag{2.11}$$

By substituting equality (2.11) into formula (2.8), we finally obtain

$$f(t) = \iint\limits_{R_{u(t)}} \mu(\alpha,\beta)\hat{\gamma}_{\alpha,\beta}u(t)d\alpha d\beta \; + \; \frac{1}{2}\left(f^+_{u(t)} + f^-_{u(t)}\right). \tag{2.12}$$

The last expression is formally equivalent to the classical formula (2.1). However, in this expression the integration is performed not over the fixed

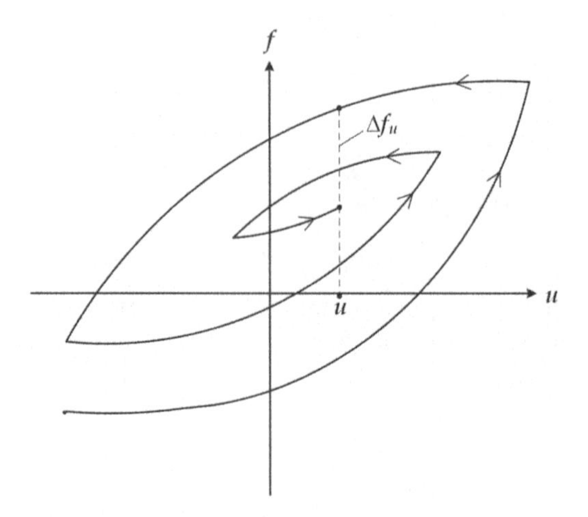

Fig. 2.2

limiting triangle T but over the rectangle $R_{u(t)}$ which changes along with input variations. For this reason, the expression (2.12) is termed here as a "moving" Preisach model. It is also clear from formula (2.12) that $\frac{1}{2}(f^{+}_{u(t)} + f^{-}_{u(t)})$ represents a fully reversible component of hysteresis nonlinearity described by the classical Preisach model. In this respect, the first term in the right-hand side of formula (2.12) can be construed as irreversible component of the classical Preisach model. To make the last point transparent, consider some output increment Δf_u corresponding to some input value u (see Fig. 2.2). This increment depends on a particular history of input variations and can be regarded as a measure of irreversibility of hysteresis nonlinearity for this particular history. It is clear from the diagram shown in Fig. 2.3 and the expression (2.12) that the above increment is given by

$$\Delta f_u = 2 \iint_{\Omega} \mu(\alpha, \beta) d\alpha d\beta. \tag{2.13}$$

The region of integration Ω belongs to $R_{u(t)}$ and depends on past history of input variations. This fact clearly suggests that the first term in the right-hand side of formula (2.12) describes irreversible processes. Thus, the expression (2.12) gives the decomposition of hysteresis nonlinearity described by classical Preisach model into irreversible and reversible components.

It is stressed in the above discussion that the expression (2.12) is mathematically equivalent to the classical definition (2.1). However, it is apparent

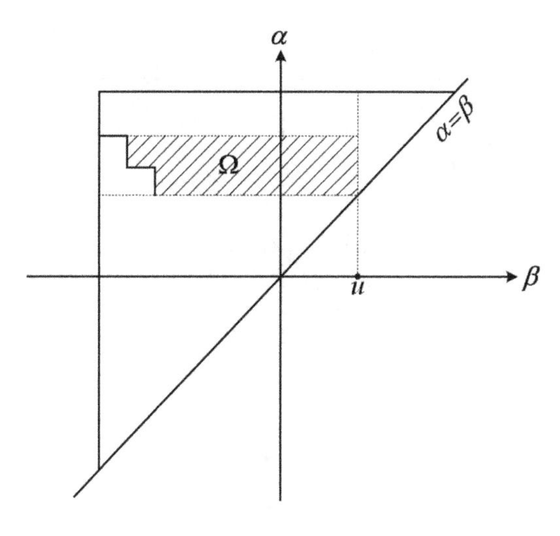

Fig. 2.3

that this equivalence holds only for input and output variations confined to the region enclosed by major hysteresis loop. Outside this region, the classical Preisach model prescribes flat saturation values for output, while the moving model (2.12) prescribes the actual experimentally observed values $f^+_{u(t)}$ and $f^-_{u(t)}$, for the states of negative and positive saturation, respectively. This is the case because for these states ascending and descending branches merge together and consequently $f^+_{u(t)} = f^-_{u(t)}$. As far as the first term in (2.12) is concerned, it is clear from formula (2.3) that this term vanishes. Thus, the moving model (2.12) can be regarded as a generalization of the classical model as far as the description of hysteresis nonlinearities beyond the limits of major loops is concerned.

It is instructive to consider directly the identification problem for the model (2.12) without invoking our previous discussion of this problem for the classical model (2.1). The essence of this problem is in determining the function μ by fitting the model (2.12) to some experimental data. Suppose that, starting from the state of negative saturation, the input $u(t)$ is monotonically increased until it reaches some value α. Then the input is monotonically decreased until it reaches some value β. The corresponding diagram is shown in Fig. 2.4. By using (2.12) and this diagram, we find that the output value corresponding to the final value $f_{\alpha\beta}$ of output is given

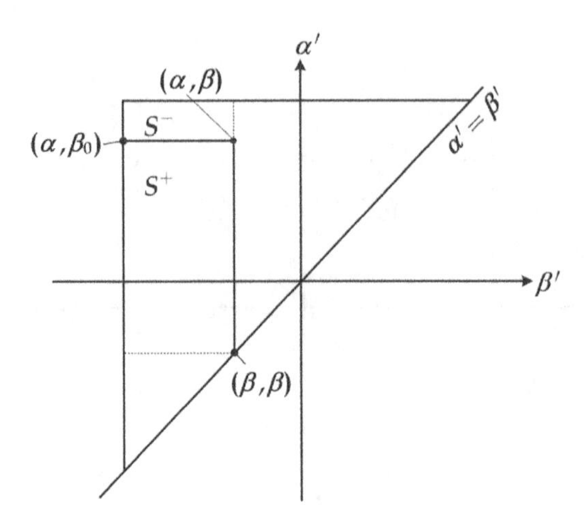

Fig. 2.4

by

$$f_{\alpha\beta} = \iint_{R(\alpha,\beta_0,\beta,\beta)} \mu(\alpha',\beta')d\alpha' d\beta' - \iint_{R(\alpha_0,\beta_0,\alpha,\beta)} \mu(\alpha',\beta')d\alpha' d\beta' + \frac{1}{2}\left(f_\beta^+ + f_\beta^-\right) . \tag{2.14}$$

Here, $R(\alpha_0, \beta_0, \alpha, \beta)$ is the rectangle whose opposite vertices are the points (α_0, β_0) and (α, β); the notation $R(\alpha, \beta_0, \beta, \beta)$ has a similar meaning.

Now suppose that, starting from the state of positive saturation, the input $u(t)$ is monotonically decreased until it reaches the value β. The corresponding $\alpha - \beta$ diagram is shown in Fig. 2.5. From this diagram and formula (2.12) we find the following expression for the resulting value of output:

$$f_\beta^- = \iint_{R(\alpha_0,\beta_0,\beta,\beta)} \mu(\alpha',\beta')d\alpha' d\beta' + \frac{1}{2}\left(f_\beta^+ + f_\beta^-\right) . \tag{2.15}$$

Next, we introduce the function

$$T(\alpha,\beta) = f_\beta^- - f_{\alpha\beta} , \tag{2.16}$$

which is equal to output increments between the limiting descending branch and first-order reversal curves. From formulas (2.14), (2.15) and (2.16), we

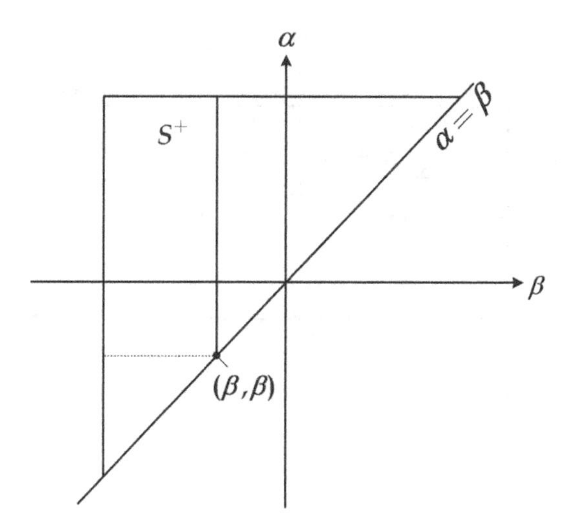

Fig. 2.5

find

$$
\begin{aligned}
T(\alpha, \beta) &= 2 \iint\limits_{R(\alpha_0, \beta_0, \alpha, \beta)} \mu(\alpha', \beta') d\alpha' d\beta' \\
&= 2 \int_{\alpha}^{\alpha_0} \left(\int_{\beta_0}^{\beta} \mu(\alpha', \beta') d\beta' \right) d\alpha'.
\end{aligned}
\tag{2.17}
$$

By differentiating the last expression two times, we obtain

$$
\mu(\alpha, \beta) = -\frac{1}{2} \frac{\partial^2 T(\alpha, \beta)}{\partial \alpha \partial \beta}. \tag{2.18}
$$

By recalling formula (2.16) for $T(\alpha, \beta)$, from equation (2.18) we derive

$$
\mu(\alpha, \beta) = \frac{1}{2} \frac{\partial^2 f_{\alpha\beta}}{\partial \alpha \partial \beta}, \tag{2.19}
$$

which coincides with the expression obtained for the classical Preisach model in the previous chapter.

Next, we show that the integration in (2.12) can be avoided and that the explicit expression for $f(t)$ in terms of experimentally measured function $T(\alpha, \beta)$ can be derived. To start the derivation, consider the $\alpha - \beta$ diagram

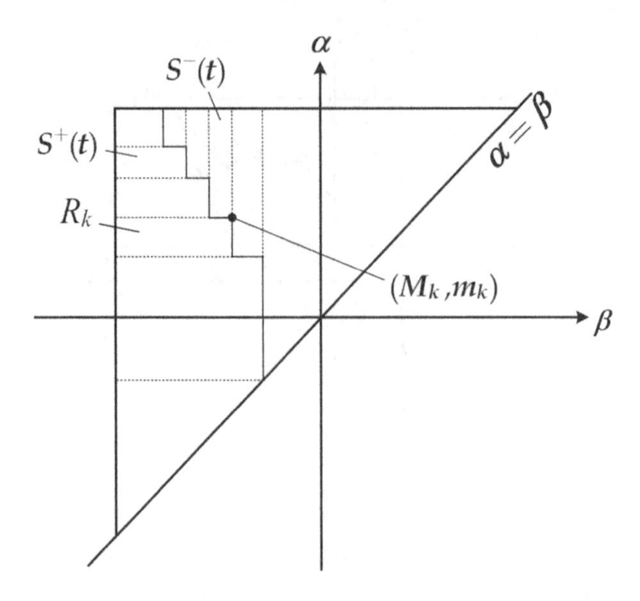

Fig. 2.6

shown in Fig. 2.6. Then, according to formula (2.12), we have

$$\begin{aligned} f(t) &= \iint_{S^+(t)} \mu(\alpha,\beta)d\alpha d\beta - \iint_{S^-(t)} \mu(\alpha,\beta)d\alpha d\beta + \frac{1}{2}\left(f^+_{u(t)} + f^-_{u(t)}\right) \\ &= 2\iint_{S^+(t)} \mu(\alpha,\beta)d\alpha d\beta - \iint_{R_{u(t)}} \mu(\alpha,\beta)d\alpha d\beta + \frac{1}{2}\left(f^+_{u(t)} + f^-_{u(t)}\right) . \end{aligned} \tag{2.20}$$

To evaluate the integral over $R_{u(t)}$ in the last formula, we consider a monotonic increase of input from the state of negative saturation to some value $u(t)$. Then from the expression (2.12) we find

$$f^+_{u(t)} = -\iint_{R_{u(t)}} \mu(\alpha,\beta)d\alpha d\beta + \frac{1}{2}\left(f^+_{u(t)} + f^-_{u(t)}\right) . \tag{2.21}$$

By substituting the last expression into formula (2.20), we conclude

$$f(t) = 2\iint_{S^+(t)} \mu(\alpha,\beta)d\alpha d\beta + f^+_{u(t)} . \tag{2.22}$$

It is clear that the moving model (2.12) is equivalent to the classical Preisach model as far as description of purely hysteretic behavior is concerned. For

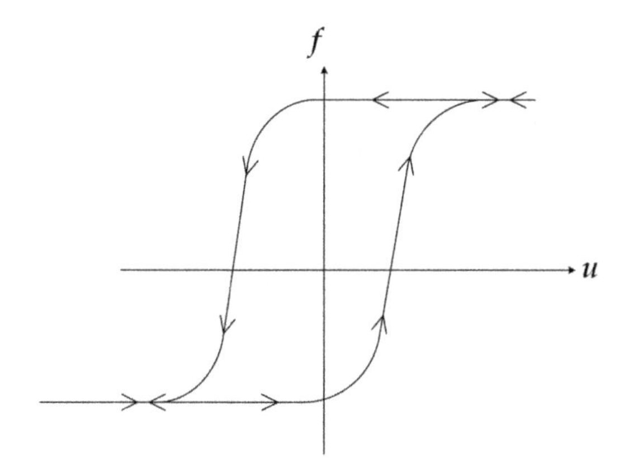

Fig. 2.7

this reason, the erasure property and congruency property of minor loops are valid for the moving model. According to the erasure property, the staircase interface $L(t)$ in Fig. 2.6 has vertices whose α and β coordinates are equal to M_k and m_k, respectively, and, as before, numbers M_k and m_k form the alternating series of past dominant input extrema. Now we subdivide $S^+(t)$ into rectangles R_k and represent the integral in formula (2.22) as

$$\iint_{S^+(t)} \mu(\alpha,\beta)d\alpha d\beta = \sum_{k=1}^{n(t)} \iint_{R_k} \mu(\alpha,\beta)d\alpha d\beta \,. \tag{2.23}$$

It is easy to see from the expression (2.17) for the function $T(\alpha,\beta)$ that the integrals over R_k can be represented in the form

$$2\iint_{R_k} \mu(\alpha,\beta)d\alpha d\beta = T(M_k,m_k) - T(M_{k+1},m_k). \tag{2.24}$$

From formulas (2.22)–(2.24) we obtain

$$f(t) = \sum_{k=1}^{n(t)} \Big[T(M_k,m_k) - T(M_{k+1},m_k)\Big] + f^+_{u(t)}. \tag{2.25}$$

This is the final result which expresses the output $f(t)$ in terms of experimentally measured function T.

Up to this point, we have discussed the modeling of "counter-clockwise" hysteresis (see Fig. 2.7). For this type of hysteresis, the positive saturation state is achieved for a larger input value than the negative saturation

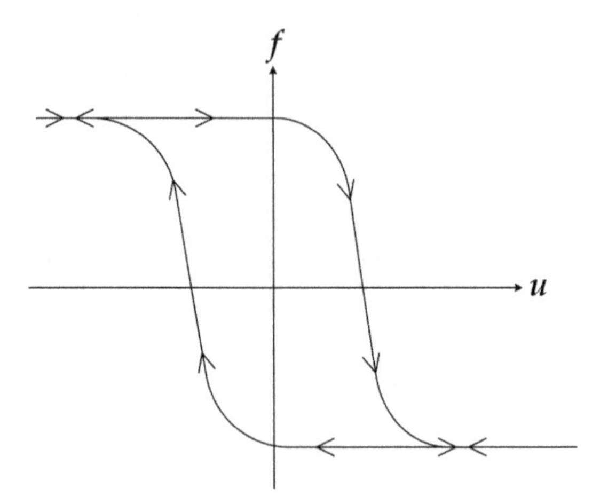

Fig. 2.8

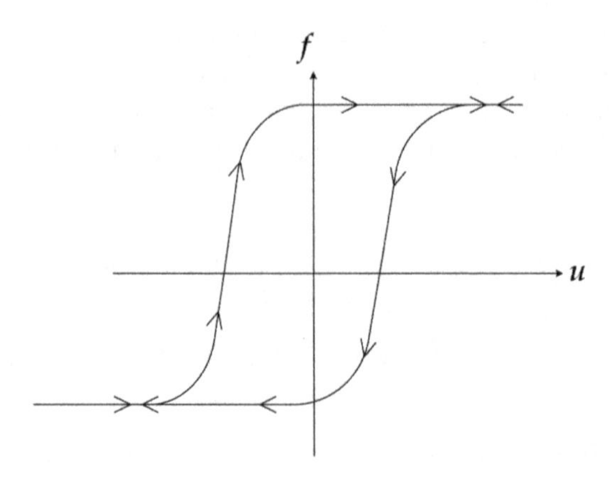

Fig. 2.9

state, and for any two consecutive descending and ascending branches the descending branch is above the corresponding ascending branch (see, for instance, Fig. 2.2). This type of hysteresis is typical (for instance) for magnetic materials and it can be modelled by using the classical Preisach model with positive measure $\mu(\alpha, \beta)$. There exists, however, "clock-wise" hysteresis (see Fig. 2.8). It is apparent that the classical Preisach model with negative measure can be used for the modeling of "clock-wise" hysteresis when the positive saturation state is achieved for a smaller input value than the negative saturation state. This type of hysteresis occurs (for instance) in superconductors due to their diamagnetic nature. The modeling of superconducting hysteresis is discussed in the last section of this chapter. There exists, however, the "clock-wise" hysteresis with the property that the positive saturation state is achieved for a larger input value than the negative saturation state (see Fig. 2.9). This is typical for hysteresis that occurs for certain front propagation problems in nonlinear diffusion of electromagnetic fields in magnetically nonlinear conductors. The modeling of this type of hysteresis is not readily available within the framework of the classical Preisach model. However, it can be easily accomplished by using the "moving" Preisach model (2.12). Indeed, the proper saturation states can be modelled by the appropriate choice of the reversible terms $\frac{1}{2}(f^+_{u(t)} + f^-_{u(t)})$ while the "clock-wise" nature of hysteresis is imposed by choosing a negative measure $\mu(\alpha, \beta)$ in the irreversible component. In other words, the decomposition (2.12) of hysteresis nonlinearity on reversible and irreversible components makes it possible to separately control the (clock-wise or counter clock-wise) orientation of hysteresis and the location of saturation states.

2.2 Preisach Model of Hysteresis with Input-Dependent Measure

The Preisach model with input-dependent measure is discussed in this section. It has the following advantages over the classical model. First, the congruency property of minor loops is relaxed for this model. This results in a broader area of applicability of this model as compared with the classical model. Second, the model with input-dependent measure allows one to fit experimentally measured first- and second-order reversal curves. Since higher-order reversal curves are "sandwiched" between first- and second-order reversal curves, it is natural to expect that this model will be more accurate than the classical one.

The Preisach model with input-dependent measure can be mathematically defined as

$$f(t) = \iint_{R_{u(t)}} \mu(\alpha, \beta, u(t)) \hat{\gamma}_{\alpha,\beta} u(t) d\alpha d\beta \; + \; \frac{1}{2}(f^+_{u(t)} + f^-_{u(t)}). \tag{2.26}$$

It is clear that a new feature of this model in comparison with the "moving" model (2.12) is the dependence of the distribution function μ on the current value of input, $u(t)$. For this reason, the model (2.26) can also be termed as

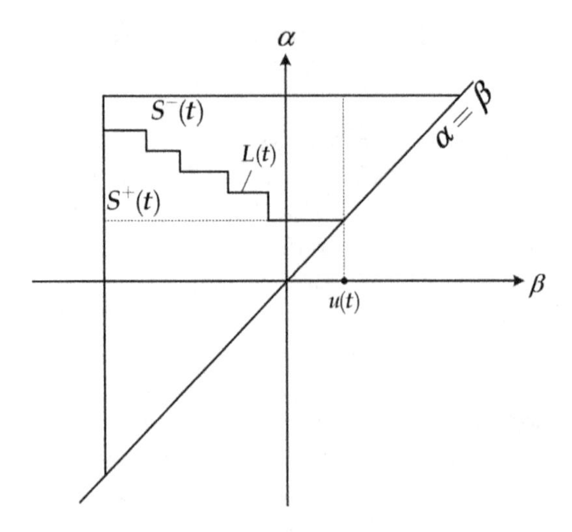

Fig. 2.10

the "nonlinear" Preisach model. Due to the new feature mentioned above, the first term in the right-hand side of (2.26) can be construed as a partially reversible component of hysteresis nonlinearity. Indeed, for each pair (α, β), the integrand $\mu(\alpha, \beta, u(t))\hat{\gamma}_{\alpha,\beta}u(t)$ is reversible for input variations between α and β. The Preisach model (2.26) admits a geometric interpretation which is similar to that for the classical model. In other words, it could be easily demonstrated that at any instant of time t the rectangle $R_{u(t)}$ is subdivided into two sets (see Fig. 2.10): $S^+(t)$ and $S^-(t)$ consisting of points (α, β) for which $\hat{\gamma}_{\alpha,\beta}u(t) = +1$ and $\hat{\gamma}_{\alpha,\beta}u(t) = -1$, respectively. The interface $L(t)$ between $S^+(t)$ and $S^-(t)$ is a staircase line whose vertices have α and β coordinates equal (respectively) to past dominant extrema M_k and m_k. Using the above geometric interpretation, the model (2.26) can be represented in the form

$$f(t) = \iint_{S^+(t)} \mu(\alpha, \beta, u(t))d\alpha d\beta - \iint_{S^-(t)} \mu(\alpha, \beta, u(t))d\alpha d\beta + \frac{1}{2}(f^+_{u(t)} + f^-_{u(t)}). \tag{2.27}$$

It can be shown that the following properties are valid for the "non-linear" model.

PROPERTY A (Erasure Property) *Only the alternating series of dominant global extrema M_k and m_k are stored by the "nonlinear" Preisach model (2.26).*

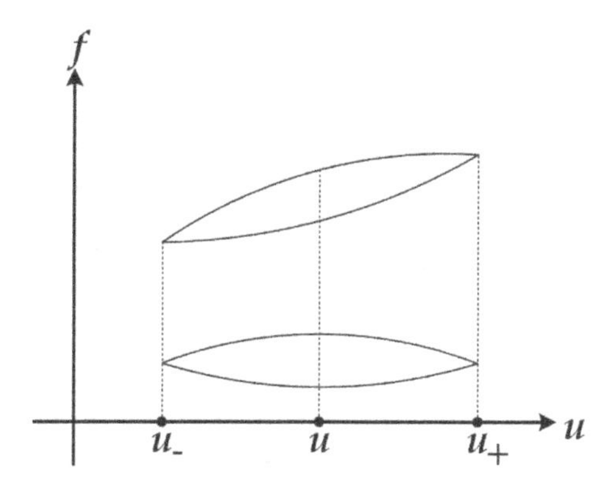

Fig. 2.11

The proof of this property is completely identical to that for the classical model.

PROPERTY B (Property of Equal Vertical Chords) *All minor loops resulting from back-and-forth input variations between the same two consecutive extrema have equal vertical chords (output increments) for the same input values* (see Fig. 2.11).

PROOF Consider a minor loop formed as a result of back-and-forth input variations between u_+ and u_- (Fig. 2.12). Let $f_u^{''}$ and $f_u^{'}$ be output values along descending and ascending branches of this loop, respectively. These values correspond to the same value of input u from the interval $u_- < u < u_+$. By using the expression (2.27), $f_u^{''}$ and $f_u^{'}$, can be computed as

$$f_u^{'} = \iint\limits_{S_+^{'}} \mu(\alpha,\beta,u)d\alpha d\beta \; - \iint\limits_{S_-^{'}} \mu(\alpha,\beta,u)d\alpha d\beta \; + \; \frac{1}{2}(f_u^+ + f_u^-) \qquad (2.28)$$

$$f_u^{''} = \iint\limits_{S_+^{''}} \mu(\alpha,\beta,u)d\alpha d\beta \; - \iint\limits_{S_-^{''}} \mu(\alpha,\beta,u)d\alpha d\beta \; + \; \frac{1}{2}(f_u^+ + f_u^-), \qquad (2.29)$$

where the sets $S_+^{'}$, $S_-^{'}$, $S_+^{''}$ and $S_-^{''}$, are as shown in the diagram presented in Fig. 2.13. It is clear from these diagrams that

$$S_+^{''} - S_+^{'} = R(u_+, u, u_-), \quad S_-^{'} - S_-^{''} = R(u_+, u, u_-). \qquad (2.30)$$

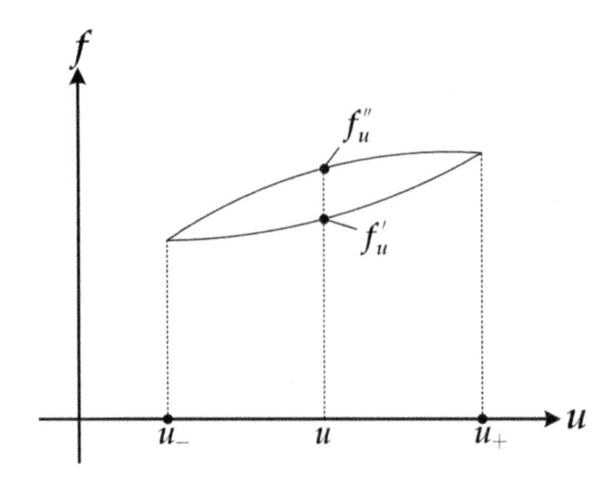

Fig. 2.12

From formulas (2.28), (2.29) and (2.30) we derive

$$f''_u - f'_u = 2 \iint\limits_{R(u_+,u,u_-)} \mu(\alpha,\beta,u)d\alpha d\beta \ . \tag{2.31}$$

According to (2.31), we find that for any $u \in (u_+, u_-)$ the corresponding vertical chord does not depend on a particular past history preceding the formation of minor loop. This proves that all comparable minor loops, that is the loops with the same reversal input values u_+ and u_-, have equal vertical chords.

It is left to the reader as a useful exercise to prove that comparable minor loops described by the nonlinear model (2.26) are not necessarily congruent.

Now we turn to the identification problem of determining the distribution function $\mu(\alpha, \beta, u)$ by fitting the model (2.26) to some experimental data. It turns out that for the solution of this identification problem the sets of first- and second-order reversal curves are required. These curves can be measured experimentally as follows. We first decrease the input, $u(t)$, to such a negative value that the outputs of all operators $\hat{\gamma}_{\alpha,\beta}$ are equal to -1(state of negative saturation). Then, we monotonically increase the input until it reaches some value α As we do this, we will follow along the ascending branch of the major loop (see Fig. 2.14). As we already know, the first-order reversal curves are attached to this ascending branch and they are formed when the above monotonic increase of $u(t)$ is followed by a subsequent monotonic decrease. The notation $f^+_{\alpha u}$ will be used for

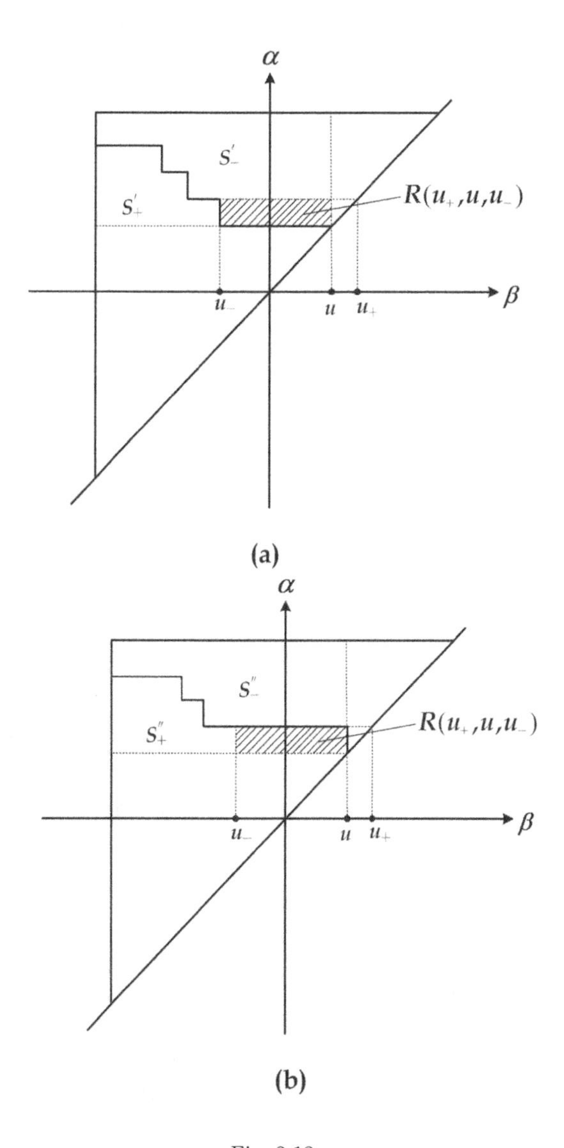

Fig. 2.13

the output values on the first-order reversal curve attached to the ascending branch of the major loop at the point f^+_α. The second-order reversal curves are attached to the first-order reversal curves, and they are formed when the above monotonic decrease is followed by a monotonic increase. The notation $f_{\alpha\beta u}$ will be used for the output values on the second-order

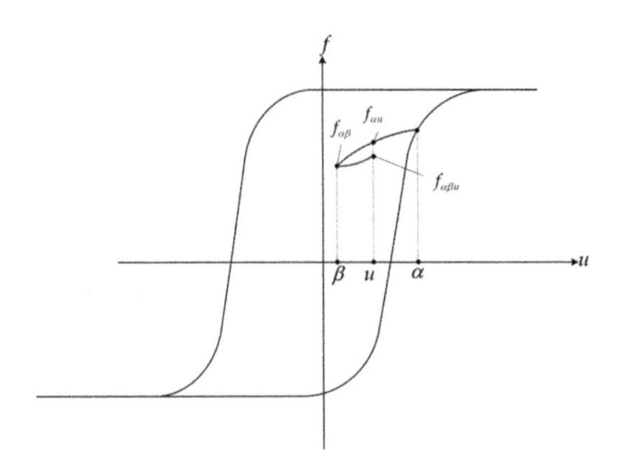

Fig. 2.14

reversal curve attached to the first-order reversal curve $f_{\alpha u}$ at the point $f_{\alpha\beta}$ (Fig. 2.14).

Consider the function

$$P(\alpha,\beta,u) = f_{\alpha u} - f_{\alpha\beta u} \tag{2.32}$$

which has the physical meaning of output increments between the first- and second-order reversal curves.

It is clear from the definition of this function that

$$P(\alpha,u,u) = P(u,\beta,u) = P(u,u,u) = 0\ . \tag{2.33}$$

This property will be employed later in our discussion. Now we will try to relate the function $P(\alpha,\beta,u)$ to the distribution function $\mu(\alpha,\beta,u)$. To this end, we will use the diagrams shown in Fig. 2.15. From these diagrams and formula (2.27) we conclude that

$$\begin{aligned} f_{\alpha u} &= \iint\limits_{\tilde{S}_+} \mu(\alpha',\beta',u)d\alpha' d\beta' \; - \iint\limits_{\tilde{S}_-} \mu(\alpha',\beta',u)d\alpha' d\beta' \; + \frac{1}{2}(f_u^+ + f_u^-)\ , \\ f_{\alpha\beta u} &= \iint\limits_{\tilde{\tilde{S}}_+} \mu(\alpha',\beta',u)d\alpha' d\beta' \; - \iint\limits_{\tilde{\tilde{S}}_-} \mu(\alpha',\beta',u)d\alpha' d\beta' \; + \frac{1}{2}(f_u^+ + f_u^-)\ , \end{aligned} \tag{2.34}$$

$$\tilde{\tilde{S}}_+ - \tilde{S}_+ = R(\alpha,\beta,u), \quad \tilde{\tilde{S}}_- - \tilde{S}_- = R(\alpha,\beta,u)\ . \tag{2.35}$$

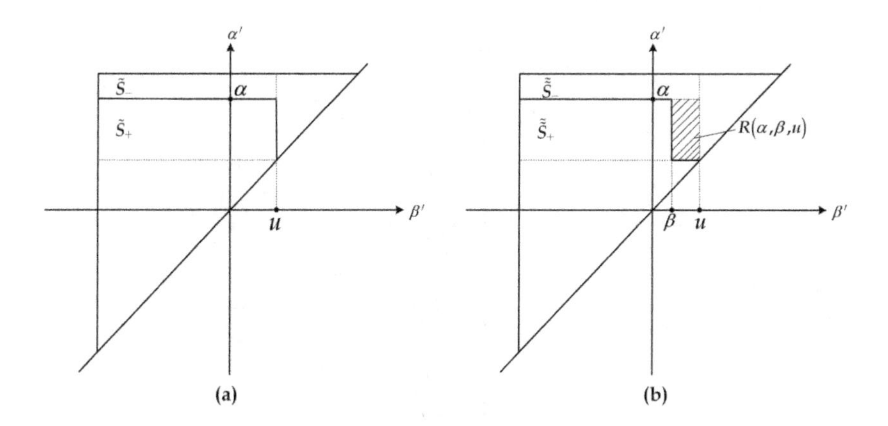

Fig. 2.15

By using equations (2.32), (2.34) and (2.35), we derive

$$
\begin{aligned}
P(\alpha,\beta,u) &= 2 \iint\limits_{R(\alpha,\beta,u)} \mu(\alpha',\beta',u)d\alpha' d\beta' \\
&= 2\int_u^\alpha \left(\int_\beta^u \mu(\alpha',\beta',u)d\beta' \right) d\alpha' .
\end{aligned} \tag{2.36}
$$

By differentiating the last expression twice, we obtain

$$\mu(\alpha,\beta,u) = -\frac{1}{2}\,\frac{\partial^2 P(\alpha,\beta,u)}{\partial\alpha\partial\beta} . \tag{2.37}$$

By recalling the definition (2.32) of $P(\alpha,\beta,u)$, from the last equation we find

$$\mu(\alpha,\beta,u) = \frac{1}{2}\,\frac{\partial^2 f_{\alpha\beta u}}{\partial\alpha\partial\beta} . \tag{2.38}$$

It is clear from the above derivation, that the expression (2.37) and (2.38) are valid if $\beta < u < \alpha$. If $u \leq \beta$ or $u \geq \alpha$, then we define

$$\mu(\alpha,\beta,u) \equiv 0 , \tag{2.39}$$

which is consistent with formula (2.33).

Thus, if the distribution function, $\mu(\alpha,\beta,u)$, is determined from (2.36) or (2.38), then the model (2.26) will match the increments between first- and second-order reversal curves. Next we shall show that the limiting ascending branch will be matched by this model, as well. Indeed, it is easy

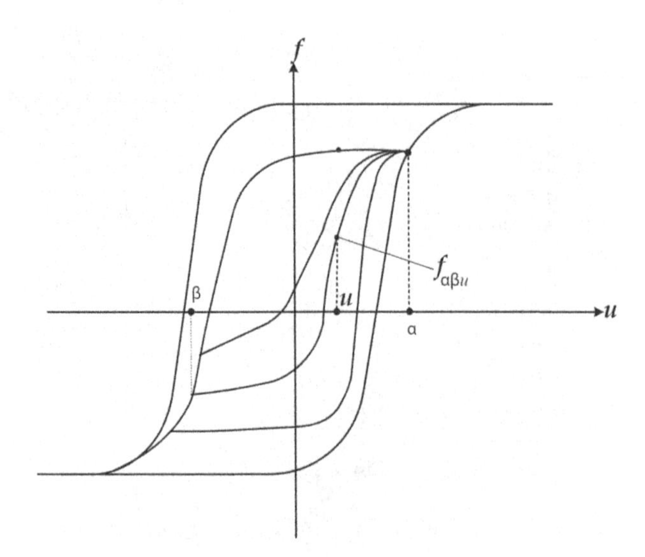

Fig. 2.16

to see that the output values f_u on the limiting ascending branch predicted by the nonlinear model (2.26) are equal to

$$f_u = -\iint_{R(\alpha_0,\beta_0,u)} \mu(\alpha',\beta',u)d\alpha' d\beta' + \frac{1}{2}(f_u^+ + f_u^-) . \tag{2.40}$$

According to formulas (2.36) and (2.32), we have

$$\iint_{R(\alpha_0,\beta_0,u)} \mu(\alpha',\beta',u)d\alpha' d\beta' = \frac{1}{2}P(\alpha_0,\beta_0,u) = \frac{1}{2}(f_{\alpha_0 u} - f_{\alpha_0\beta_0 u}) = \frac{1}{2}(f_u^- - f_u^+). \tag{2.41}$$

By substituting (2.41) in (2.40), we find

$$f_u = f_u^+ . \tag{2.42}$$

Thus, if the function, $\mu(\alpha, \beta, u)$, is determined according to formula (2.38), then the model (2.26) fits: (a) the output increments between the first- and second-order reversal curves, (b) the ascending branch of the major loop. Since the ascending branch of the major loop can be construed as a second-order reversal curve, we conclude that the model (2.26) fits the sets of first- and second-order reversal curves.

In the above discussion, we have used second-order *increasing* reversal curves (see Fig. 2.13) in order to determine the distribution function

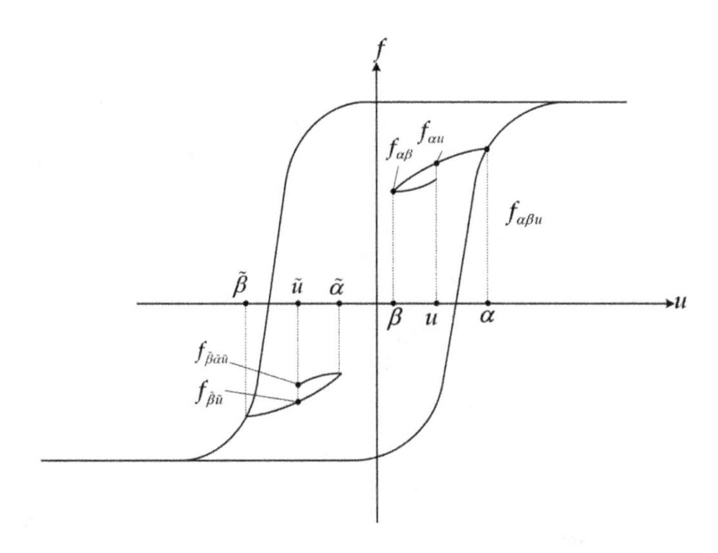

Fig. 2.17

$\mu(\alpha, \beta, u)$. However, by almost literally repeating the previous line of reasoning, a similar expression can be found for $\mu(\alpha, \beta, u)$ by using second-order *decreasing* reversal curves $f_{\tilde{\beta}\tilde{\alpha}\tilde{u}}$. One of these curves is shown in Fig. 2.17. By using this figure, we can introduce the function

$$P(\tilde{\beta}, \tilde{\alpha}, \tilde{u}) \;=\; f_{\tilde{\beta}\tilde{\alpha}\tilde{u}} - f_{\tilde{\beta}\tilde{u}} \,. \tag{2.43}$$

In the same way as before, we can show that

$$P(\tilde{\beta}, \tilde{\alpha}, \tilde{u}) \;=\; 2 \iint\limits_{R(\tilde{\alpha}, \tilde{\beta}, \tilde{u})} \mu(\alpha', \beta', \tilde{u})\, d\alpha'\, d\beta' \tag{2.44}$$

and

$$\mu(\tilde{\alpha}, \tilde{\beta}, \tilde{u}) = -\frac{1}{2}\,\frac{\partial^2 P(\tilde{\alpha}, \tilde{\beta}, \tilde{u})}{\partial\tilde{\alpha}\partial\tilde{\beta}} \,. \tag{2.45}$$

If

$$\tilde{\beta} = -\alpha, \quad \tilde{\alpha} = -\beta, \quad \tilde{u} = -u \,, \tag{2.46}$$

then due to the symmetry between increasing and decreasing second-order reversal curves (see Fig. 2.17) we find

$$P(\tilde{\beta}, \tilde{\alpha}, \tilde{u}) \;=\; P(\alpha, \beta, u) \,. \tag{2.47}$$

By using formulas (2.46) and (2.47) in equation (2.45), we derive

$$\mu(-\beta, -\alpha, u) = -\frac{1}{2}\,\frac{\partial^2 P(\alpha, \beta, u)}{\partial\alpha\partial\beta} \,. \tag{2.48}$$

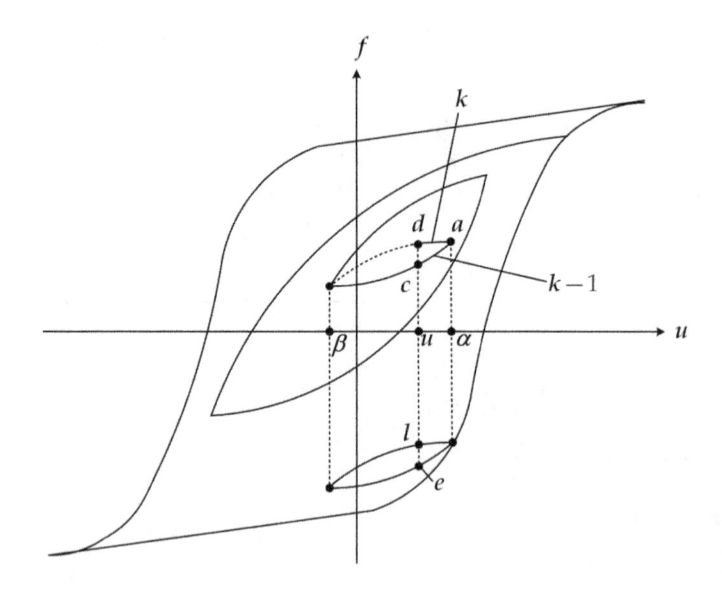

Fig. 2.18

From formulas (2.28) and (2.37), we conclude that

$$\mu(\alpha, \beta, u) = \mu(-\beta, -\alpha, u) \ . \tag{2.49}$$

The last formula can be regarded as a generalization of the mirror symmetry previously established for the classical Preisach model.
We next proceed to the proof of the following important result.

REPRESENTATION THEOREM *The erasure property and the property of equal vertical chords for comparable minor loops constitute the necessary and sufficient conditions for the representation of a hysteresis nonlinearity by the Preisach model (2.26).*

PROOF Necessity: If a hysteresis nonlinearity is representable by the Preisach model (2.26), then this nonlinearity should have the same properties as the model. This means that this nonlinearity should exhibit the erasure property and the property of equal vertical chords for comparable minor loops.
Sufficiency: Consider a hysteresis nonlinearity which has both the erasure property and the property of equal vertical chords. For this nonlinearity we find the distribution function $\mu(\alpha, \beta, u)$ by using formula (2.37) (or (2.38)). Then the Preisach model (2.26) will match exactly the sets of all first- and second-order reversal curves. We intend to prove that this model will match

all possible higher-order reversal curves, as well. The proof is based on the induction argument. Let us assume that the above statement is true for all possible reversal curves up to the order $k-1$. Then, for the induction inference to take place, we need to prove that the same statement holds for any reversal curve of order k. Let a be a point at which a reversal curve of order k is attached to a reversal curve of order $k-1$ (see Fig. 2.18). According to the induction assumption, the output values for the actual hysteresis nonlinearity and for nonlinear Preisach model coincide at each point of the reversal curve of order $k-1$. Thus, it remains to be proved that the output increments between the reversal curves of orders k and $k-1$ are the same for the actual hysteresis non-linearity and for the model (2.26). It is here that the erasure property and the property of equal vertical chords will be used. According to the erasure property, the kth reversal curve should meet the $(k-1)^{\text{th}}$ reversal curve at some point b, which is the point of inception of the latter curve. As a result, a minor loop is formed. Consider a comparable minor loop (loop with the same reversal input values), which is attached to the limiting ascending branch (Fig. 2.18). This loop is formed by some first- and second-order transition curves. According to the property of equal vertical chords, this loop has the same vertical chords as the loop formed by $(k-1)^{\text{th}}$ and k^{th} reversal curves. Consider an arbitrary value u of input such that $\beta < u < \alpha$. Using the diagram shown in Fig. 2.19, it is easy to derive the following expression for the output increment

$$f_u^{(k)} - f_u^{(k-1)} = 2 \iint_{R(\alpha,\beta,u)} \mu(\alpha', \beta', u) d\alpha' d\beta' , \tag{2.50}$$

where $f_u^{(k)}$ and $f_u^{(k-1)}$ are the output values on the kth and $(k-1)^{\text{th}}$ reversal curves, respectively, corresponding to the input value u, as predicted by the model (2.26). From formula (2.36), we find that the right-hand side of equation (2.50) is equal to the output increment el between the first- and second-order transition curves. Consequently,

$$f_u^{(k)} - f_u^{(k-1)} = el . \tag{2.51}$$

According to the property of vertical chords, we have

$$el = cd . \tag{2.52}$$

From the last two formulas, we conclude that

$$f_u^{(k)} - f_u^{(k-1)} = cd . \tag{2.53}$$

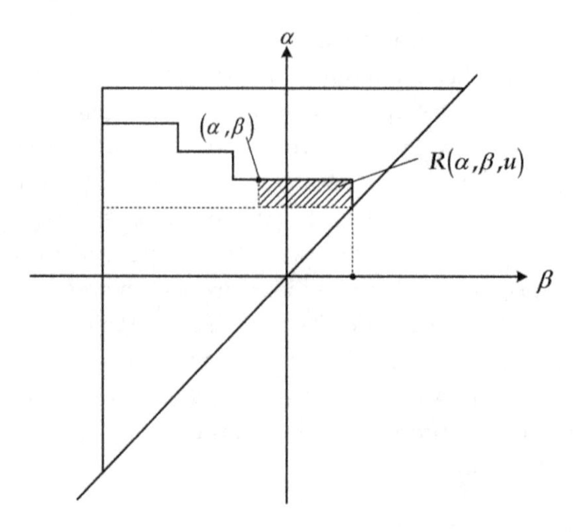

Fig. 2.19

Thus the nonlinear model predicts the correct output increments between the kth and $(k-1)^{\mathrm{th}}$ reversal curves. From this fact and the above induction assumption we conclude that the nonlinear model predicts the correct output values on the reversal curve of order k. This concludes the proof of the theorem.

The proved theorem establishes the exact bounds of applicability of the Preisach model (2.26). It is apparent that the property of equal vertical chords is more general than the congruency property. Indeed, if comparable minor loops are congruent, then they have equal vertical chords. However, if comparable minor loops have equal vertical chords, they are not necessarily congruent. This clearly shows that the Preisach model (2.26) has a broader area of applicability than the classical Preisach model. Next we shall show that the model (2.26) contains the classical Preisach model as a particular case. The exact statement of this fact is given by the following theorem.

REDUCTION THEOREM *If all comparable minor loops of hysteresis nonlinearity are congruent, then the Preisach model (2.26) for this nonlinearity coincides with the classical Preisach model.*

PROOF: Since all comparable minor loops are congruent, these loops have equal vertical chords. Assuming also that the erasure property holds, we can represent the mentioned hysteresis nonlinearity by the Preisach model (2.26). We intend to show next that, because of congruency property, the distribution function μ in (2.26) does not depend on u. It is clear from Fig. 2.20 that the congruency property results in the congruency of second-order reversal curves $f_{\alpha'\beta u}$, $f_{\alpha\beta u}$ and $f_{\alpha''\beta u}$. This means that the derivative $\partial f_{\alpha\beta u}/\partial u$ does not depend on α. Consequently,

$$\frac{\partial^3 f_{\alpha\beta u}}{\partial\alpha\partial\beta\partial u} \equiv 0 \, . \tag{2.54}$$

From formulas (2.54) and (2.38), we find

$$\frac{\partial\mu(\alpha,\beta,u)}{\partial u} \equiv 0. \tag{2.55}$$

Thus, μ does not depend on u and is only a function of α and β:

$$\mu(\alpha,\beta,u) = \upsilon(\alpha,\beta) \, . \tag{2.56}$$

From formulas (2.56) and (2.26), we obtain

$$f(t) = \iint\limits_{R_{u(t)}} \upsilon(\alpha,\beta)\hat{\gamma}_{\alpha,\beta}u(t)d\alpha d\beta + \frac{1}{2}(f^{+}_{u(t)} + f^{-}_{u(t)}) \, . \tag{2.57}$$

It remains to be proven that $\upsilon(\alpha,\beta)$ in the last equation coincides with $\mu(\alpha,\beta)$ in formula (2.37). The proof is straightforward. By using relations (2.37) and (2.57), we find that for any α, β and u, such that $\beta \le u \le \alpha$ we have

$$P(\alpha,\beta,u) = f_{\alpha u} - f_{\alpha\beta u} = 2\iint\limits_{R_{u(t)}} \mu(\alpha',\beta')d\alpha' d\beta' \, , \tag{2.58}$$

$$P(\alpha,\beta,u) = f_{\alpha u} - f_{\alpha\beta u} = 2\iint\limits_{R_{u(t)}} \upsilon(\alpha',\beta')d\alpha' d\beta' \, . \tag{2.59}$$

From the last two formulas, as before, we derive

$$\mu(\alpha,\beta) = \upsilon(\alpha,\beta) = -\frac{1}{2}\frac{\partial^2 P(\alpha,\beta,u)}{\partial\alpha\partial\beta} \, . \tag{2.60}$$

Thus, it is proved that under the congruency condition, the Preisach model (2.26) coincides with the moving Preisach model (2.37). On the other hand, the moving model coincides with the classical Preisach model as far as the description of purely hysteretic behavior is concerned. From here we conclude that under the congruency condition the model (2.26) coincides with the classical Preisach model, and this concludes the proof of the theorem.

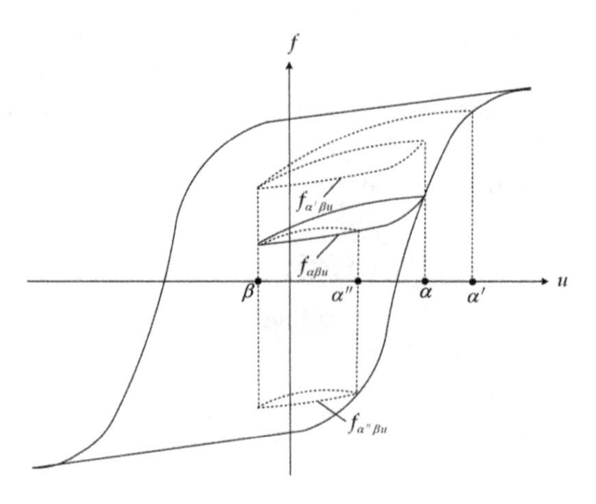

Fig. 2.20

We next turn to the discussion of numerical implementation of the model (2.26). We intend to show that double integration in (2.26) can be completely avoided and that explicit expressions for the output $f(t)$ in terms of experimentally measured function $P(\alpha, \beta, u)$ can be derived. The starting point of our derivation is the expression (2.27) that can be modified as follows:

$$f(t) = \iint_{R_{u(t)}} \mu(\alpha, \beta, u(t))d\alpha d\beta - 2 \iint_{S^-(t)} \mu(\alpha, \beta, u(t))d\alpha d\beta + \frac{1}{2}(f^+_{u(t)} + f^-_{u(t)}) . \tag{2.61}$$

According to formula (2.41), we have

$$\iint_{R_{u(t)}} \mu(\alpha, \beta, u(t))d\alpha d\beta = \frac{1}{2}(f^-_{u(t)} - f^+_{u(t)}) . \tag{2.62}$$

By substituting (2.62) in (2.61), we obtain

$$f(t) = f^-_{u(t)} - 2 \iint_{S^-(t)} \mu(\alpha, \beta, u(t))d\alpha d\beta . \tag{2.63}$$

We next subdivide $S^-(t)$ into rectangles R_k (see Fig. 2.21) and represent the integral (2.63) as

$$\iint_{S^-(t)} \mu(\alpha, \beta, u(t))d\alpha d\beta = \sum_{k=1}^{n(t)} \iint_{R_k} \mu(\alpha, \beta, u(t))d\alpha d\beta . \tag{2.64}$$

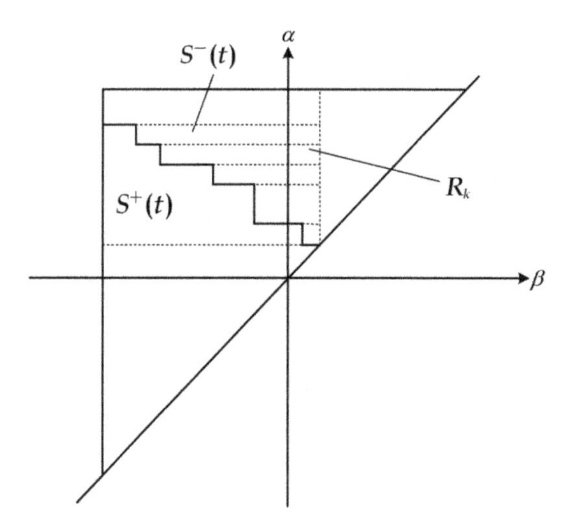

Fig. 2.21

It is easy to see that

$$R_k = R\big(M_k, m_k, u(t)\big) - R\big(M_{k+1}, m_k, u(t)\big) . \tag{2.65}$$

From formulas (2.65) and (2.36), we conclude that

$$\begin{aligned}
&\iint\limits_{R_k} \mu\big(\alpha, \beta, u(t)\big) d\alpha d\beta \\
&= \iint\limits_{R(M_k, m_k, u(t))} \mu\big(\alpha, \beta, u(t)\big) d\alpha d\beta - \iint\limits_{R(M_{k+1}, m_k, u(t))} \mu\big(\alpha, \beta, u(t)\big) d\alpha d\beta \\
&= \frac{1}{2}\Big[P(M_k, m_k, u(t)) - P(M_{k+1}, m_k, u(t))\Big] .
\end{aligned} \tag{2.66}$$

By substituting the last equation into (2.64) and then into (2.63), we obtain

$$f(t) = f^-_{u(t)} - \sum_{k=1}^{n(t)} \Big[P(M_k, m_k, u(t)) - P(M_{k+1}, m_k, u(t))\Big] . \tag{2.67}$$

This is the final formula which expresses explicitly the output $f(t)$ in terms of the experimentally measured function P. This formula has been used to develop a digital code which numerically implements the Preisach model (2.26).

We conclude this section by the discussion of two facts which may further reveal the advantages of the nonlinear Preisach model over the classical

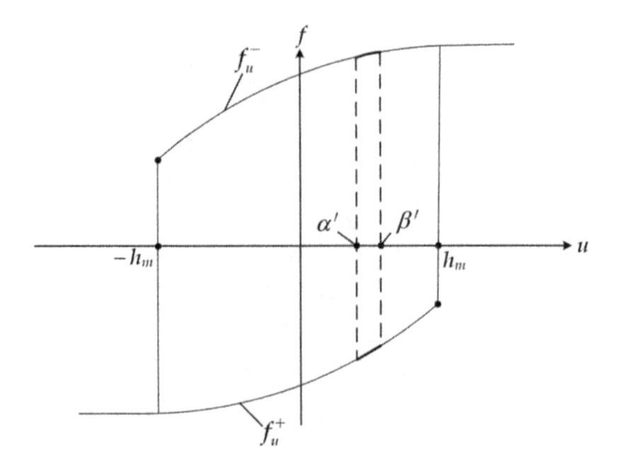

Fig. 2.22

one. Consider the hysteresis nonlinearities shown in Fig. 2.22. It is pointed out in Chapter 1 that these nonlinearities cannot be described by the classical Preisach model. The reason is that degenerate minor loops traced as the input varies back and forth between α' and β' are not congruent. It is easy to see that the hysteresis nonlinearities can be described by the Preisach model (2.26). First, this is clear from the fact that the property of equal vertical chords is satisfied because all minor loops are degenerate and, consequently, they have equal (zero) vertical chords. Second, the explicit representation for this hysteresis nonlinearity can be found. Indeed, it can be shown that

$$\mu(\alpha, \beta, u(t)) = \frac{1}{2}(f^-_{u(t)} - f^+_{u(t)})\delta(\alpha - h_m, \beta + h_m) , \tag{2.68}$$

where δ is the Dirac function.

By substituting the last formula into equation (2.26), we find

$$f(t) = \frac{1}{2}(f^-_{u(t)} - f^+_{u(t)})\hat{\gamma}_{h_m, -h_m} u(t) + \frac{1}{2}(f^+_{u(t)} + f^-_{u(t)}) . \tag{2.69}$$

It can be easily checked that the last expression indeed represents the hysteresis nonlinearity depicted in Fig. 2.22.

Finally, the following observation is helpful in order to appreciate the extent to which the Preisach model (2.26) is more general than the classical one. The classical Preisach model represents hysteresis non-linearities that, for any *reversal* point, have (regardless of past history) only one branch starting from this point (see Fig. 2.25). This branch is congruent to one of the first-order reversal curves. This is apparent from formula (1.73), and

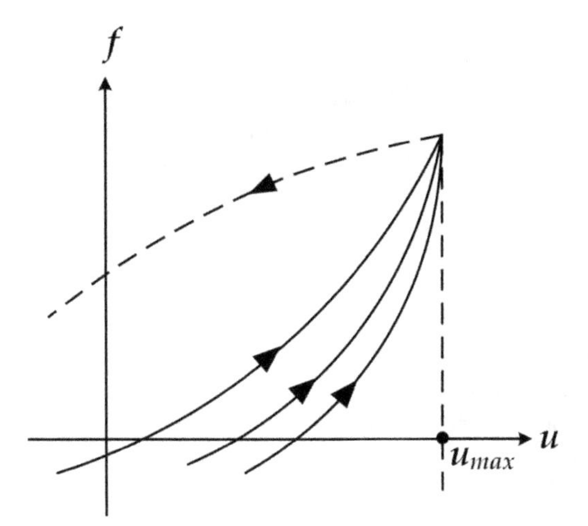

Fig. 2.23

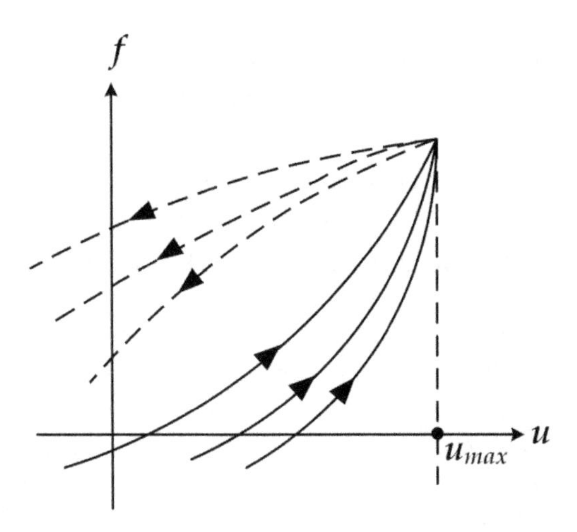

Fig. 2.24

is a consequence of the congruency property of the classical model. On the other hand, the Preisach model (2.26) describes hysteresis non-linearities with the property that for any reversal point there are infinite possible branches starting at this point (see Fig. 2.24). A particular realization of these branches is determined by a particular past history. This property follows, for instance, from the expression (2.67) where all terms are input-dependent. For the classical model, the similar expressions (1.70) and (1.73) have only the last terms which are input-dependent. The above observation shows that the model (2.26) is endowed with a much more general mechanism of branching than the classical model.

2.3 "Restricted" Preisach Models of Hysteresis

In the previous section we have discussed the hysteresis Preisach model (2.26) which is a far-reaching generalization of the classical Preisach model. This generalization has been achieved by assuming that the distribution function μ is dependent of the current value of input $u(t)$. Another approach to the generalization of the classical Preisach model is to assume that the function μ depends on stored past extremum values of input, $\{M_k, m_k\}$. This approach was briefly explored in [13]. Here, we shall follow this approach as well, however, our treatment of the model itself and the identification problem for this model will deviate appreciably from the discussion in [13].

We begin with the simplest case when the function μ depends only on the first global maximum, M_1. Thus, we define the new Preisach type model as

$$f(t) = \iint\limits_{T_{M_1}} \mu(\alpha, \beta, M_1)\hat{\gamma}_{\alpha,\beta}u(t)d\alpha d\beta \; + \; C_{M_1} \; , \tag{2.70}$$

where M_1 is the largest input maximum since the departure from the state of negative saturation, and the support of $\mu(\alpha, \beta, M_1)$ is the triangle T_{M_1} defined by inequalities $\beta_0 \leq \alpha \leq \beta \leq M_1$ (see Fig. 2.25). We shall use the following interpretation of the above model. For any fixed extremum M_1, the model (2.70) will be used to describe hysteresis behavior in the region confined between an ascending branch $f^+_{u(t)}$, and a first-order reversal curve $f_{M_1\beta}$ (see Fig. 2.26). For this reason, the model (2.70) can be termed as a "restricted" Preisach model of hysteresis. However, the above "restriction" does not diminish at all the region of applicability of the model. This is because M_1 may assume any value between β_0 and α_0. The constant in (2.70) can be easily determined from the condition that the model matches the output values $f^+_{M_1}$ for $u(t) = M_1$ and f_- for $u(t) = \beta_0$. Indeed, from (2.70) we easily derive

$$f^+_{M_1} = \iint\limits_{T_{M_1}} \mu(\alpha, \beta, M_1)\hat{\gamma}_{\alpha,\beta}u(t)d\alpha d\beta \; + \; C_{M_1} \; , \tag{2.71}$$

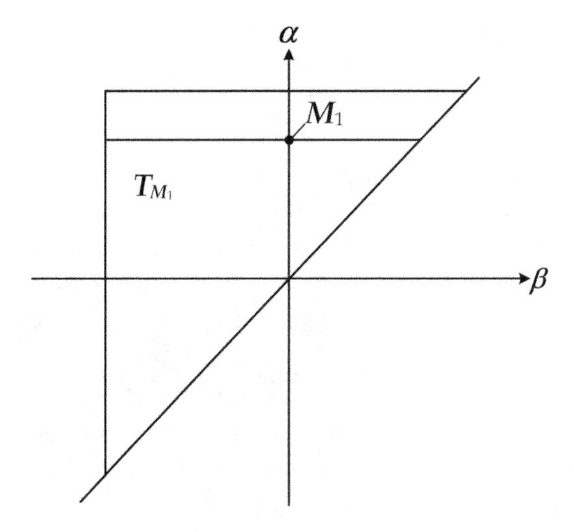

Fig. 2.25

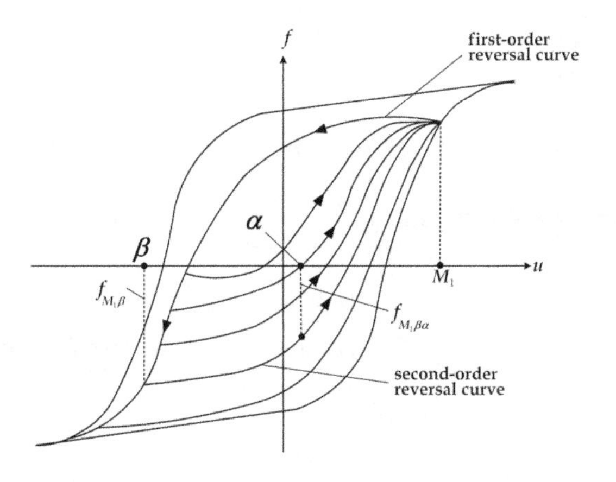

Fig. 2.26

$$f_- = - \iint_{T_{M_1}} \mu(\alpha, \beta, M_1) \hat{\gamma}_{\alpha,\beta} u(t) d\alpha d\beta \ + \ C_{M_1} \ . \tag{2.72}$$

From the last two equations, we find

$$C_{M_1} = \frac{1}{2}\left(f^+_{M_1} + f_-\right) , \tag{2.73}$$

which leads to the following representation for the model (2.70):

$$f(t) = \iint_{T_{M_1}} \mu(\alpha, \beta, M_1)\hat{\gamma}_{\alpha,\beta}u(t)d\alpha d\beta + \frac{1}{2}\left(f_{M_1}^+ + f_-\right). \tag{2.74}$$

Next, we shall be concerned with the solution of the identification problem. The essence of this problem is in determining the function $\mu(\alpha, \beta, M_1)$ by fitting the model to some experimental data. It turns out that $\mu(\alpha, \beta, M_1)$ can be found by matching second-order reversal curves $f_{M_1\beta\alpha}$ shown in Fig. 2.26. To do this, we introduce the function

$$F(\alpha, \beta, M_1) = \frac{f_{M_1\beta\alpha} - f_{M_1\beta}}{2}. \tag{2.75}$$

This function is equal to one half of the output increments along the second-order reversal curves. To relate this function to $\mu(\alpha, \beta, M_1)$, consider diagrams shown in Fig. 2.27. By using exactly the same line of reasoning as in the case of the classical Preisach model (see Section 4 of Chapter 1), from these diagrams and we derive

$$\begin{aligned} F(\alpha, \beta, M_1) &= \iint_{T(\alpha,\beta)} \mu(\alpha', \beta', M_1)d\alpha' d\beta' \\ &= \int_\beta^\alpha \left(\int_{\beta'}^\beta \mu(\alpha', \beta', M_1)d\alpha' \right) d\beta'. \end{aligned} \tag{2.76}$$

By differentiating twice in the last equation, we obtain

$$\mu(\alpha, \beta, M_1) = -\frac{1}{2}\frac{\partial^2 F(\alpha, \beta, M_1)}{\partial\alpha\partial\beta}. \tag{2.77}$$

By recalling the definition of $F(\alpha, \beta, M_1)$, from the last formula we find

$$\mu(\alpha, \beta, M_1) = -\frac{1}{2}\frac{\partial^2 f_{M_1\beta\alpha}}{\partial\alpha\partial\beta}. \tag{2.78}$$

Thus, if the distribution function μ is determined from (2.77) or (2.78), then the restricted Preisach model will match the output increments along second-order reversal curves $f_{M_1\beta\alpha}$ attached to the first-order reversal curve $f_{M_1\beta}$. This implies that the limiting ascending branch f^+ will be matched because this branch coincides with the second-order reversal curves $f_{M_1\beta_0\alpha}$ and because the value f_- is matched by the model. From (2.75) we also find that the output increments along the first-order reversal curve $f_{M_1\beta}$ will be matched because these increments are twice of $F(M_1, \beta, M_1)$. Since the limiting ascending branch output increments along the first-order transition curves $f_{M_1\beta}$ and the output increment along the second-order reversal

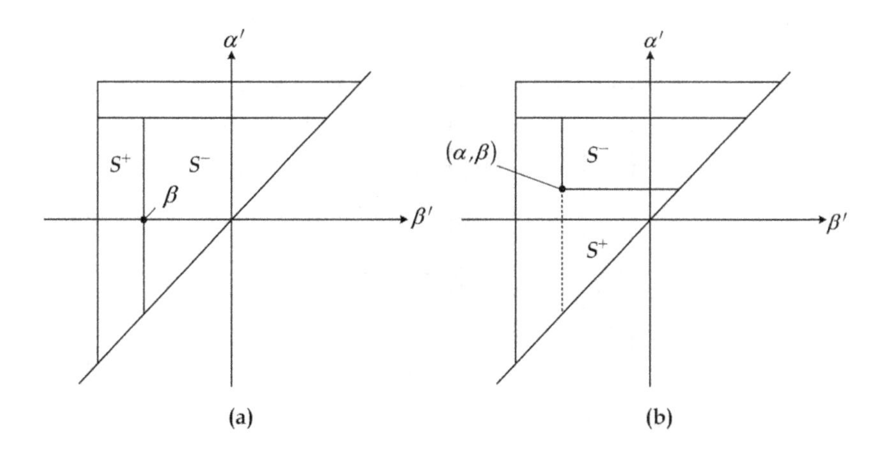

Fig. 2.27

curves $f_{M_1\beta\alpha}$ will all be matched, we conclude that the second-order transition curves $f_{M_1\beta\alpha}$ themselves will be matched.

Up to this point it has been tacitly assumed that input variations are started from the state of negative saturation $\big(u(t) \leq \beta_0\big)$. This is a natural assumption because the state of negative saturation is a well-defined state. However, another well-defined state is the state of positive saturation $\big(u(t) \geq \alpha_0\big)$. If input variations start from this state, then it is natural to assume that the distribution function depends on the first global minimum m_1. This leads us to the following restricted Preisach model:

$$f(t) = \iint\limits_{T_{m_1}} \tilde{\mu}(\alpha, \beta, m_1)\hat{\gamma}_{\alpha,\beta}u(t)d\alpha d\beta \; + \; C_{m_1} \,, \tag{2.79}$$

where the support of $\tilde{\mu}(\alpha, \beta, m_1)$ is the triangle T_{m_1} defined by inequalities $m_1 \leq \beta \leq \alpha \leq \alpha_0$ (see Fig. 2.28).

The model (2.79) can be regarded as a counterpart of the model (2.70) and our immediate goal is to establish some connections between distribution functions μ and $\tilde{\mu}$. To this end, we first find the constant C_{m_1} in formula (2.79) by matching the output values $f^-_{m_1}$ and f_+:

$$f^-_{m_1} = -\iint\limits_{T_{m_1}} \mu(\alpha, \beta, m_1)d\alpha d\beta \; + \; C_{m_1} \,, \tag{2.80}$$

$$f_+ = \iint\limits_{T_{m_1}} \mu(\alpha, \beta, m_1)d\alpha d\beta \; + \; C_{m_1} \,. \tag{2.81}$$

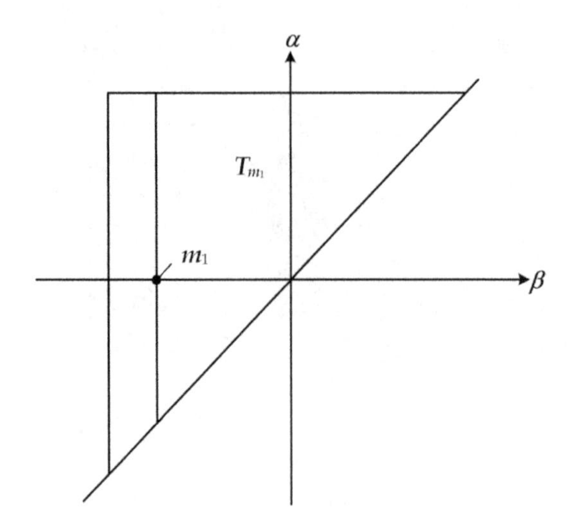

Fig. 2.28

From the last two equations, we find

$$C_{m_1} = \frac{1}{2}(f^-_{m_1} + f_+) \ . \tag{2.82}$$

And the restricted model (2.79) can be represented as

$$f(t) = \iint\limits_{T_{m_1}} \tilde{\mu}(\alpha, \beta, m_1)\hat{\gamma}_{\alpha,\beta}u(t)d\alpha d\beta \ + \ \frac{1}{2}(f^-_{m_1} + f_+) \ . \tag{2.83}$$

To determine the distribution function $\tilde{\mu}(\alpha, \beta, m_1)$ we shall use the decreasing second-order reversal curves $f_{m_1\tilde{\alpha}\tilde{\beta}}$ which are attached to the increasing first-order reversal curves $f_{m_1\tilde{\alpha}}$ (see Fig. 2.29). As before, we can introduce the function

$$\tilde{F}(\tilde{\alpha}, \tilde{\beta}, m_1) = \frac{1}{2}(f_{m_1\tilde{\alpha}} - f_{m_1\tilde{\alpha}\tilde{\beta}}) \tag{2.84}$$

and show that

$$\tilde{F}(\tilde{\alpha}, \tilde{\beta}, m_1) = \iint\limits_{T(\tilde{\alpha},\tilde{\beta})} \tilde{\mu}(\alpha', \beta', m_1)d\alpha' d\beta' \ . \tag{2.85}$$

From formula (2.84), we derive

$$\tilde{\mu}(\tilde{\alpha}, \tilde{\beta}, m_1) = - \ \frac{\partial^2 \tilde{F}(\tilde{\alpha}, \tilde{\beta}, m_1)}{\partial\tilde{\alpha}\partial\tilde{\beta}} \ . \tag{2.86}$$

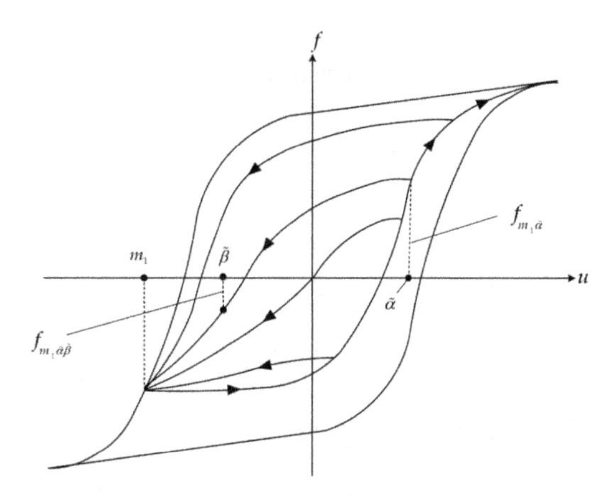

Fig. 2.29

By invoking relation (2.84) in the last equation, we obtain

$$\tilde{\mu}(\tilde{\alpha}, \tilde{\beta},) = \frac{1}{2} \frac{\partial^2 f_{m_1 \tilde{\alpha}\tilde{\beta}}}{\partial \tilde{\alpha} \partial \tilde{\beta}} \, . \tag{2.87}$$

Next, we will utilize the symmetry between the ascending and descending second-order reversal curves. In mathematical terms, this symmetry means that if

$$m_1 = -M_1 \, , \quad \tilde{\alpha} = -\beta \, , \quad \tilde{\beta} = -\alpha \, , \tag{2.88}$$

then

$$\tilde{F}(\tilde{\alpha}, \tilde{\beta}, m_1) = F(\alpha, \beta, M_1) \, . \tag{2.89}$$

The last formula can also be expressed as

$$\tilde{F}(-\beta, -\alpha, -M_1) = F(\alpha, \beta, M_1) \, . \tag{2.90}$$

By substituting formulas (2.89) and (2.90) into (2.86) and taking into account (2.78), we derive

$$\tilde{\mu}(\tilde{\alpha}, \tilde{\beta}, m_1) = - \frac{\partial^2 F(\alpha, \beta, M_1)}{\partial \alpha \partial \beta} = \mu(\alpha, \beta, M_1) \, . \tag{2.91}$$

From formulas (2.88) and (2.91), we finally obtain

$$\mu(\alpha, \beta, M_1) = \tilde{\mu}(-\tilde{\beta}, -\tilde{\alpha}, -M_1) \, . \tag{2.92}$$

The last expression can be regarded as a generalization of the mirror symmetry property previously derived for the classical Preisach model. Indeed, if $M_1 = \alpha_0$ and $m_1 = \beta_0$ ($\beta_0 = -\alpha_0$), then the models and (2.83) coincide, respectively, with the classical Preisach model. Consequently, we have

$$\mu(\alpha, \beta, \alpha_0) = \mu(\alpha, \beta) , \quad \tilde{\mu}(\tilde{\alpha}, \tilde{\beta}, -\alpha_0) = \mu(\alpha, \beta) , \tag{2.93}$$

and the equality (2.92) can be rewritten as

$$\mu(\alpha, \beta) = \mu(- \beta, -\alpha) , \tag{2.94}$$

which is the property of mirror symmetry of the classical Preisach model.

The formula (2.92) also shows that, having determined the function $\mu(\alpha, \beta, M_1)$, we have solved the identification problem for the model (2.74) and its counterpart (2.83). This suggests that the model (2.83) is not independent of the model (2.74), but rather complements the latter model. In a way, we deal here with the same model which is written in two different forms. These two different forms correspond to two different initial states (states of positive or negative saturation, respectively). For this reason, in our subsequent discussion we will not draw any distinction between the models (2.74) and (2.83). In the sequel, all results will be discussed for the model (2.74), and it will be tacitly implied that they are also valid for the model (2.83).

It is clear that the model (2.74) has almost identical structure with the classical Preisach model. For this reason, it is apparent that the erasure property holds for the restricted model (2.74). However, the congruency property of minor hysteresis loops undergoes some modification. This modification can be described as follows. We call minor hysteresis loops comparable if they are formed as a result of back-and-forth input variations between the same consecutive reversal values and these input variations occur at some time after the same largest input maximum was achieved. The given definition of comparable minor loops implies the possibility of different past input histories between the time when the largest maximum was achieved and the time when the above mentioned back-and-forth input variations commence. By using the same reasoning as in Section 3 of Chapter 1, we can prove that all comparable minor loops described by the restricted model (2.74) are congruent. It is clear from the above statement that the congruency of minor hysteresis loops prescribed by the model (2.74) for the same input reversal values are to a certain extent history dependent. This is not the case for the classical Preisach model.

It turns out that the erasure property and the modified congruency property are characteristic for the restricted model (2.74) in a sense that the following result is valid.

REPRESENTATION THEORM *The erasure property and the congruency property of comparable minor loops constitute necessary and sufficient conditions for the representation of actual hysteresis nonlinearities by the restricted Preisach model (2.74).*

The proof of this theorem is very similar to the proof of the representation theorem for the classical Preisach model. For this reason, this proof is omitted.

It is clear that the modified congruency property is less restricted than the congruency property of the classical Preisach model. Thus, the model (2.74) is more general than the classical one. In addition, the model (2.74) allows one to fit experimentally measured first- and second-order reversal curves, while the classical Preisach model is able to fit only first-order reversal curves. Since higher-order reversal curves are "sandwiched" between first- and second-order reversal curves, it is natural to expect that the model (2.74) will be more accurate than the classical Preisach model.

We next turn to the discussion of numerical implementation of the restricted model (2.74)). As before, we will show that double integration in (2.74) can be completely avoided and that an explicit expression for the output, $f(t)$ in terms of the experimentally measured function, $F(\alpha, \beta, M_1)$, can be derived. The derivation proceeds as follows. From (2.74), by means of simple transformations, we find

$$\begin{aligned} f(t) &= \iint\limits_{S^+_{M_1}(t)} \mu(\alpha,\beta,M_1)d\alpha d\beta - \iint\limits_{S^-_{M_1}(t)} \mu(\alpha,\beta,M_1)d\alpha d\beta + \frac{1}{2}\left(f^+_{M_1} + f_-\right) \\ &= 2 \iint\limits_{S^+_{M_1}(t)} \mu(\alpha,\beta,M_1)d\alpha d\beta - \iint\limits_{T_{M_1}} \mu(\alpha,\beta,M_1)d\alpha d\beta + \frac{1}{2}\left(f^+_{M_1} + f_-\right) . \end{aligned} \tag{2.95}$$

By invoking formulas (2.71) and (2.72), we derive

$$\iint\limits_{T_{M_1}} \mu(\alpha,\beta,M_1)d\alpha d\beta = \frac{1}{2}\left(f^+_{M_1} - f_-\right) . \tag{2.96}$$

By substituting the last formula into equation (2.95), we obtain

$$f(t) = 2 \iint\limits_{S^+_{M_1}(t)} \mu(\alpha,\beta,M_1)d\alpha d\beta + f_- . \tag{2.97}$$

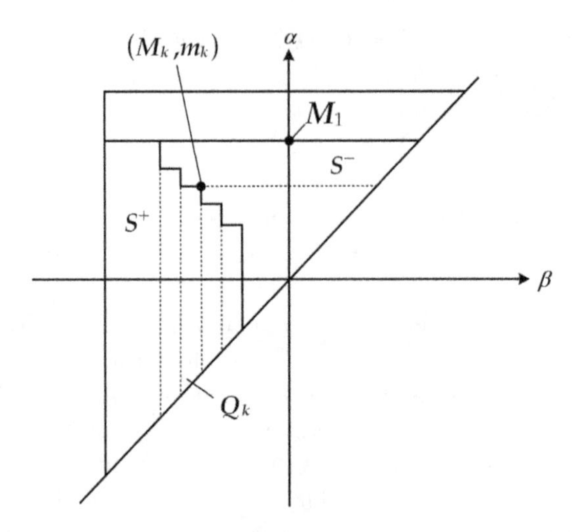

Fig. 2.30

The set $S^+_{M_1}(t)$ can be subdivided into n trapezoids Q_k shown in Fig. 2.30. As a result, we have

$$\iint\limits_{S^+_{M_1}(t)} \mu(\alpha, \beta, M_1) d\alpha d\beta = \sum_{k=1}^{n(t)} \iint\limits_{Q_k} \mu(\alpha, \beta, M_1) d\alpha d\beta . \tag{2.98}$$

Each integral in the right-hand side of the last equation can be represented as

$$\begin{aligned} \iint\limits_{Q_k} \mu(\alpha, \beta, M_1) d\alpha d\beta = & \iint\limits_{T(M_k, m_{k-1})} \mu(\alpha, \beta, M_1) d\alpha d\beta \\ & - \iint\limits_{T(M_k, m_k)} \mu(\alpha, \beta, M_1) d\alpha d\beta . \end{aligned} \tag{2.99}$$

By recalling equation (2.76), from the last formula we find

$$\iint\limits_{Q_k} \mu(\alpha, \beta, M_1) d\alpha d\beta = F(M_k, m_{k-1}, M_1) - F(M_k, m_k, M_1) . \tag{2.100}$$

From equations (2.99), (2.98) and (2.97), we finally obtain

$$f(t) = 2 \sum_{k=1}^{n(t)} \Big[F(M_k, m_{k-1}, M_1) - F(M_k, m_k, M_1) \Big] + f_- . \tag{2.101}$$

Thus, the formula (2.101) expresses the output, $f(t)$, explicitly in terms of experimentally measured second-order reversal curves which are related to the function F by formula (2.75). This formula has a two-fold advantage over the expression (2.74). First, double integration is avoided. Second, the determination of $\mu(\alpha, \beta, M_1)$ through differentiation of experimentally obtained data is completely circumvented. This is a welcome feature because the above differentiation may amplify noise inherently present in any experimental data.

So far we have discussed the restricted Preisach model for which the distribution function μ depends only on the first global extrema M_1 or m_1. It is natural to call it a first-order restricted Preisach model. It turns out that further generalizations in this direction are possible. In these generalizations, the function μ is assumed to be dependent on some finite sequence of past dominant extrema: $\mu(\alpha, \beta, M_1, m_1, M_2, m_2, \dots, M_k, m_k)$. It is natural to call these models as high-order restricted Preisach models. To make the general idea of these models clear, consider a second-order restricted Preisach model. In this model, the function μ is assumed to be dependent on M_1 and m_1, and the model itself is defined as

$$f(t) = \iint\limits_{T_{M_1 m_1}} \mu(\alpha, \beta, M_1, m_1)\hat{\gamma}_{\alpha,\beta} u(t) d\alpha d\beta \;+\; C_{M_1 m_1}\,, \tag{2.102}$$

where the support of μ is the triangle $T_{M_1 m_1}$ specified by inequalities $m_1 \leq \alpha \leq \beta \leq M_1$ (see Fig. 2.31).

For any fixed extrema M_1 and m_1, the model (2.102) will be used to describe hysteresis behavior in the region confined between the first-order reversal curve $f_{M_1 \alpha}$ and the second-order reversal curve $f_{M_1 m_1 \alpha}$ (see Fig. 2.32). This explains the origin of the term "restricted" used for the name of this model. However, the described restriction does not narrow at all the region of applicability of this model. This is because M_1 and m_1 are free parameters which may assume any values between β_0 and α_0. These values depend on a particular past input history and may even change with time when the previous extrema M_1 and m_1 are erased by subsequent input variations.

The constant $C_{M_1 m_1}$ in formula (2.102) can be determined from the condition that the model matches the output values $f^+_{M_1}$ and $f_{M_1 m_1}$:

$$f^+_{M_1} = \iint\limits_{T_{M_1 m_1}} \mu(\alpha, \beta, M_1, m_1) d\alpha d\beta \;+\; C_{M_1 m_1}\,, \tag{2.103}$$

$$f_{M_1 m_1} = -\iint\limits_{T_{M_1 m_1}} \mu(\alpha, \beta, M_1, m_1) d\alpha d\beta \;+\; C_{M_1 m_1}\,. \tag{2.104}$$

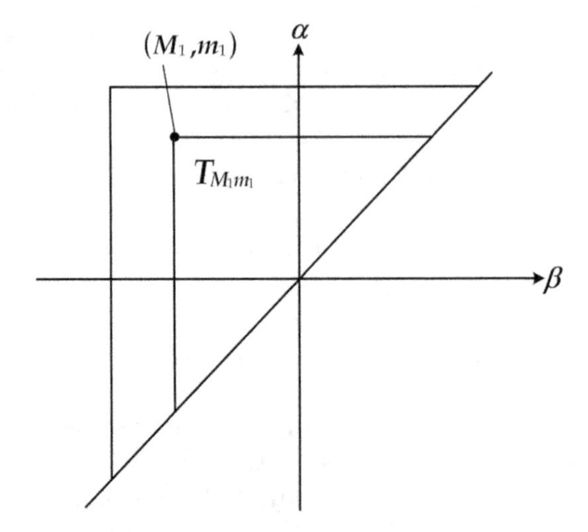

Fig. 2.31

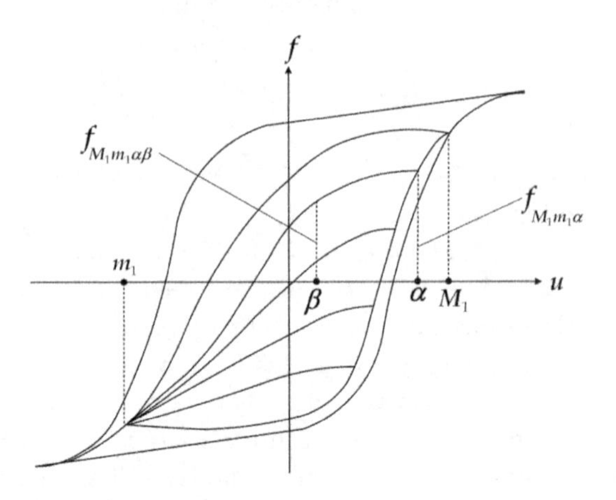

Fig. 2.32

From the last two formulas we find

$$C_{M_1 m_1} = \frac{f_{M_1}^{+} + f_{M_1 m_1}}{2}\,, \tag{2.105}$$

which leads to the following expression for the model (2.102)

$$f(t) = \iint\limits_{T_{M_1 m_1}} \mu(\alpha, \beta, M_1, m_1)\hat{\gamma}_{\alpha,\beta} u(t) d\alpha d\beta \; + \; \frac{f_{M_1}^{+} + f_{M_1 m_1}}{2}\,. \tag{2.106}$$

To determine the distribution function, the experimentally measured third-order reversal curve $f_{M_1 m_1 \alpha\beta}$ (Fig. 2.32) should be employed. By using these curves we can introduce the function

$$F(\alpha, \beta, M_1, m_1) = \frac{1}{2}\left(f_{M_1 m_1 \alpha} - f_{M_1 m_1 \alpha\beta}\right) . \tag{2.107}$$

Exactly in the same way as before it can be shown that the second-order restricted Preisach model will fit the third-order reversal curves if the function $F(\alpha, \beta, M_1, m_1)$ is related to the function $\mu(\alpha, \beta, M_1, m_1)$ by the equation

$$F(\alpha, \beta, M_1, m_1) = \iint\limits_{T(\alpha,\beta)} \mu(\alpha', \beta', M_1, m_1) d\alpha' d\beta' . \tag{2.108}$$

From the last equation, we easily derive

$$\mu(\alpha, \beta, M_1, m_1) = -\frac{\partial^2 F(\alpha, \beta, M_1, m_1)}{\partial\alpha\partial\beta} \tag{2.109}$$

and

$$\mu(\alpha, \beta, M_1, m_1) = \frac{1}{2}\frac{\partial^2 f_{M_1 m_1 \alpha\beta}}{\partial\alpha\partial\beta} . \tag{2.110}$$

By its design, the model (2.102) is valid under the condition that the initial state of hysteresis transducer is the state of negative saturation. If the initial state is the state of positive saturation, then the following counterpart of the model (2.102) can be used:

$$f(t) = \iint\limits_{T_{\tilde{M}_1 \tilde{m}_1}} \tilde{\mu}(\alpha, \beta, \tilde{m}_1, \tilde{M}_1)\hat{\gamma}_{\alpha,\beta} u(t) d\alpha d\beta + \frac{f^{+}_{\tilde{m}_1} + f_{\tilde{m}_1 \tilde{M}_1}}{2} , \tag{2.111}$$

where $\tilde{m}_1$ is the global minimum and $\tilde{M}_1$ is a subsequent global maximum.

As before, we can establish the following relationship between the function μ and $\tilde{\mu}$:

$$\mu(\alpha, \beta, M_1, m_1) = \tilde{\mu}(-\beta, -\alpha, -M_1, -m_1) , \tag{2.112}$$

which shows that (2.106) and (2.111) are just different forms of the same model. These two different forms correspond to two different well-defined initial states of hysteresis nonlinearity.

It is apparent that the congruency property of minor hysteresis loops undergoes further modification in the case of the second-order restricted Preisach model (2.106). The essence of this modification is that for minor loops to be congruent the corresponding inputs must vary back-and-forth between the same consecutive reversal values and also assume in the past the same values of M_1 and m_1. It can be proven that the erasure property and the above-mentioned modified congruency property of minor loops constitute necessary and sufficient conditions for the representation of actual hysteresis nonlinearities by the model (2.106). This is the so-called representation theorem for the second-order restricted Preisach model. As before, it can be shown that the following expression can be used for the numerical implementation of the model (2.106):

$$f(t) = 2\sum_{k=1}^{n(t)} \Big[F(M_k, m_{k-1}, M_1, m_1) - F(M_k, m_k, M_1, m_1)\Big] + f_{M_1 m_1} \, . \tag{2.113}$$

The main advantage of this expression over the formula (2.106) is that it represents the output, $f(t)$, directly in terms of the experimentally measured third-order transition curves.

It is clear from the previous discussion that higher-order Preisach models of hysteresis can be defined as

$$f(t) = \iint\limits_{T_{M_1 m_1 \ldots M_k}} \mu(\alpha, \beta, M_1, m_1, \ldots, M_k)\hat{\gamma}_{\alpha,\beta} u(t) d\alpha d\beta \; + \; C_{M_1 m_1 \ldots M_k} \, . \tag{2.114}$$

It is also apparent now how higher-order transition curves can be used for the determination of the function $\mu(\alpha, \beta, M_1, m_1, \ldots, M_k)$. It goes without saying that by increasing the order of the Preisach model we can increase the accuracy of the model. However, this increase in accuracy is amply paid for by the increase in the amount of experimental data required for the identification of higher-order models. For this reason, the use of restricted Preisach models of order higher than two does not seem to be practically feasible or attractive.

We conclude this section with a brief discussion of another Preisach model of hysteresis that combines main features of "restricted" and "nonlinear" models. This Preisach model can be defined as follows:

$$f(t) = \iint\limits_{R_{M_1 u}} \mu(\alpha, \beta, u(t), M_1)\hat{\gamma}_{\alpha,\beta} u(t) d\alpha d\beta + \frac{1}{2}\Big(f_{M_1 u(t)} + f^{+}_{u(t)}\Big) \, , \tag{2.115}$$

where the moving support of $\mu(\alpha, \beta, u(t), M_1)$ is the rectangle $R_{M_1 u}$ specified by the inequalities $\beta_0 \le \beta \le u(t)$ and $u(t) \le \alpha \le M_1$ (see Fig. 2.33), and the meaning of $f_{M_1 u(t)}$ is clear from Fig. 2.34.

By introducing the function

$$P(\alpha, \beta, u, M_1) = f_{M_1 \beta \alpha u} - f_{M_1 \beta u} \tag{2.116}$$

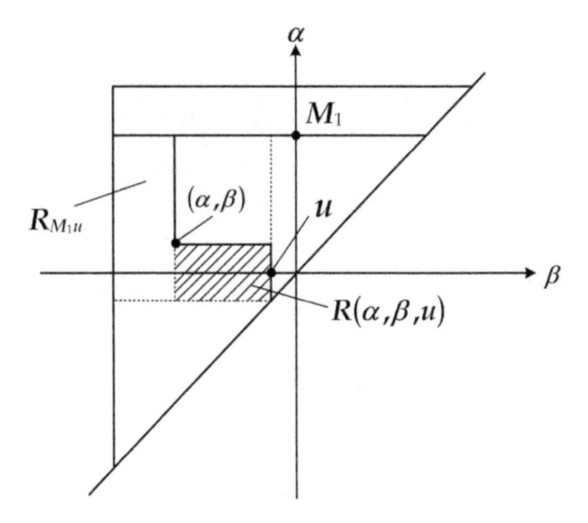

Fig. 2.33

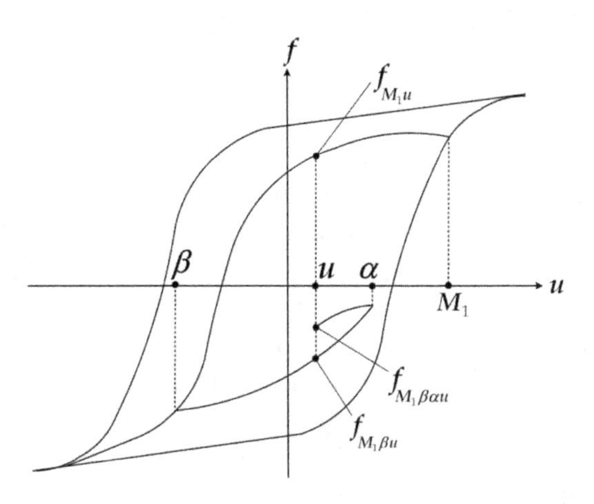

Fig. 2.34

and by using the same reasoning as in the previous section, we can establish that

$$P(\alpha, \beta, u, M_1) = 2 \iint\limits_{R(\alpha,\beta,u)} \mu(\alpha', \beta', u, M_1) d\alpha' d\beta' \ . \tag{2.117}$$

From formula (2.117) we can derive the following expressions:

$$\mu(\alpha, \beta, u, M_1) = -\ \frac{1}{2}\ \frac{\partial^2 P(\alpha, \beta, u, M_1)}{\partial\alpha\partial\beta}\ , \tag{2.118}$$

and

$$\mu(\alpha, \beta, u, M_1) = -\frac{1}{2} \frac{\partial^2 f_{M_1 \beta \alpha u}}{\partial \alpha \partial \beta} . \tag{2.119}$$

We can also derive the following explicit expression for the output, $f(t)$, of the model (2.115):

$$f(t) = f_{M_1 u(t)} + \sum_{k=1}^{n(t)} \Big[P(M_{k+1}, m_k, u(t), M_1) - P(M_k, m_k, u(t), M_1) \Big] . \tag{2.120}$$

It is worthwhile to remember here that the function $P(\alpha, \beta, u, M_1)$ is directly related to experimental data and it has the meaning of output increments between the second- and third-order reversal curves.

It is easy to formulate and to prove the representation theorem for the model (2.115). This is left to the reader as a useful exercise.

2.4 "Dynamic" Preisach Models of Hysteresis

All our previous discussion has been centered around the classical and generalized Preisach models of hysteresis that are rate-independent in nature. The term "rate-independent" implies that in these models only past input extrema leave their mark upon the future values of output, while the speed of input and output variations has no influence on branching. The intent of this section is to relax the "rate-independence property" of Preisach type models. For this reason, new Preisach type models that are applicable to the description of dynamic hysteresis are introduced. The identification problem of fitting these models to some experimental data is then studied. Finally, some discussion is presented concerning numerical implementation of the dynamic Preisach models of hysteresis.

The main idea behind the dynamic Preisach-type models of hysteresis is to introduce the dependence of μ-functions on the speed of output variations, df/dt. This leads to the following dynamic Preisach models of hysteresis:

$$f(t) = \iint_{\alpha \geq \beta} \mu\left(\alpha, \beta, \frac{df}{dt}\right) \hat{\gamma}_{\alpha,\beta} u(t) d\alpha d\beta , \tag{2.121}$$

$$f(t) = \iint_{R_{u(t)}} \mu\left(\alpha, \beta, u(t), \frac{df}{dt}\right) \hat{\gamma}_{\alpha,\beta} u(t) d\alpha d\beta + \frac{1}{2}\left(f^+_{u(t)} + f^-_{u(t)}\right) . \tag{2.122}$$

The above models are "dynamic" generalizations of the classical Preisach model and the nonlinear Preisach model, respectively. Similar generalizations for the restricted Preisach models are apparent. They will not be discussed in this section because their treatment mostly parallels that of the model (2.121).

The direct utilization of the models (2.121) and (2.122) is associated with some untractable difficulties. First, μ-functions depend on the unknown quantity, df/dt, and this complicates numerical implementations of the models (2.121) and (2.122). Second, it is not clear how to pose the identification problems for these models. The above difficulties can be completely circumvented by using the power series expansions for μ-functions with respect to df/dt:

$$\mu\left(\alpha, \beta, \frac{df}{dt}\right) = \mu_0(\alpha, \beta) + \frac{df}{dt}\mu_1(\alpha, \beta) + \dots, \tag{2.123}$$

$$\mu\left(\alpha, \beta, u(t), \frac{df}{dt}\right) = \mu_0(\alpha, \beta, u(t)) + \frac{df}{dt}\mu_1(\alpha, \beta, u(t)) + \dots. \tag{2.124}$$

By retaining only the first two terms of the above expression, we arrive at the following dynamic models:

$$f(t) = \iint\limits_{\alpha \geq \beta} \mu_0(\alpha, \beta)\hat{\gamma}_{\alpha,\beta}u(t)d\alpha d\beta \ + \ \frac{df}{dt} \iint\limits_{\alpha \geq \beta} \mu_1(\alpha, \beta)\hat{\gamma}_{\alpha,\beta}u(t)d\alpha d\beta \ , \tag{2.125}$$

$$\begin{aligned} f(t) = & \iint\limits_{R_{u(t)}} \mu_0(\alpha, \beta, u(t))\hat{\gamma}_{\alpha,\beta}u(t)d\alpha d\beta + \frac{1}{2}\left(f^+_{u(t)} + f^-_{u(t)}\right) \\ & + \frac{df}{dt} \iint\limits_{R_{u(t)}} \mu_1(\alpha, \beta, u(t))\hat{\gamma}_{\alpha,\beta}u(t)d\alpha d\beta \ . \end{aligned} \tag{2.126}$$

It is clear that in the case of very slow output variations, the above models are reduced to the corresponding rate-independent hysteresis models. This means that the μ_0-functions in (2.125) and (2.126) should coincide with the μ-functions of rate-independent models (2.1) and (2.26), respectively. In other words, the μ_0-functions in (2.125) and (2.126) can be determined by matching first-order and second-order reversal curves, respectively.

The above reasoning suggests that the models (2.125) and (2.126) can be represented in the following equivalent forms:

$$f(t) = \tilde{f}(t) \ + \ \frac{df}{dt} \iint\limits_{\alpha \geq \beta} \mu_1(\alpha, \beta)\hat{\gamma}_{\alpha,\beta}u(t)d\alpha d\beta \ , \tag{2.127}$$

$$f(t) = \tilde{f}(t) + \frac{df}{dt} \iint\limits_{R_{u(t)}} \mu_1(\alpha, \beta, u(t)) \hat{\gamma}_{\alpha,\beta} u(t) d\alpha d\beta , \tag{2.128}$$

where the $\tilde{f}$-terms stand for the "static" (i.e. rate independent) components of hysteresis nonlinearities:

$$\tilde{f}(t) = \iint\limits_{\alpha \geq \beta} \mu_0(\alpha, \beta) \hat{\gamma}_{\alpha,\beta} u(t) d\alpha d\beta , \tag{2.129}$$

$$\tilde{f}(t) = \iint\limits_{R_{u(t)}} \mu_0(\alpha, \beta, u(t)) \hat{\gamma}_{\alpha,\beta} u(t) d\alpha d\beta + \frac{1}{2}\left(f^+_{u(t)} + f^-_{u(t)}\right) . \tag{2.130}$$

The expressions (2.127) and (2.128) are transparent from the physical point of view. They show that the instant speeds of output variations are directly proportional to the differences between instant and "static" output values.

We next turn to the identification problems of determining the μ_1-functions by fitting the models (2.127) and (2.128) to some experimental data. We first consider the identification problem for the model (2.127). The following experiments can be used to solve this problem. Starting from the state of negative saturation, the input $u(t)$ is monotonically increased until it reaches some value α at $t = t_0$ and it is kept constant for $t \geq t_0$. As the input is being kept constant, the output relaxes from its value f_α at $t = t_0$ to its static value $\tilde{f}_\alpha$. According to the model (2.127), this relaxation process is described by the differential equation

$$\tau_\alpha \frac{df}{dt} + f = \tilde{f}_\alpha , \tag{2.131}$$

where

$$\tau_\alpha = \iint\limits_{S^-_\alpha} \mu_1(\alpha', \beta') d\alpha' d\beta' - \iint\limits_{S^+_\alpha} \mu_1(\alpha', \beta') d\alpha' d\beta' , \tag{2.132}$$

and, S^-_α and S^+_α are negative and positive sets of the Preisach diagram (see Fig. 2.35) corresponding to the above input variation.

The solution to equation (2.131) is given by

$$f(t) = \left(f_\alpha - \tilde{f}_\alpha\right) e^{-t/\tau_\alpha} + \tilde{f}_\alpha . \tag{2.133}$$

Thus, τ_α has the meaning of relaxation time and can be experimentally measured.

Next, the hysteresis nonlinearity is brought back to the state of negative saturation. Starting from this state, the input is again monotonically

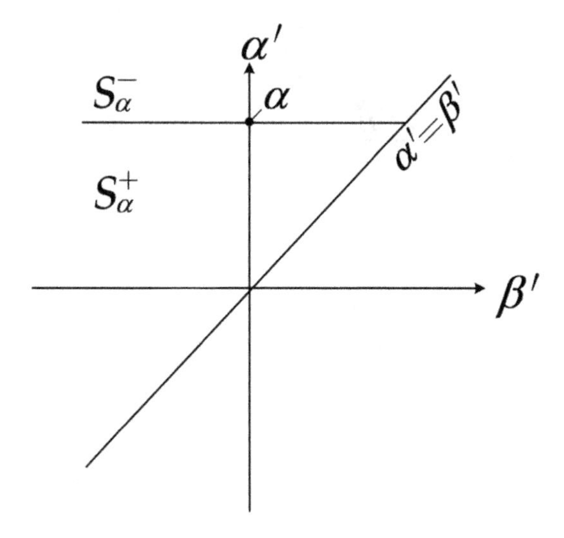

Fig. 2.35

increased until it reaches the value α. Then the input is monotonically decreased until it reaches some value β at time $t = t_0^{'}$ and it is kept constant for $t > t_0^{'}$. As the input is being kept constant, the output relaxes from its value $f_{\alpha\beta}$ at $t = t_0^{'}$ to its static value $\tilde{f}_{\alpha\beta}$. The model (2.127) yields the following differential equation for the above relaxation process:

$$\tau_{\alpha\beta}\frac{df}{dt} + f = \tilde{f}_{\alpha\beta} \ , \tag{2.134}$$

where according to the model (2.127) and the Preisach diagram shown in Fig. 2.36 the coefficient $\tau_{\alpha\beta}$ is given by the expression

$$\tau_{\alpha\beta} = \iint\limits_{S_{\alpha\beta}^{-}} \mu_1(\alpha^{'}, \beta^{'})d\alpha^{'}d\beta^{'} \ - \iint\limits_{S_{\alpha\beta}^{+}} \mu_1(\alpha^{'}, \beta^{'})d\alpha^{'}d\beta^{'} \ . \tag{2.135}$$

By solving equation (2.134) we find

$$f(t) = \Big(f_{\alpha\beta} - \tilde{f}_{\alpha\beta}\Big)e^{-t/\tau_{\alpha\beta}} + \tilde{f}_{\alpha\beta} \ . \tag{2.136}$$

Thus, $\tau_{\alpha\beta}$ has also the meaning of relaxation time and can be experimentally measured. It is apparent, that the relaxation time τ_α can be construed as the relaxation time $\tau_{\alpha\alpha}$ and, consequently, it belongs to the set $\{\tau_{\alpha\beta}\}$. We next show that by knowing these relaxation times, we can find the function $\mu_1(\alpha, \beta)$. To this end, we introduce the function

$$q(\alpha, \beta) = \tau_\alpha - \tau_{\alpha\beta} \ . \tag{2.137}$$

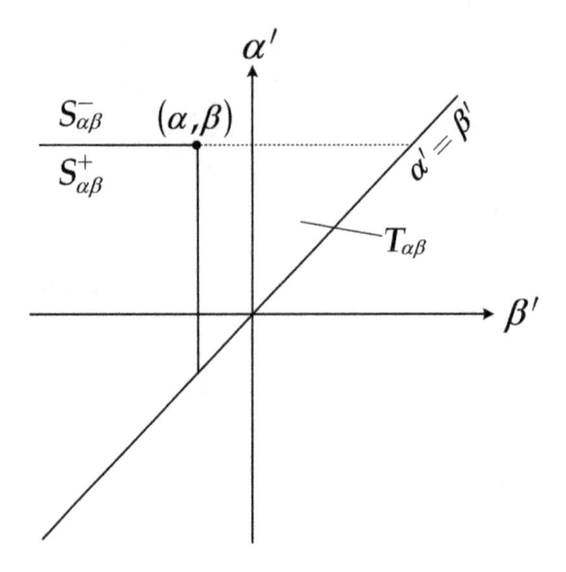

Fig. 2.36

From formulas (2.132), (2.135) and (2.137), we find

$$q(\alpha,\beta) = -2 \iint_{T_{\alpha\beta}} \mu_1(\alpha^{'},\beta^{'})d\alpha^{'}d\beta^{'} \ , \tag{2.138}$$

where $T_{\alpha\beta}$ is a triangle shown in Fig. 2.36.

From equation (2.138), we can easily derive the expression:

$$\mu_1(\alpha,\beta) = \frac{1}{2}\,\frac{\partial^2 q(\alpha,\beta)}{\partial\alpha\partial\beta} \ . \tag{2.139}$$

By recalling formula (2.137), we find

$$\mu_1(\alpha,\beta) = -\,\frac{1}{2}\,\frac{\partial^2 \tau_{\alpha\beta}}{\partial\alpha\partial\beta} \ . \tag{2.140}$$

The solution of the identification problem for the model (2.128) can be found in a similar way. For this reason, our comments will be concise. We consider two types of relaxation processes. A first type process occurs after monotonic input increase to some value α and subsequent monotonic decrease of input to some value u. According to the model (2.128), the first type of relaxation processes are described by the differential equation

$$\tau_{\alpha u}\frac{df}{dt} + f = \tilde{f}_{\alpha u} \ , \tag{2.141}$$

where

$$\tau_{\alpha u} = \iint\limits_{S^-_{\alpha u}} \mu_1(\alpha', \beta', u) d\alpha' d\beta' \; - \iint\limits_{S^+_{\alpha u}} \mu_1(\alpha', \beta', u) d\alpha' d\beta' \, . \tag{2.142}$$

From the previous differential equation, we find

$$f(t) = \left(f_{\alpha u} - \tilde{f}_{\alpha u}\right) e^{-t/\tau_{\alpha u}} + \tilde{f}_{\alpha u} \, . \tag{2.143}$$

A second type relaxation process occurs when the input is first monotonically increased to α, then decreased to β, then monotonically increased to u, and kept constant afterwards. These relaxation processes are described by the equation

$$\tau_{\alpha\beta u} \frac{df}{dt} + f = \tilde{f}_{\alpha\beta u} \, , \tag{2.144}$$

where

$$\tau_{\alpha\beta u} = \iint\limits_{S^-_{\alpha\beta u}} \mu_1(\alpha', \beta', u) d\alpha' d\beta' \; - \iint\limits_{S^+_{\alpha\beta u}} \mu_1(\alpha', \beta', u) d\alpha' d\beta' \, . \tag{2.145}$$

As before, we have

$$f(t) = \left(f_{\alpha\beta u} - \tilde{f}_{\alpha\beta u}\right) e^{-t/\tau_{\alpha\beta u}} + \tilde{f}_{\alpha\beta u} \, . \tag{2.146}$$

It is clear from formulas (2.143) and (2.146) that $\tau_{\alpha u}$ and $\tau_{\alpha\beta u}$ have the physical meaning of relaxation times and can be measured experimentally. Knowing these relaxation times, we can define the function

$$Q(\alpha, \beta, u) = \tau_{\alpha u} - \tau_{\alpha\beta u} \, . \tag{2.147}$$

From equations (2.142), (2.145) and (2.147), we derive

$$Q(\alpha, \beta, u) = -2 \iint\limits_{R(\alpha,\beta,u)} \mu_1(\alpha', \beta', u) d\alpha' d\beta' \, . \tag{2.148}$$

From the last formula, we obtain

$$\mu_1(\alpha, \beta, u) = \frac{1}{2} \frac{\partial^2 Q(\alpha, \beta, u)}{\partial\alpha\partial\beta} \, . \tag{2.149}$$

By invoking the last formula, we find the following expression for μ_1:

$$\mu_1(\alpha, \beta, u) = -\frac{1}{2} \frac{\partial^2 \tau_{\alpha\beta u}}{\partial\alpha\partial\beta} \, . \tag{2.150}$$

Consider the relaxation processes which are in some sense symmetric to those discussed above. Suppose that we start from the state of positive saturation and reduce the input to some value $\tilde{\beta}$, then increase the input to some value $\tilde{\alpha}$ and keep it constant thereafter. Suppose also that the subsequent output variations are characterized by the relaxation times $\tau_{\tilde{\beta}\tilde{\alpha}}$. If

$$\tilde{\beta} = -\alpha, \quad \tilde{\alpha} = -\beta \,, \tag{2.151}$$

then due to symmetry we have

$$\tau_{\tilde{\beta}\tilde{\alpha}} \ = \ \tau_{\alpha\beta} \ . \tag{2.152}$$

As before, we can derive

$$\mu_1(\tilde{\alpha}, \tilde{\beta}) = -\ \frac{1}{2}\ \frac{\partial^2 \tau_{\tilde{\beta}\tilde{\alpha}}}{\partial\tilde{\alpha}\partial\tilde{\beta}} \ . \tag{2.153}$$

By substituting formulas (2.152) and (2.151) into the right-hand side of equation (2.153) and by recalling relation (2.140), we obtain

$$\mu_1(\tilde{\alpha}, \tilde{\beta}) = -\ \frac{1}{2}\ \frac{\partial^2 \tau_{\beta\alpha}}{\partial\beta\partial\alpha} \ = \ -\mu_1(\alpha, \beta) \ . \tag{2.154}$$

From formula (2.151) and (2.154), we conclude

$$\mu_1\big(-\beta, -\alpha\big) \ = \ -\mu_1\big(\alpha, \beta\big) \ . \tag{2.155}$$

Similarly, we can introduce the relaxation times $\tau_{\tilde{\beta}\tilde{\alpha}\tilde{u}}$ and prove that

$$\mu_1(\tilde{\alpha}, \tilde{\beta}, \tilde{u}) = -\ \frac{1}{2}\ \frac{\partial^2 \tau_{\tilde{\beta}\tilde{\alpha}\tilde{u}}}{\partial\tilde{\alpha}\partial\tilde{\beta}} \ . \tag{2.156}$$

If

$$\tilde{\beta} = -\alpha, \quad \tilde{\alpha} = -\beta, \quad \tilde{u} = -u \,, \tag{2.157}$$

then due to symmetry we have

$$\tau_{\tilde{\beta}\tilde{\alpha}\tilde{u}} \ = \ \tau_{\alpha\beta u} \ . \tag{2.158}$$

By using the same line of reasoning as before, we derive

$$\mu_1\big(-\beta, -\alpha, -u\big) \ = \ -\mu_1\big(\alpha, \beta, u\big) \ . \tag{2.159}$$

We next proceed to the numerical implementation of the dynamic models. The models (2.127) and (2.128) can be represented as the following differential equation:

$$a\big(u(t)\big)\frac{df}{dt} + f(t) = \tilde{f}(t) \,, \tag{2.160}$$

where the hysteretic coefficient $a(u(t))$ is defined by the formulas

$$a\big(u(t)\big) = -\iint\limits_{\alpha\geq\beta} \mu_1(\alpha, \beta)\hat{\gamma}_{\alpha,\beta}u(t)d\alpha d\beta \,, \tag{2.161}$$

$$a(u(t)) = -\iint\limits_{R_{u(t)}} \mu_1(\alpha, \beta, u(t)) \hat{\gamma}_{\alpha,\beta} u(t) d\alpha d\beta \;, \tag{2.162}$$

for the models (2.127) and (2.128), respectively.

The explicit solution to equation (2.160) is well known and can be expressed as

$$f(t) \;=\; b(t)\left[f_0 + \int_0^t \frac{\tilde{f}(\xi)}{a(\xi)b(\xi)} d\xi \right] , \tag{2.163}$$

where f_0 is the initial output value, and $b(t)$ is given by the formula

$$b(t) = \exp\left(-\int_0^t \frac{d\xi}{a(\xi)} \right) . \tag{2.164}$$

The expressions (2.163) and (2.164) can be used for computing $f(t)$, if $\tilde{f}(t)$ and $a(t)$ are known. The calculation of rate-independent $\tilde{f}$-components in the case of the classical Preisach model as well as the Preisach model with input dependent distribution function has been discussed in detail in the previous sections. Since the mathematical structure of $a(t)$ is similar to the mathematical structure of the rate-independent Preisach models, similar explicit formulas can be derived for the numerical evaluation of $a(t)$. In particular, it can be shown that the following formulas are valid for $a(t)$ in the case of models (2.127) and (2.128), respectively:

$$a(u(t)) = 2q(\alpha_0, \beta_0) \;-\; 4\sum_{k=1}^{n(t)} \left[q(M_k, m_{k-1}) - q(M_k, m_k) \right] , \tag{2.165}$$

$$a(u(t)) = -\frac{1}{2}Q(\alpha_0, \beta_0, u(t)) - \sum_{k=1}^{n(t)} \left[Q(M_k, m_k, u(t)) - Q(M_{k+1}, m_k, u(t)) \right] . \tag{2.166}$$

The above formulas are convenient not only because they give explicit expressions for integrals in (2.161) and (2.162), but also because these expressions are presented in terms of experimentally measured data.

It has been tacitly assumed in the foregoing discussion that the relaxation processes used in the identification procedures are well characterized by single relaxation times. If this is not the case and several relaxation times have to be employed to describe the above relaxation processes, then the discussed dynamic models must be generalized. The natural way to generalize these models is to use higher-order differential equations with hysteretic coefficients in order to account for several relaxation times. We demonstrate such a generalization for the second-order dynamic model:

$$a^{(2)}(u(t))\frac{d^2f}{dt^2} + a^{(1)}(u(t))\frac{df}{dt} + f(t) = \tilde{f}(t) , \tag{2.167}$$

where

$$\tilde{f}(t) = \iint\limits_{\alpha\geq\beta} \mu_0(\alpha,\beta)\hat{\gamma}_{\alpha,\beta}u(t)d\alpha d\beta , \tag{2.168}$$

$$a^{(1)}(u(t)) = \iint\limits_{\alpha\geq\beta} \mu_1(\alpha,\beta)\hat{\gamma}_{\alpha,\beta}u(t)d\alpha d\beta , \tag{2.169}$$

$$a^{(2)}(u(t)) = \iint\limits_{\alpha\geq\beta} \mu_2(\alpha,\beta)\hat{\gamma}_{\alpha,\beta}u(t)d\alpha d\beta . \tag{2.170}$$

To find $\mu_1(\alpha,\beta)$ and $\mu_2(\alpha,\beta)$, we shall use the same two relaxation processes as for the identification of the model (2.127). In the first process, we start from the state of negative saturation and monotonically increase input to some value α and keep it constant thereafter. As the input is being kept constant, the output relaxes. According to (2.167), this relaxation is described by the equation

$$a_\alpha^{(2)}\frac{d^2f}{dt^2} + a_\alpha^{(1)}\frac{df}{dt} + f = \tilde{f}_\alpha . \tag{2.171}$$

A solution to this equation has the form

$$f(t) = C_\alpha^{(1)}e^{-t/\tau_\alpha^{(1)}} + C_\alpha^{(2)}e^{-t/\tau_\alpha^{(2)}} + \tilde{f}_\alpha , \tag{2.172}$$

where $\tau_\alpha^{(1)}$ and $\tau_\alpha^{(2)}$ are the roots of the characteristic equation

$$a_\alpha^{(2)}\tau^2 + a_\alpha^{(1)}\tau + 1 = 0 . \tag{2.173}$$

These roots are assumed to be real and distinct. Consequently,

$$a_\alpha^{(2)} = \frac{1}{\tau_\alpha^{(1)}\tau_\alpha^{(2)}} , \tag{2.174}$$

$$a_\alpha^{(1)} = -\frac{\tau_\alpha^{(1)} + \tau_\alpha^{(2)}}{\tau_\alpha^{(1)}\tau_\alpha^{(2)}} . \tag{2.175}$$

The constants $\tau_\alpha^{(1)}$ and $\tau_\alpha^{(2)}$ have the physical meaning of relaxation times and can be measured experimentally. This leads to the experimental determination of $a_\alpha^{(2)}$ and $a_\alpha^{(1)}$ according to formulas (2.174) and (2.175).

Now, we consider the second relaxation process. In this case, we start from the state of negative saturation, increase input to some value α, then decrease input to some value β and keep it constant thereafter. As the input is being kept constant, the output relaxes and this relaxation is governed by the equation

$$a^{(2)}_{\alpha\beta}\frac{d^2 f}{dt^2} + a^{(1)}_{\alpha\beta}\frac{df}{dt} + f = \tilde{f}_{\alpha\beta} \ , \tag{2.176}$$

whose solution is given by

$$f(t) = C^{(1)}_{\alpha\beta}e^{-t/\tau^{(1)}_{\alpha\beta}} + C^{(2)}_{\alpha\beta}e^{-t/\tau^{(2)}_{\alpha\beta}} + \tilde{f}_{\alpha\beta} \ . \tag{2.177}$$

The constants $\tau^{(1)}_{\alpha\beta}$ and $\tau^{(2)}_{\alpha\beta}$ have the meaning of relaxation times and can be measured experimentally. As soon as this is done, we can find $a^{(1)}_{\alpha\beta}$ and $a^{(2)}_{\alpha\beta}$:

$$a^{(2)}_{\alpha\beta} = \frac{1}{\tau^{(1)}_{\alpha\beta}\tau^{(2)}_{\alpha\beta}} \ , \tag{2.178}$$

$$a^{(1)}_{\alpha\beta} = -\frac{\tau^{(1)}_{\alpha\beta} + \tau^{(2)}_{\alpha\beta}}{\tau^{(1)}_{\alpha\beta}\tau^{(2)}_{\alpha\beta}} \ . \tag{2.179}$$

Next, we introduce the functions

$$q^{(1)}_{\alpha\beta} = a^{(1)}_{\alpha} - a^{(1)}_{\alpha\beta} \ , \tag{2.180}$$

$$q^{(2)}_{\alpha\beta} = a^{(2)}_{\alpha} - a^{(2)}_{\alpha\beta} \ , \tag{2.181}$$

which are directly related to the above-mentioned experimental data. Using the same reasoning that we used many times before, we can establish the formulas

$$q^{(1)}_{\alpha\beta} = 2\iint\limits_{T(\alpha,\beta)} \mu_1(\alpha',\beta')d\alpha' d\beta' \ , \tag{2.182}$$

$$q^{(2)}_{\alpha\beta} = 2\iint\limits_{T(\alpha,\beta)} \mu_2(\alpha',\beta')d\alpha' d\beta' \ , \tag{2.183}$$

from which we derive

$$\mu_1(\alpha,\beta) = -\frac{1}{2}\frac{\partial^2 q^{(1)}_{\alpha\beta}}{\partial\alpha\partial\beta} \ , \tag{2.184}$$

$$\mu_2(\alpha,\beta) = -\frac{1}{2}\frac{\partial^2 q^{(2)}_{\alpha\beta}}{\partial\alpha\partial\beta} \ . \tag{2.185}$$

Thus, the identification problem for the second-order model (2.167)–(2.170) is solved. Extensions to higher-order dynamic models are straightforward.

2.5 Nonlinear Diffusion and Preisach Model

In this section, the application of the Preisach model to nonlinear diffusion is discussed. Nonlinear diffusion has qualitative features which are not observed for linear diffusion. In particular, linear diffusion exhibits infinite speed of propagation of zero front. Whereas in certain problems of nonlinear diffusion wave phenomena are exhibited, and the speed of propagation of zero front is finite. It turns out that the Preisach model of hysteresis is useful for the analysis of such problems of nonlinear diffusion. It is also worthwhile to mention that similar problems of nonlinear diffusion are encountered in neural science and are related to the propagation of action potentials in neurons (see Section 3.3). To make our presentation physically and practically meaningful, the case of nonlinear diffusion in type-II superconductors with sharp resistive transitions is discussed.

It is well known that high field (hard) type-II superconductors are actually not ideal conductors of electric current. It is also known that these superconductors exhibit magnetic hysteresis. Finite resistivity and magnetic hysteresis in these superconductors appear because the motion of flux filaments is pinned by defects such as voids, normal inclusions, dislocations, grain boundaries, and compositional variations. This pinning results in the multiplicity of metastable states, which manifest themselves in hysteresis. When the flux filaments depin by thermal activation or because a current density exceeds some critical value, their motion induces an electric field. As a result, superconductors exhibit "current-voltage" laws $E(J)$, which are strongly nonlinear. Thus, the very phenomenon (pinning) that makes type-II superconductors useful in practical applications is also responsible for their magnetic hysteresis and nonzero resistivity.

From the point of view of phenomenological electrodynamics, type-II superconductors can be treated as electrically nonlinear conductors, and the process of electromagnetic field penetration in such superconductors is the process of nonlinear diffusion. Analysis of nonlinear diffusion in type-II superconductors is of practical and theoretical importance because it can be useful for the evaluation of magnetic hysteresis in these superconductors, as well as for the study of creep phenomena.

We consider the case of sharp resistive transition shown in Fig. 2.37. This transition implies that persistent currents up to a critical current density J_c are always induced in superconducts. We consider nonlinear diffusion of linearly polarized electromagnetic fields. This diffusion is described

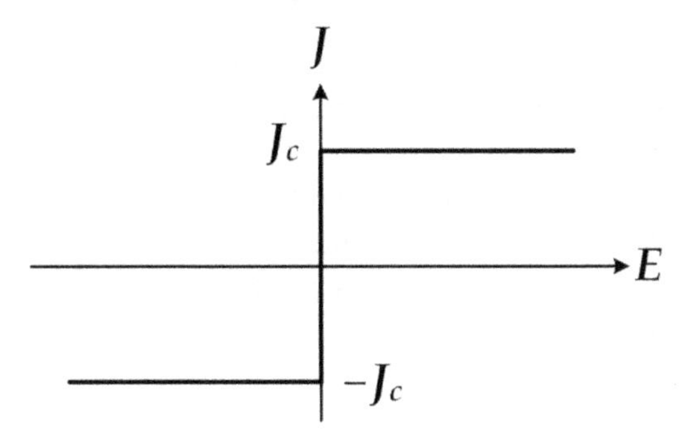

Fig. 2.37

by the following nonlinear partial differential equation:

$$\frac{\partial^2 E}{\partial z^2} = \mu_o \frac{\partial J(E)}{\partial t} , \tag{2.186}$$

where according to the Fig. 2.37

$$J(E) = J_c \text{sign} E , \tag{2.187}$$

while E is the electric field, μ_o is the magnetic permeability of free space, and z-axis is the direction of propagation of electromagnetic field.

Since magnetic field H at the boundary is usually specified, it is natural to analyze nonlinear diffusion in terms of this field. This can be done by representing nonlinear diffusion equation (2.186) as two coupled first order partial differential equations

$$\frac{\partial E}{\partial z} = -\mu_o \frac{\partial H}{\partial t} , \tag{2.188}$$

$$\frac{\partial H}{\partial z} = -J(E) . \tag{2.189}$$

It is easy to see that partial differential equations (2.188) and (2.189) are formally equivalent to equation (2.186). Indeed, by differentiating equation (2.188) with respect to z and equation (2.189) with respect to t and then subtracting the results, we derive equation (2.186). However, equations (2.188) and (2.189) have some mathematical advantages over equation (2.186). First, equation (2.186) contains the time derivative of the discontinuous function $J(E)$, which is not rigorously defined. Equations (2.188) and (2.189) are free of this formal difficulty. Actually, a solution to nonlinear diffusion equation (2.186) can be defined as a solution of coupled equations (2.188) and (2.189). Second and more importantly, coupled equations (2.188) and (2.189) are easy to solve.

The sharp resistive transition (see Fig. 2.37) along with formula (2.188) form the basis for the critical state model for magnetic hysteresis of type-II superconductors. This model was first proposed by C. P. Bean [14]–[15], (see also [16]). The critical state type model has been tested experimentally and has proved to be fairly accurate for simple specimen geometries (plane slabs, circular cross-section cylinders). It has also been realized that the critical state type model has some intrinsic limitations. The main of them is that this model leads to explicit analytical results only for very simple specimen geometries.

Next, we shall briefly describe some basic facts concerning the critical state (Bean) model for superconducting hysteresis. Then, we shall demonstrate that the critical state type models are particular cases of the Preisach model of hysteresis. By using this fact, we shall make the case for the Preisach model as an efficient tool for the description of superconducting hysteresis.

Consider a plane superconducting slab subject to an external time-varying magnetic field $H_0(t)$. We will be interested in the B vs. H_0 relation. Here, B is an average magnetic flux density that is defined as

$$B = \frac{\mu_o}{\Delta} \int_{-\frac{\Delta}{2}}^{+\frac{\Delta}{2}} H(z)dz \ , \tag{2.190}$$

and $H(z)$ is the magnetic field within the slab.

In practice, B and H_0 are quantities that are experimentally measured and it is their relation that exhibits hysteresis.

It follows from formula (2.190) that in order to compute B for any H_0, we have to find a magnetic field profile (magnetic field distribution) within the superconducting slab. This is exactly what we shall do next.

Suppose that no magnetic field was present prior to the instant of time t_0. It is assumed that for times $t > t_0$, the external magnetic field $H_0(t)$ is monotonically increased until it reaches some maximum value H_m. The monotonic increase in the external magnetic field induces persisting electric currents of density J_c.. According to formula (2.189), this results in the formation of linear profiles of the magnetic field shown in Fig. 2.38. The corresponding distribution of persisting electric currents is shown in Fig. 2.39. It is easy to see that the instantaneous depth of penetration of the magnetic field is given by the formula

$$z_0(t) = \frac{H_0(t)}{J_c} \ . \tag{2.191}$$

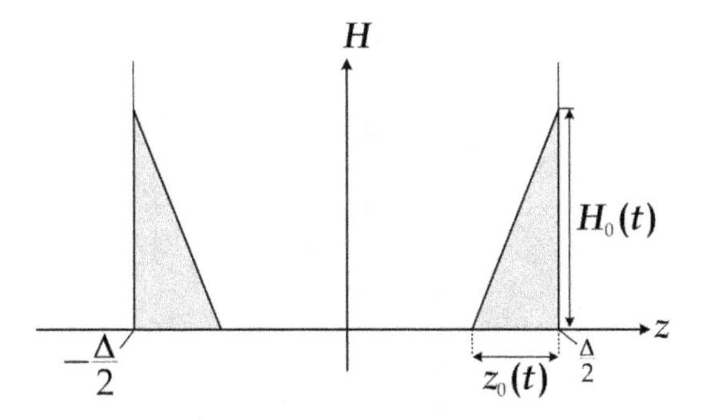

Fig. 2.38

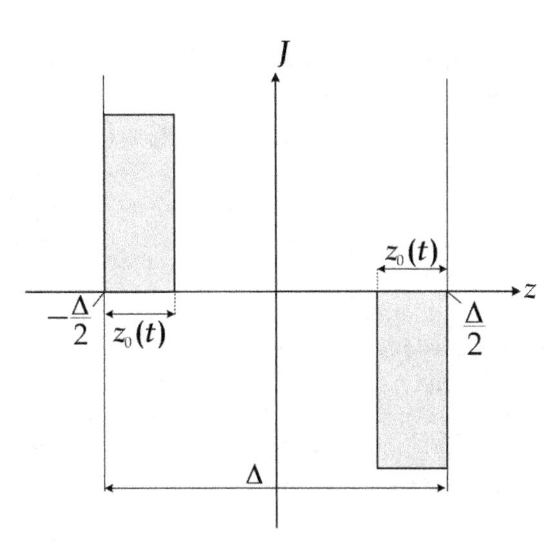

Fig. 2.39

It is also clear that

$$z_0(t) \leq \frac{\Delta}{2} , \tag{2.192}$$

if

$$H_0(t) \leq \frac{J_c \Delta}{2} = H^* . \tag{2.193}$$

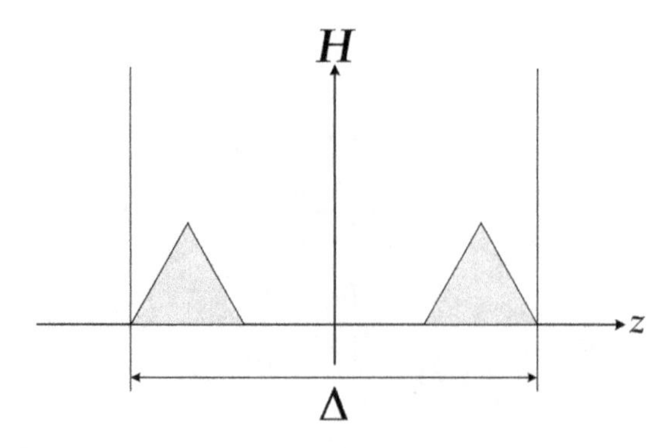

Fig. 2.40

By using Fig. 2.38 and formulas (2.190), (2.191) and (2.192), we find the average value of the magnetic flux density

$$B(t) = \frac{\mu_o z_0(t) H_0(t)}{\Delta} = \frac{\mu_o (H_0(t))^2}{2H^*} \; . \tag{2.194}$$

Suppose now that after achieving the maximum value, H_m, the external magnetic field is monotonically decreased to zero. As soon as the maximum value H_m is achieved, the motion of the previous linear profile is terminated and a new moving linear profile of magnetic field is formed. Due to the previously induced persisting currents, the previous profile stays still and is partially erased by the motion of the new profile. The distribution of the magnetic field within the slab at the instant of time when the external magnetic field is reduced to zero is shown in Fig. 2.40. This figure shows that there is nonzero (positive) average magnetic flux density, which is given by the formula

$$\tilde{B} = \frac{\mu_o H_m^2}{4H^*} > 0 \; . \tag{2.195}$$

This clearly suggests that the B vs. H_0 relation exhibits hysteresis. We next demonstrate the validity of this statement by computing the hysteresis loop for the case of back-and-forth variation of the external magnetic field between $-H_m$ and $+H_m$. For the sake of simplicity of our computations, we shall assume that

$$H_m \leq H^* \; . \tag{2.196}$$

We first consider the half-period when the external magnetic field is monotonically decreased. A typical magnetic field distribution for this half-period is shown in Fig. 2.41. For penetration depths z_0 and δ shown in this

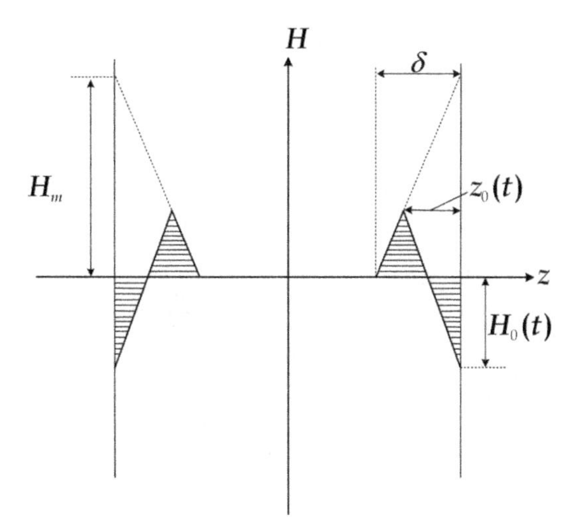

Fig. 2.41

figure, we have

$$\delta = \frac{H_m}{J_c}\,, \qquad z_0(t) = \frac{H_m - H_0(t)}{2J_c}\,. \tag{2.197}$$

By using Fig. 2.41 and formula (2.197), we find the increment of the average magnetic flux density:

$$\Delta B = \frac{2\mu_o}{\Delta}\,\frac{(H_m - H_0(t))z_0(t)}{2} \;=\; \mu_o\frac{(H_m - H_0)^2}{4H^*}\,. \tag{2.198}$$

This leads to the following expression for the average magnetic flux density on the descending branch of the hysteresis loop:

$$B = B_m - \Delta B = \frac{\mu_o H_m^2}{2H^*} - \frac{\mu_o(H_m - H_0)^2}{4H^*}\,. \tag{2.199}$$

Consider now the half-period during which the external magnetic field is monotonically increased from $-H_m$ and $+H_m$. A typical magnetic field distribution for this half-period is shown in Fig. 2.42. By using this figure, as before we find

$$\Delta B = \frac{\mu_o(H_m + H_0)^2}{4H^*}\,, \tag{2.200}$$

and

$$B = -B_m + \Delta B = -\frac{\mu_o H_m^2}{2H^*} + \frac{\mu_o(H_m + H_0)^2}{4H^*}\,. \tag{2.201}$$

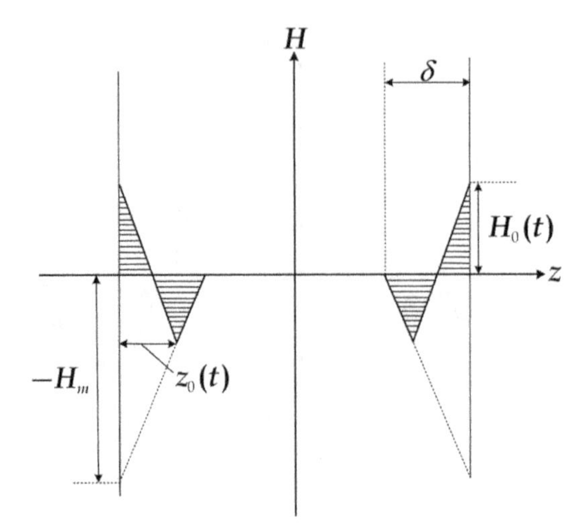

Fig. 2.42

The expressions (2.199) and (2.201) can be combined into one formula:

$$B = \pm\, \mu_o \left[\frac{H_m^2}{2H^*} - \frac{(H_m \mp H_0)^2}{4H^*} \right], \tag{2.202}$$

where the upper signs correspond to the descending branch of the loop, while the lower signs correspond to the ascending branch.

On the basis of the previous discussion, the essence of the Bean model can now be summarized as follows. Each reversal of the magnetic field $H_0(t)$ at the boundary of the superconducting slab results in the formation of a linear profile of the magnetic field. The zero front of this profile extends inward into the superconductor until another reversal value of the magnetic field at the boundary is reached. At this point, the motion of the previous front is terminated and a new moving linear front is formed. Due to the previously induced persisting currents, the previous linear fronts remain still. These remaining fronts represent past history, which leaves its mark upon future values of average magnetic flux density. These persisting linear fronts of the magnetic field may be partially or completely erased by new moving fronts.

Next, we shall establish the connection between the critical state (Bean) model for superconducting hysteresis and the Preisach model [17]. To do this, we shall establish that the erasure property and congruency property hold for the Bean model. Indeed, a moving linear front of the magnetic field will erase those persisting linear fronts if they correspond to the previous extremum values of $H_0(t)$, which are exceeded by a new extremum value. In this way, the effect of those previous extremum values of $H_0(t)$ on the future average values of magnetic flux density B will be completely eliminated. This means that the erasure property holds. It can also be shown that the congruency property of minor loops corresponding to the same reversal values of $H_0(t)$ holds as well. Indeed, consider two variations of external magnetic field $H_0^{(1)}(t)$ and $H_0^{(2)}(t)$. Suppose that these external fields may have different past histories, but starting from some instant of time t_0 they vary back-and-forth between the same reversal values. It is apparent from the previous description of the Bean model that these back-and-forth variations will affect in the *identical* way the same surface layers of superconductors. Consequently, these variations will result in equal increments of B, which is tantamount to the congruency of the corresponding minor loops.

It was established in Chapter 1 that the erasure property and congruency property constitute necessary and sufficient conditions for the representation of actual hysteresis nonlinearity by the Preisach model. Thus, we conclude that the Bean model is a particular case of the Preisach model:

$$B(t) = \iint\limits_{\alpha \geq \beta} \mu(\alpha, \beta)\hat{\gamma}_{\alpha,\beta}H_0(t)d\alpha d\beta \ . \tag{2.203}$$

It is instructive to find such a function $\mu(\alpha, \beta)$ for which the Preisach model coincides with the Bean model. To do this, consider a "major" loop formed when the external magnetic field varies back-and-forth between $+H_m$ and $-H_m$. Consider first-order reversal curves $B_{\alpha\beta}$ attached to the ascending branch of the previously mentioned loop. We recall that the curves $B_{\alpha\beta}$ are formed when, after reaching the value $-H_m$, the external magnetic field is monotonically increased to the value α and subsequently monotonically decreased to the value β. Depending on particular values of α and β, we may have three typical field distributions shown in Figs. 2.43, 2.44 and 2.45. We will use these figures to evaluate the function

$$F(\alpha, \beta) = \frac{1}{2}\left(B_\alpha - B_{\alpha\beta}\right) . \tag{2.204}$$

Figure 2.43 is valid under the condition

$$H_m + \alpha \leq 2H^* \ . \tag{2.205}$$

From this figure we find

$$F(\alpha, \beta) = \frac{\mu_o(\alpha - \beta)^2}{8H^*} \ . \tag{2.206}$$

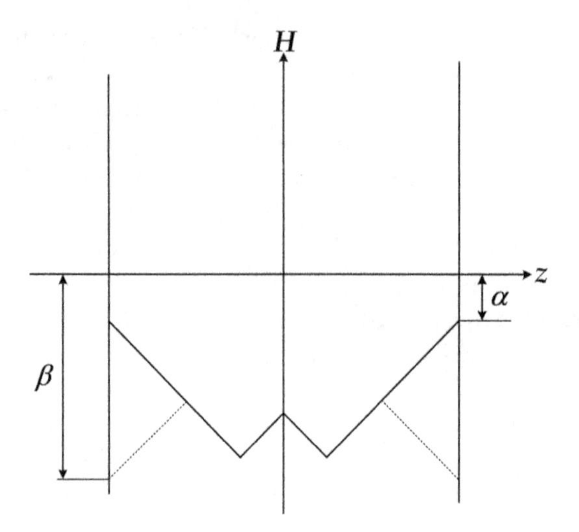

Fig. 2.43

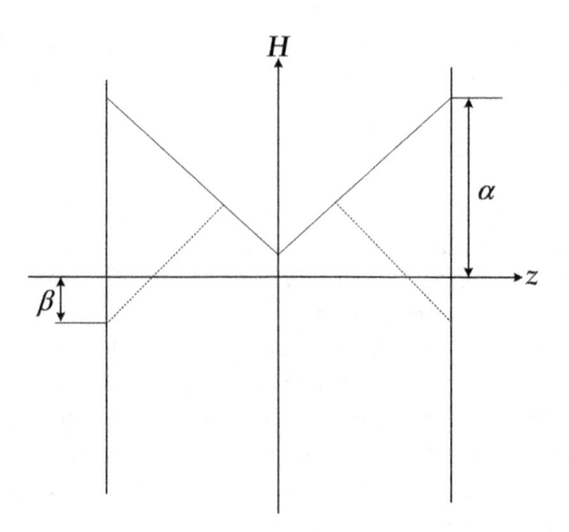

Fig. 2.44

Figure 2.44 holds when

$$H_m + \alpha \geq 2H^*, \qquad \alpha - \beta \leq 2H^* \ . \tag{2.207}$$

By using this figure, we derive

$$F(\alpha, \beta) = \frac{\mu_o(\alpha - \beta)^2}{8H^*} \ . \tag{2.208}$$

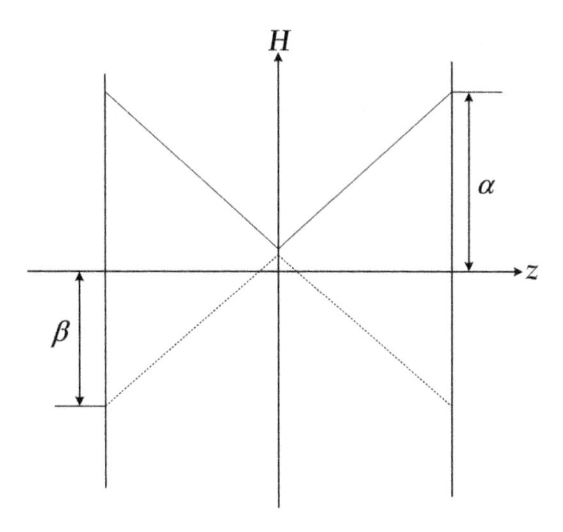

Fig. 2.45

Finally, the distribution of the magnetic field shown in Fig. 2.45 occurs when

$$H_m + \alpha \geq 2H^*, \quad \alpha - \beta \geq 2H^* . \tag{2.209}$$

From this figure, we obtain

$$F(\alpha, \beta) = \frac{\mu_o}{2}\left(\alpha - \beta - H^*\right) . \tag{2.210}$$

The expressions (2.206), (2.208) and (2.210) can be combined into one formula:

$$F(\alpha, \beta) = \begin{cases} \frac{\mu_o(\alpha-\beta)^2}{8H^*} & \text{if } 0 < \alpha - \beta \leq 2H^*, \ |\alpha| \leq H_m, \ |\beta| \leq H_m, \\ \frac{\mu_o}{2}\left(\alpha - \beta - H^*\right) & \text{if } \alpha - \beta \geq 2H^*, \ |\alpha| \leq H_m, \ |\beta| \leq H_m. \end{cases} \tag{2.211}$$

By using the formula (2.211) as well as the formula (see Chapter 1)

$$\mu(\alpha, \beta) = -\frac{\partial^2 F(\alpha, \beta)}{\partial\alpha\partial\beta} , \tag{2.212}$$

we find

$$\mu(\alpha, \beta) = \begin{cases} \frac{\mu_o}{4H^*} & \text{if } 0 < \alpha - \beta \leq 2H^*, \ |\alpha| \leq H_m, \ |\beta| \leq H_m, \\ 0 & \text{if } \alpha - \beta \geq 2H^*, \ |\alpha| \leq H_m, \ |\beta| \leq H_m. \end{cases} \tag{2.213}$$

The trapezoidal support of $\mu(\alpha, \beta)$ given by formula (2.213) is illustrated in Fig. 2.46.

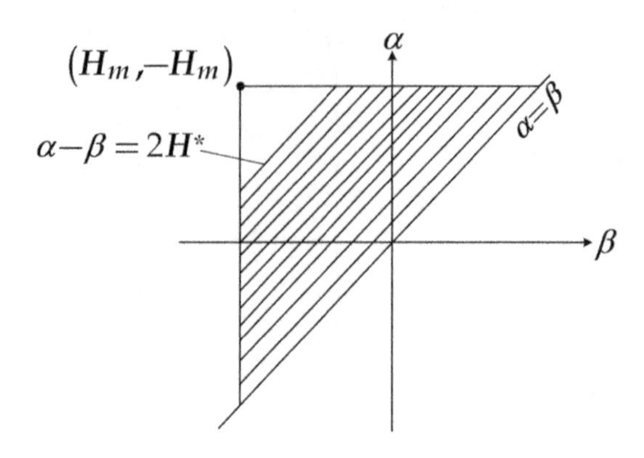

Fig. 2.46

Thus, it has been shown that the critical state model for superconducting hysteresis is a very particular case of the Preisach model. This result has been established for one-dimensional flux distributions and specimens of simple shapes (plane slabs). For these cases, explicit analytical expressions for magnetic field distributions within the superconductors are readily available, and they have been instrumental in the discussion just presented.

Next, we shall demonstrate that the critical state model is a particular case of the Preisach model for specimens of arbitrary shapes and complex flux distributions [18]. For these specimens, analytical machinery for the calculation of magnetic fields within the superconductors does not exist. Nevertheless, it will be shown next that the superconducting hysteresis (as described by the critical state model) still exhibits the erasure property and the congruency property of minor hysteresis loops.

To start the discussion, consider a superconducting cylinder of arbitrary cross-section subject to a uniform external field $B_0(t)$ whose direction does not change with time and lies in the plane of superconductor cross-section (Fig. 2.47). We will choose this direction as the direction of axis x. As the time-varying flux enters the superconductor, it induces screening (shielding) currents of density $\pm J_c$. The distribution of these superconducting screening currents is such that they create the magnetic field, which at any instant of time completely compensates for the change in the external field $B_0(t)$. Mathematically, this can be expressed as follows:

$$\delta B_0(t) + B_i(t) = 0 \ . \tag{2.214}$$

Here, $\delta B_0(t)$ is the change in $B_0(t)$, while $B_i(t)$ is the field created by superconducting screening currents, and equally (2.214) holds in the region interior to these currents.

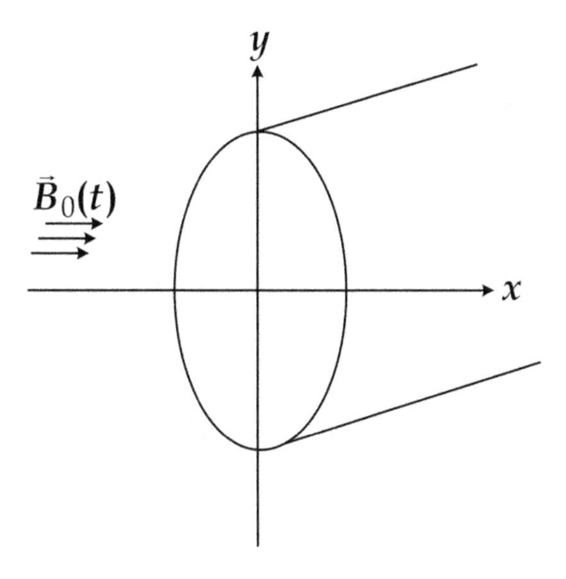

Fig. 2.47

It is clear that $\delta B_0(t) \geq 0$ when $B_0(t)$ is monotonically increased, and $\delta B_0(t) \leq 0$ when $B_0(t)$ is monotonically decreased. By using this fact and (2.214), it can be concluded that there is a reversal in the direction (polarity) of superconducting screening currents as $B_0(t)$ goes through its maximum or minimum values.

With these facts in mind, consider how the distribution of superconducting currents is generically modified in time by temporal variations of the external magnetic field. Suppose that, starting from zero value, the external field is monotonically increased until it reaches its maximum value M_1 at some time $t = t_1^+$. This monotonic variation of $B_0(t)$ induces a surface layer of superconducting screening currents. The interior boundary of this current layer extends inwards as $B_0(t)$ is increased [see Fig. 2.48a], and at any instant of time this boundary is uniquely determined by the instantaneous values of $B_0(t)$. Next, we suppose that this monotonic increase is followed by a monotonic decrease until $B_0(t)$ reaches its minimum value m_1 at some time $t = t_1^-$. For the time being it is assumed that $|m_1| < M_1$. As soon as the maximum value M_1 is achieved, the inward extension of the previous current layer is terminated and a new surface current layer of reversed polarity (direction) is induced [see Fig. 2.48b]. This new current layer creates field $B_i(t)$, which compensates for monotonic decrease in $B_0(t)$ in the region interior to this current layer. For this reason, it is clear that

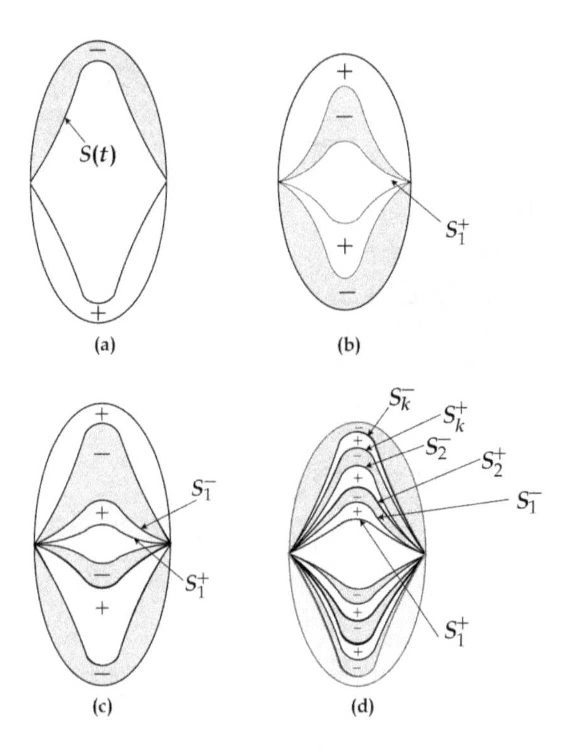

Fig. 2.48

the interior boundary of the new current layer extends inwards as $B_0(t)$ is monotonically decreased. It is also clear that this boundary is uniquely determined by the instantaneous value of $\delta B_0(t)$, and, consequently, by the instantaneous value of $B_0(t)$ for any specific (given) value of M_1. Now suppose that the monotonic decrease is followed by a monotonic increase until $B_0(t)$ reaches its new maximum value M_2 at some time $t = t_2^+$. For the time being, it is assumed that $M_2 < |m_1|$. As soon as the minimum value m_1 is achieved, the inward extension of the second layer of superconducting screening currents is terminated and a new surface current layer of reversed polarity is introduced to counteract the monotonic increase of the external field [see Fig. 2.48c]. This current layer extends inwards until the maximum value M_2 is achieved; at this point the inward extension of the current layer is terminated. As before, the instantaneous position of the interior boundary of this layer is uniquely determined by the instantaneous value of $\delta B_0(t)$, and, consequently, by the instantaneous value of $B_0(t)$ for a specific (given) value of m_1.

Thus, it can be concluded that at any instant of time there may exist several (many) layers of persisting superconducting currents [see Fig. 2.48d]. These persisting currents have opposite polarities (directions) in adjacent layers. The interior boundaries S_k^+ and S_k^- of all layers (except the last one) remain still and they are uniquely determined by the past extremum values M_k and m_k of $B_0(t)$, respectively. The last induced current layer extends inward as the external field changes in time monotonically.

The magnetic moment $\vec{M}$ of the superconductor is related to the distribution of the superconducting screening currents as follows:

$$\vec{M}(t) = \int_S \left[\vec{r} \times \vec{j}(t)\right] ds \ , \tag{2.215}$$

where the integration is performed over the superconductor cross-section.

In general, this magnetic moment has x and y components. According to formula (2.215), these components are given by the expressions

$$M_x(t) = \int_S y \ j(t) \ ds \ , \tag{2.216}$$

$$M_y(t) = -\int_S x \ j(t) \ ds \ . \tag{2.217}$$

It is clear that if the superconductor cross-section is symmetric with respect to the x-axis, then only the x component of the magnetic moment is present. In the absence of this symmetry, two components of the magnetic moments exist.

It is apparent from the previous discussion that the instantaneous values of $M_x(t)$ and $M_y(t)$ depend not only on the current instantaneous value of the external field $B_0(t)$ but on the past extremum values of $B_0(t)$, as well. This is because the overall distribution of persisting superconducting currents depends on the past extrema of $B_0(t)$. Thus, it can be concluded that relationships $M_x(t)$ vs. $B_0(t)$, and $M_y(t)$ vs. $B_0(t)$ exhibit discrete memories that are characteristic and intrinsic of the rate-independent hysteresis. It is worthwhile to note that it is the hysteretic relationship $M_x(t)$ vs. $B_0(t)$ that is typically measured in experiments by using, for instance, a vibrating sample magnetometer (VSM) with one pair of pickup coils. By using a VSM equipped with two pairs of orthogonal pickup coils, the hysteretic relation between $M_y(t)$ vs. $B_0(t)$ can be measured, as well.

It is important to stress here that the origin of rate independence of superconducting hysteresis can be traced back to the assumption of sharp resistive transitions. This connection is especially apparent for superconducting specimens of simple shapes (plane slabs). For such specimens, the explicit and single-valued relations between the increments of the external field and the location of inward boundaries of superconducting layers can be found by resorting only to Ampere's Law.

It is clear from the presented discussion that a newly induced and inward-extending layer of superconducting currents will erase (replace) some layers of persisting superconducting currents if they correspond to the previous extremum values of $B_0(t)$, which are exceeded by a new extremum value. In this way, the effect of those previous extremum values of $B_0(t)$ on the overall future current distributions will be completely eliminated. According to formulas (2.216) and (2.217), the effect of those past extremum values of the external magnetic field on the magnetic moment will be eliminated as well. This is the erasure property of the superconducting hysteresis as described by the critical state model.

Next, we proceed with the discussion of the congruency property. Consider two distinct variations of the external field, $B_0^{(1)}(t)$ and $B_0^{(2)}(t)$. Suppose that these two external fields have different past histories and, consequently, different sequences of local past extrema, $\{M_k^{(1)}, m_k^{(1)}\}$ and $\{M_k^{(2)}, m_k^{(2)}\}$. However, starting from some instant of time they vary back-and-forth between the same reversal values. It is apparent from the description of the critical state model and expressions (2.216) and (2.217) that these two identical back-and-forth variations of the external field will result in the formation of two minor loops for the hysteretic relation $M_x(t)$ vs. $B_0(t)$ [or $M_y(t)$ vs. $B_0(t)$]. It is also apparent from the same description of the critical state model that these two back-and-forth variations of the external field will affect in the *identical* way the *same* surface layers of a superconductor. Unaffected layers of the persistent superconducting currents will be different because of different past histories of $B_0^{(1)}(t)$ and $B_0^{(2)}(t)$. According to formulas (2.216) and (2.217), these unaffected layers of persistent currents result in constant-in-time ("background") components of the magnetic moment. Consequently, it can be concluded that the same *incremental* variations of $B_0^{(1)}(t)$ and $B_0^{(2)}(t)$ will result in equal *increments* of M_x (and M_y). This is tantamount to the congruency of the corresponding minor loops. Thus, the congruency property is established for the superconducting hysteresis as described by the critical state model.

It has been previously established that the erasure property and the congruency property constitute the necessary and sufficient conditions for the representation of actual hysteresis nonlinearities by the Preisach model.

Thus, the description of the superconducting hysteresis by the critical state model is equivalent to the description of the same hysteresis by the Preisach model.

The question can be immediately asked, "What is to be gained from this result?" The answer to this question can be stated as follows. There is no readily available analytical machinery for the calculation of the interior boundaries of superconducting current layers for specimens of arbitrary shapes. For this reason, the critical state model does not lead to mathematically explicit results. The application of the Preisach model allows one to circumvent these difficulties by using some experimental data. Namely, for any superconducting specimen, the "first-order reversal" curves can be measured and used for the identification of the Preisach model for the given specimen. By using these curves, complete prediction of hysteretic behavior of the specimen can be given at least at the same level of accuracy and physical legitimacy as in the case of the critical state model. In particular, cyclic and "ramp" losses can be explicitly expressed in terms of the first-order reversal curves (see Chapter 1).

As an aside, we point out that the presented discussion can also be useful whenever numerical implementation of the Bean model is attempted. Indeed, the numerical implementation of the Bean model can be appreciably simplified by computing only the "first-order transition" curves and then by using these curves for the prediction of hysteretic behavior for arbitrary piece wise monotonic variations of the external field. The latter is possible because, whenever the congruency and erasure properties are valid, all hysteretic data can be compressed (collapsed) into the "first-order reversal" curves.

After it was realized [17] that the critical state (Bean) model is a particular case of the classical Preisach model, several attempts have been made to test the accuracy of Preisach modeling of superconducting hysteresis. First, experimental testing of the congruency and erasure properties for type-II superconductors has been carried out by G. Friedman, L. Liu, and J. S. Kouvel [19]. In the reported experiments, two superconducting samples were used. One was a high temperature superconductor $Ba_{0.575}K_{0.425}BiO_3$, while the other was niobium (Nb). The erasure property was checked by observing the closure of minor loops at the end of the first cyclic variation of the magnetic field. To examine the congruency property, minor hysteresis loops were compared for identical cyclic variations of the magnetic field with different prior histories. The performed experiments suggest that the erasure and congruency properties fairly accurate for these superconductors.

More extensive experimental testings of the accuracy of the Preisach modeling of superconducting hysteresis have been reported in [20]. In these experiments, higher-order reversal curves predicted by the Preisach model were compared with actual higher-order reversal curves measured for the same past extremum values of the external magnetic field as used in Preisach predictions. This comparison is the basis for the assessment of the accuracy of the Preisach model because the history dependent branching is the phenomenological essence of hysteresis.

The testing was performed for $YBa_2Cu_3O_x$ superconducting samples by using a vibrating sample magnetometer (VSM) equipped with a cryostat (model MicroMag 3900 of Princeton Measurements Corporation). The specimens were sintered disk shaped samples about 4 mm in diameter and 2 mm in thickness. These samples were procured from Angstrom Sciences, Inc. The experiments were conducted in the wide range of temperatures (varying from 14 to 80 K). In these experiments, the first-order reversal curves were measured for each temperature. These curves were used for the identification of the Preisach model as discussed in Chapter 1. Then, higher-order reversal curves (up to the eighth order) were measured at each temperature for various sequences of reversal values of the applied magnetic field, that is, for various past histories. These measured higher-order reversal curves were compared with the predictions of those curves by the Preisach model computed for the same past histories as in the experiments. Sample results of these comparisons are shown in Figs. 2.49, 2.50, and 2.51 for temperatures of 14, 30, and 60 K, respectively. These sample results of the comparison between the experimental data and the Preisach model predictions are representatives of what we have observed for other temperatures. The above figures demonstrate the remarkable accuracy of the classical Preisach model in predicting various branches of superconducting hysteresis for various past histories and in the wide range of temperatures. Since history dependent branching is the essence of phenomenological manifestation of hysteresis, the above comparison suggests that the Preisach model may have a remarkable prediction power as far as the description of superconducting hysteresis is concerned. This comparison also suggests that the set of first-order reversal curves may eventually emerge as the standard experimental data that can be used for the complete phenomenological characterization of superconducting hysteresis. These first-order reversal curves can be useful not only for the prediction of branching but for calculation of cyclic and "ramp" losses, as well.

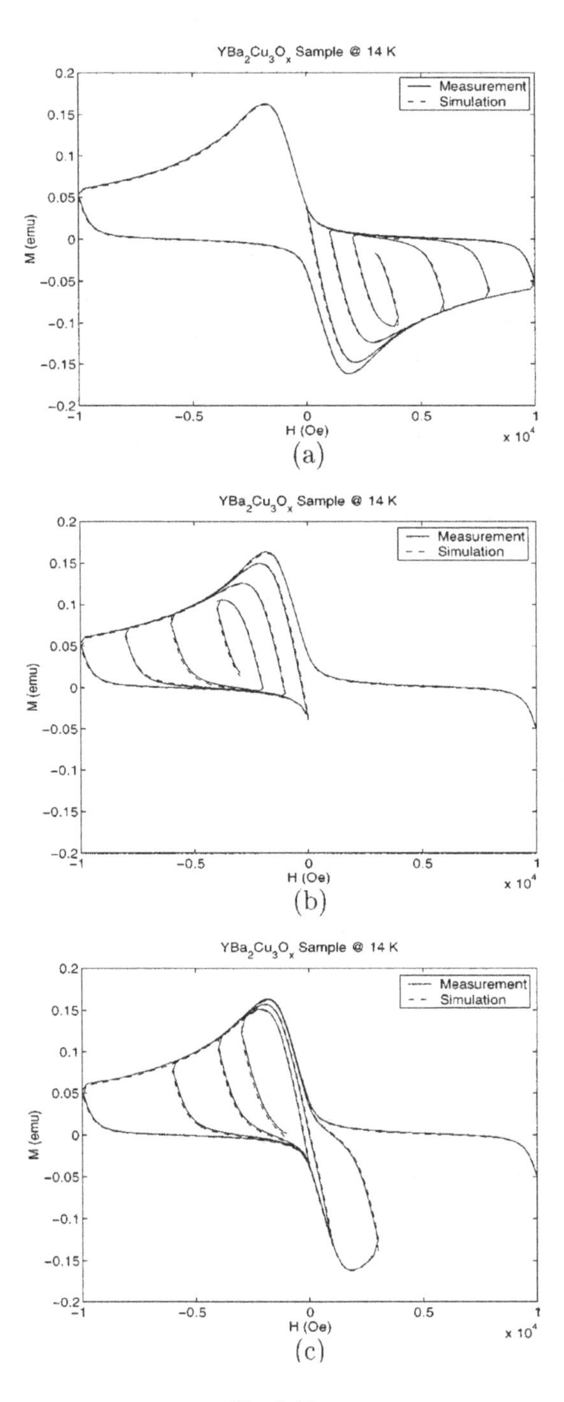
YBa2Cu3Ox Sample @ 14 K
Measurement
Simulation
M (emu)
H (Oe)
x 10^4
(a)
YBa2Cu3Ox Sample @ 14 K
Measurement
Simulation
M (emu)
H (Oe)
x 10^4
(b)
YBa2Cu3Ox Sample @ 14 K
Measurement
Simulation
M (emu)
H (Oe)
x 10^4
(c)

Fig. 2.49

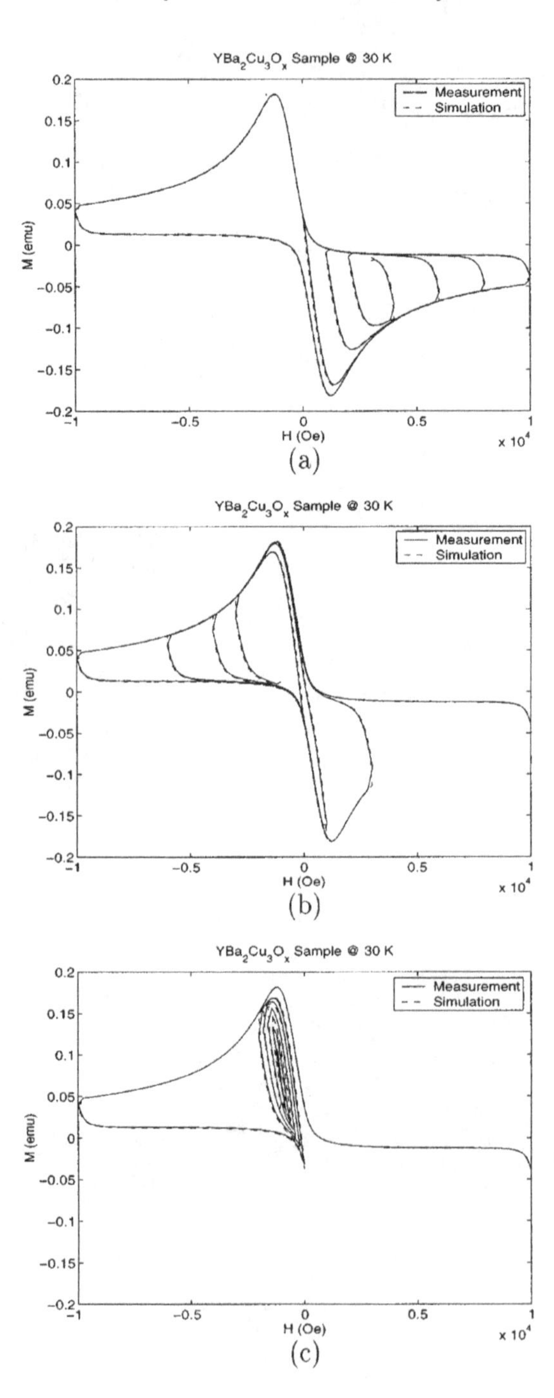

YBa2Cu3Ox Sample @ 30 K
Measurement
Simulation
M (emu)
H (Oe)
x 10^4
(a)
YBa2Cu3Ox Sample @ 30 K
Measurement
Simulation
M (emu)
H (Oe)
x 10^4
(b)
YBa2Cu3Ox Sample @ 30 K
Measurement
Simulation
M (emu)
H (Oe)
x 10^4
(c)

Fig. 2.50

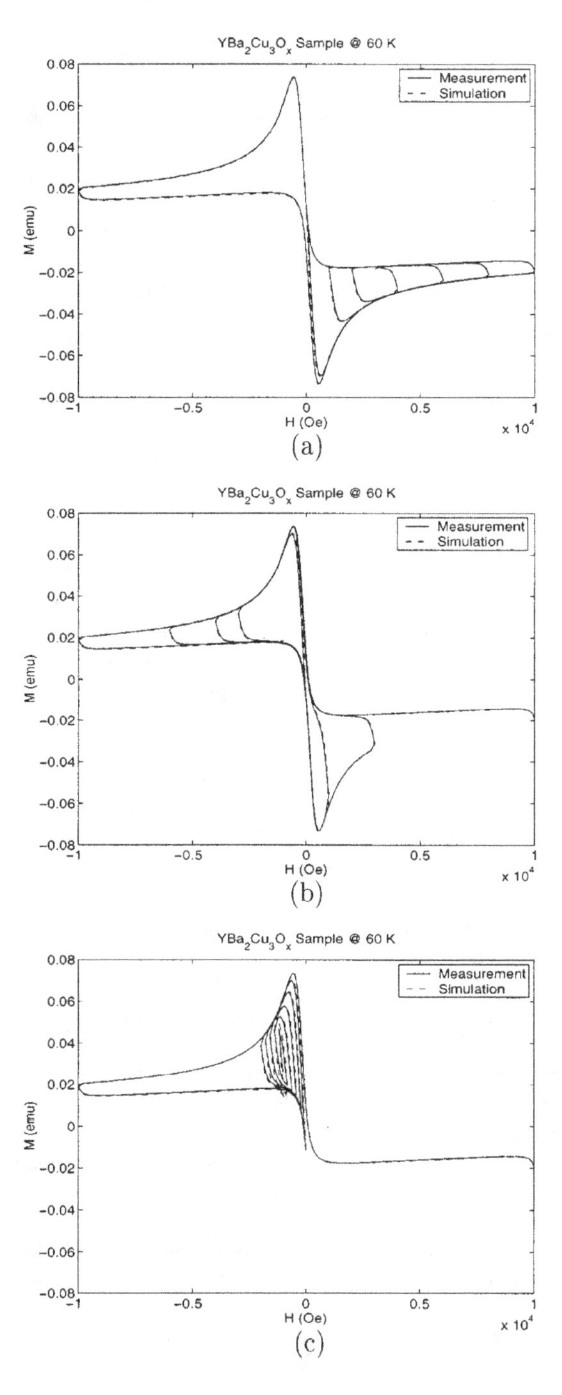
YBa2Cu3Ox Sample @ 60 K
Measurement
Simulation
M (emu)
H (Oe)
x 10^4
(a)
YBa2Cu3Ox Sample @ 60 K
Measurement
Simulation
M (emu)
H (Oe)
x 10^4
(b)
YBa2Cu3Ox Sample @ 60 K
Measurement
Simulation
M (emu)
H (Oe)
x 10^4
(c)

Fig. 2.51

As an aside, it is worth noting that there is mounting experimental and theoretical evidence that the classical Preisach model may be much more accurate for the description of superconducting hysteresis than for the description of hysteresis of magnetic materials. This is quite ironic because historically the Preisach model was first developed as a model for magnetic hysteresis and was first phrased in purely magnetic terms. This irony supports the point of view that it is beneficial to consider the Preisach model as a general mathematical tool whose usefulness extends far beyond the area of modeling of magnetic hysteresis.

References

[1] I. Mayergoyz, "Mathematical Models of Hysteresis and Their Applications," Academic Press (an imprint of Elsevier), 2003.
[2] I. D. Mayergoyz, "Mathematical Models of Hysteresis," Phys. Rev. Lett., Vol. 56, pp. 1518-1521, 1986.
[3] I. D. Mayergoyz and G. Friedman, "Generalized Preisach model of hysteresis," IEEE Transactions on Magnetics, Vol. 24, pp. 212-217, 1988.
[4] I. D. Mayergoyz, "Dynamic Preisach models of hysteresis," IEEE Transactions on Magnetics, Vol. 24 (6), pp. 2925-2927, 1988.
[5] I. D. Mayergoyz, G. Friedman and C. Salling, "Comparison of the classical and generalized Preisach hysteresis models with experiments," IEEE Transactions on Magnetics, Vol. 25 (5), pp. 3925-3927, 1989.
[6] I. D. Mayergoyz, G. Friedman and A. Adly, "New Preisach-type models of hysteresis and their experimental testing," Journal of Applied Physics, Vol. 67, pp. 5373-5375, 1990.
[7] I. D. Mayergoyz, "Input-dependent Preisach model and hysteretic energy losses," Journal of Applied Physics, Vol. 69, pp. 4611-4613, 1991.
[8] A. A. Adly, I. D. Mayergoyz and A. Bergqvist, "Preisach modeling of magnetostrictive hysteresis," Journal of Applied Physics, Vol. 69 (8), pp. 5777-5779, 1991.
[9] G. Friedman and I. D. Mayergoyz, "Input-dependent Preisach model and hysteretic energy losses", J. Appl. Phys., Vol. 69 (8), pp. 4611-4613, 1991.
[10] A. A. Adly and I. D. Mayergoyz, "Experimental testing of the average Preisach model of hysteresis," IEEE Transactions on Magnetics, Vol. 28 (5), pp. 2268-2270, 1992.
[11] I. D. Mayergoyz and A. A. Adly, "Numerical implementation of the feedback Preisach model," IEEE Transactions on Magnetics, Vol. 28 (5), pp. 2605-2607, 1992.
[12] I. D. Mayergoyz and P. Andrei, "Preisach modeling of clockwise hysteresis and its application to front propagation problems," Journal of Applied Physics, Vol. 91, pp. 7645-7647, 2002.
[13] K. Wiesen and S. H. Charap, "A better scalar Preisach algorithm," IEEE Transactions on Magnetics, Vol. 24, pp. 2491-2493, 1988.

[14] C. P. Bean, "Magnetization of Hard Superconductors," Phys. Rev. Lett., Vol. 8, pp. 250-253, 1962.
[15] C. P. Bean, "Magnetization of High-Field Superconductors," Rev. Modern Phys., Vol. 36, pp. 31-39, 1964.
[16] H. London, "Alternating current losses in superconductors of the second kind," Physics Letters, Vol. 6, pp. 162-165, 1963.
[17] I. D. Mayergoyz and T. A. Keim. "Superconducting hysteresis and the Preisach model," Journal of Applied Physics, Vol. 67, pp. 5466-5468, 1990.
[18] I. D. Mayergoyz, "Superconducting hysteresis and the Preisach model," Journal of Applied Physics, Vol. 79, pp. 6473-6475, 1996.
[19] G. Friedman, L. Liu and J. S. Kouvel, "Experimental testing of applicability of the Preisach hysteresis model to superconductors," Journal of Applied Physics, Vol. 75 (10), pp. 5683-5685, 1994.
[20] I. D. Mayergoyz, A. A. Adly, M. W. Huang and C. Kraft, "Experimental testing of the Preisach modeling of superconducting hysteresis," Journal of Applied Physics, Vol. 87 (9), pp. 5552-5554, 2000.

Chapter 3

Neural Memory and Hysteresis

3.1 Neuron

In this and the following sections, a brief review of the very basic and selected facts from neural science is presented. The detailed discussion of these and many other important facts can be found in the books on neural science [1]–[6]. This list of books is not exhaustive but rather suggestive.

It is well-known that memory is a function of the brain, which is realized due to its special structure. Neurons are the main building components of this structure. According to the existing estimates, there are about 100 billion neurons in the human brain and around 10^5 neurons in 1 mm^3 volume of cortical tissue.

Neurons (as any cells) are defined by their membranes which separate their interior from the exterior environment. Membranes are formed by phospholipid molecules. These molecules have two-long hydrophobic ("water-repeling") fatty acid tails and hydrophilic ("water-attracting") phosphorous containing heads. In water, these molecules align themselves in double layers in such a way that hydrophobic fatty tails are inside these layers (i.e. away from water), while hydrophilic heads point outwards into the water on both exterior and interior sides of neuron boundaries formed by these double layers. This lipid bilayer arrangement is illustrated in Fig. 3.1 for a small patch of a closed membrane.

The described lipid bilayer formation is achieved by self-assembly process because it corresponds to the lowest energy and, for this reason, this formation is most stable. These lipid bilayers are of 3 to 5 nm thickness, and they represent insulating barriers separating conducting water solutions on interior and exterior sides of neurons. In the case when electric potential differences between internal and external conducting solutions vary with

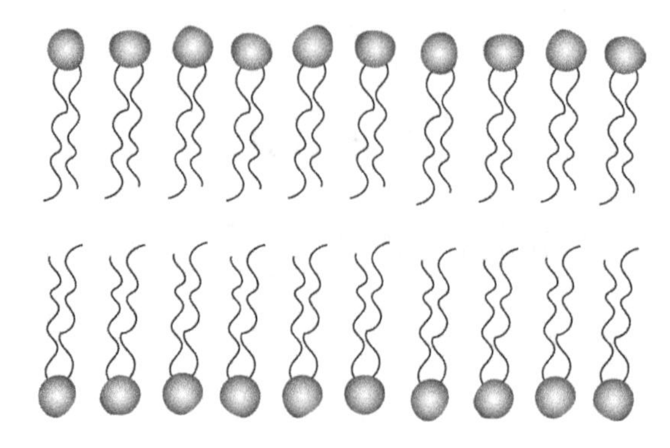

Fig. 3.1

time, displacement currents through lipid bilayers appear. These currents are usually modelled by introducing local capacitances for small patches of membranes. Along with displacement currents, there are ionic currents through neuron membranes which are due to the presence of ion channels and pumps embedded in the membranes. The walls of these channels and pumps are specific protein molecules, which may form protein pores. In the case of ion channels, the transport of specific ions is always down their concentration gradients. In other words, specific ions always flow to where their concentrations are the lowest. The ion channels play the central role in electrical signaling in neurons, and they will be discussed in some detail in the next section. In contrast with ion channels, ion pumps move ions against their concentration gradients. This means that pumps execute the active ion transport towards locations of higher concentration. This active transport requires some energy which is usually supplied by special ATP (Adenosine Triphosphate) molecules. It is apparent that active pump transport restores the gradients of ion concentrations. This makes possible the operation of ion channels.

There are many different types of neurons, and within each type there are many structurally distinguishable subtypes. It is estimated [2] that the number of anatomically distinguishable subtypes of cortical neurons is between 50 and 500. This is the reflection of ubiquitous biological diversity; the diversity which is at the very foundation of neural systems. Below, for the sake of brevity, mostly pyramidal type neurons are discussed. These neurons are abundant in the cerebral cortex and the hippocampus, which are the parts of the brain involved in neural memory formation and cognition. Pyramidal neurons were first discovered and extensively studied by

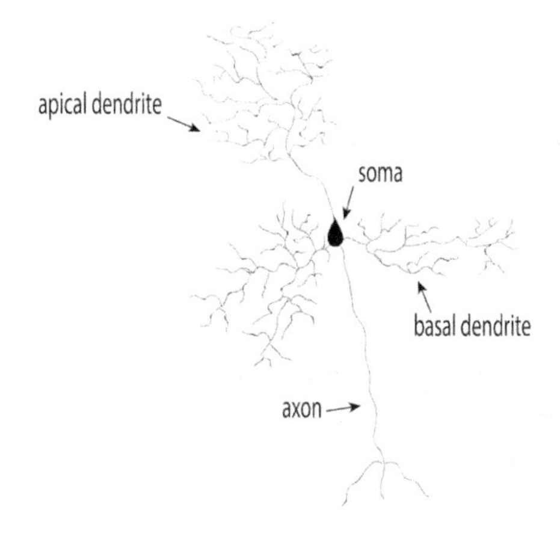

Fig. 3.2

Spanish neuroscientist Santiago Ramon y Cajal at the turn of the nineteenth century.

A schematic diagram of pyramidal neuron is shown in Fig. 3.2. Like in most neurons, three main structures can be identified in pyramidal cells. They are the cell body or soma, axon and dendritic trees. Generally speaking, these three distinct structures are respectively involved in information processing and information output/input transmission, executed by neurons.

The soma of pyramidal cells has a conic (pyramidal) shape which is reflected in the name of these neurons. Inside of the bilipid membranes of soma, there is the cell nucleus. This nucleus contains genetic materials (DNA and RNA) which control the synthesis of proteins necessary for neuron functioning. The lone axon (see Fig. 3.2) emerges from the base of the pyramidal soma at the specific site which is called an axon hillock. The axon hillocks usually have high density of voltage-controlled ion-channels utilized in the generation of action potentials. This matter is further discussed in the third section of this chapter. Pyramidal cells are among the largest in the brain and on average their soma is about 20 μm in length.

Axons conduct electrical signals (known as action potentials) away from cell bodies to other neurons. In this sense, the axons can be viewed as transmission lines of the nervous systems, and their bundles form nerves. Anatomically, an axon is a tubular type protrusion emanating at the axon hillock site of soma and extending away for long distances. A schematic of axon is presented in Fig. 3.3.

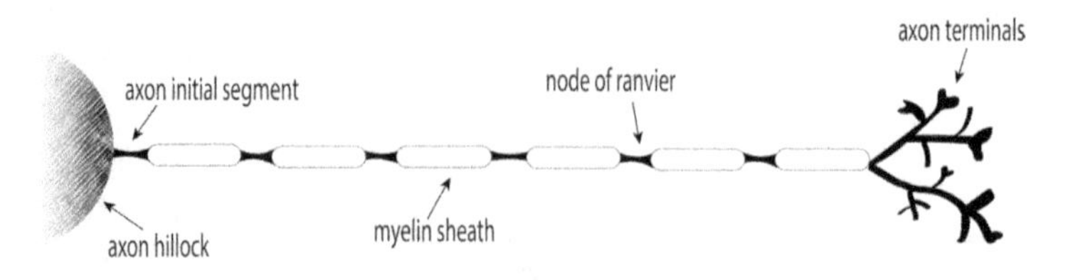

Fig. 3.3

Axon dimensions vary appreciably among neurons. Some axons may extend up to one meter while others extend only over a few millimeters. The diameter of axons is typically about one micrometer. However, for some cells it may reach 20 μm.

Long axons of the vertebrate neurons system are usually covered with myelin. This term was coined by the famous German physician, biologist and polyglot Rudolf Virchow. The myelin is a tight many layer wrapping of insulating glial cell membrane, which is usually called myelin sheath. This insulation results in faster signal speed as well as the reduction of signal decay. About every millimeter, the myelin sheath is periodically interrupted by exposing naked excitable axon membrane to the extracellular fluids. These unmyelinated spots of axons are called nodes of Ranvier, and they are about 1 μm long. Such myelin sheath gaps were first discovered by the French anatomist Louis-Antoine Ranvier in the second part of the nineteenth century. Myelin insulation prevents ions from entering or leaving the axon along myelinated segments. This implies that the ion-transport through axon membrane is strongly localized at the nodes of Ranvier. The realization of this localization of ion transport is achieved due to high concentration of ion channels in axon membrane at nodes of Ranvier. Another location with high concentration of ion-channels is the axon initial segment. It is relatively thick, unmyelinated part of the axon that emanates directly from the cell body. It is about 25 μm in length, and at this site the initiation of action potential occurs. This action potential moves very fast (leaps) through myelinated segments of axon being sequentially regenerated and properly enhanced at the nodes of Ranvier. This "hopping" of action potential from one node of Ranvier to another is known as "saltatory" conduction. At the end, an axon is divided into many unmyelinated branches, which serve as axon terminals. These terminals (also called terminal boutons) form synaptic connections with dendrites of other neurons. It is through these conducting synaptic connections that electrical signal communication between different neurons is established.

It is worthwhile to mention that axons of neuron cells in invertebrates are unmyelinated. This results in a different physical mechanism of action potential propagation. Such a mechanism is based on nonlinear diffusion which is supported by relatively uniform (i.e. homogeneous) distribution of ion-channels along axon membranes. The nonlinear diffusion mechanism has been extensively (experimentally and theoretically) studied in the case of squid giant axons. This study was initiated by Alan Hodgkin and Andrew Huxley in Cambridge, England in the middle of the last century. The above study resulted in the creation of Hodgkin-Huxley model of action potential generation and propagation. This model is widely regarded as one of the greatest achievements in neural science and has been very influential in the subsequent research in this field.

Next, we shall discuss neuron dendrites. Anatomically, dendrites are expansive and elaborate protrusions emanating from the cell body of neurons. They usually branch extensively and form tree-like arborization around neurons, called dendritic trees. It is evident from Fig. 3.2 that in the case of pyramidal neurons there are apical and basal dendrites. An apical dendrite emerges from the apex of pyramidal soma, and it can be viewed as one of the distinguishing features of pyramidal neurons. There are two types of apical dendrites: distal and proximal. The distal apical dendrites are longer than proximal, and they extend from the pyramidal cell apex in the direction opposite from the axon. As a result, the distal apical dendrites may form synaptic connections with remote neurons. In contrast, shorter proximal apical dendrites establish synaptic connections with neighboring neural cells. In pyramidal neurons, there is usually a single apical dendrite, but there are several basal dendrites. They emerge from the base of the neuron soma, which is reflected in their name. These dendrites extend in the directions somewhat opposite or perpendicular to the direction of apical dendrites, and they are a major target for synaptic inputs. It must be stressed that the structure of dendritic trees varies appreciably among neurons. This is especially apparent from the comparison of dendritic arbor of pyramidal neurons and Purkinje cells. The latter cells are schematically represented in Fig. 3.4. They are among the largest neurons in the human brain, and they are found within the Purkinje layer in the cerebellum. Their functioning is related to the regulation and coordination of motor movements and, consequently, it is related to the foundation of procedural memory.

Dendrites are irregularly and (in some cases) sparsely decorated (studded) by tiny spines. These are sub-micrometer scale membranous

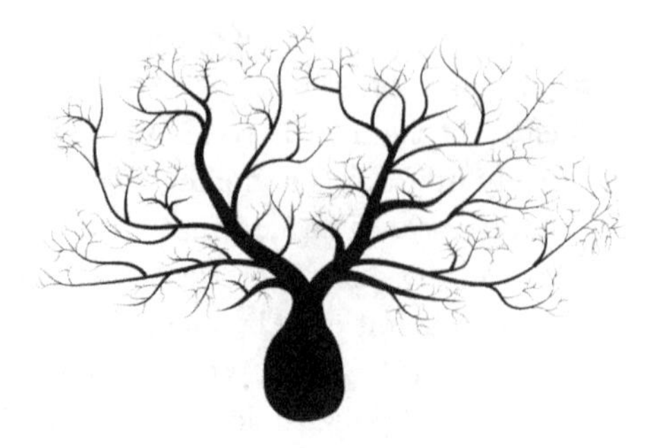

Fig. 3.4

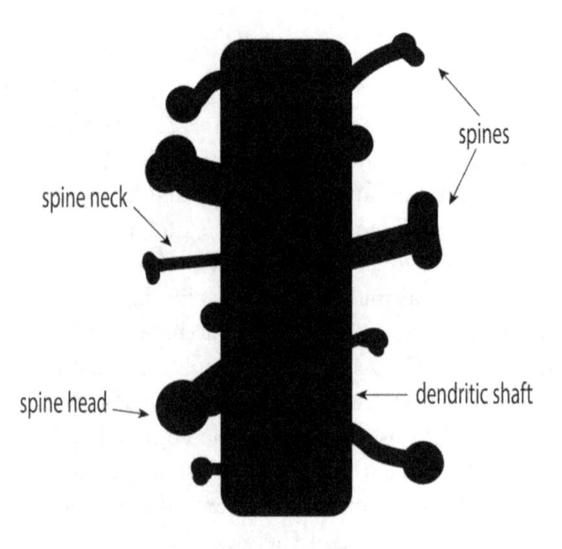

Fig. 3.5

protrusions from neuron dendrites with a wide variety of shapes (see Fig. 3.5). Most spines exhibit a bulging head and a thin neck that connects the spine head to the dendrite shaft. Spines are numerous in the case of pyramidal neurons of the neo-cortex and Purkinje cells of the cerebellum. They may occur at a density of up to five spines per one micrometer of dendrite stretch. The dendrites of a single neuron may contain thousands of spines. One of the main functions of spines is to establish electrical (electrochemical) synaptic connections with axons of other neurons and, in this way, to realize the transmission of signals from an axon of one neuron to a dendrite (and eventually, to a soma) of another neuron cell. A remarkable fact is that spines exhibit plasticity. The essence of this plasticity is to strengthen or weaken over time the synaptic connection in response to the increase or decrease of synaptic connection activity, respectively. Spine plasticity manifests itself in appreciable and sufficiently rapid changes in spine shapes, their volumes, and numbers.

Historically, dendrites were first viewed as passive cables used for transmission of synaptic inputs. Accordingly, this transmission has been described by the linear cable equations in which the dendrite membrane has been modelled by a conductance connected in parallel with a capacitance. Various techniques for the solution of these equations for passive dendritic trees have been developed. Thus, the traditional view was that dendrites receive signals from other neurons and pass them to the cell body without performing any further processing. Over the past few decades, the new experimental evidence has emerged, which suggests that dendrites are not entirely passive and that their functioning is much more complex than what was previously envisioned. Namely, it was found that voltage-controlled and calcium-gated ion channels are abundant in dendrites. These channels affect the shape, propagation, and integration of synaptic signals. The existence of such channels requires local protein production. It turns out that dendrites (and, possibly, their spines) contain the necessary machinery for local protein synthesis. The study of active properties of dendrites and their spines which lead to their plasticity driven by previous experience is currently a very promising area of intense research in neuroscience.

3.2 Channels and Synapses

From a physics point of view, neurons are highly complex and intricate electric systems. Ion channels of neurons are at the very foundation of the functioning of these systems. The ion channels are ubiquitous. They are present in somas, axons, and dendrites of neural cells. These channels are crucial for establishing and maintaining the membrane voltage, for generation and propagation of action potentials and for strengthening or weakening of synaptic connections between neurons.

Ion channels are formed by specialized proteins embedded in phospholipid bilayers of membranes. A schematic picture of an embedded ion channel is shown in Fig. 3.6.

Generally, ion channels are composed of several protein subunits which under certain conditions form pores. These pores can be viewed as narrow salt-water filled tunnels that permit specific ions to pass through. Ions

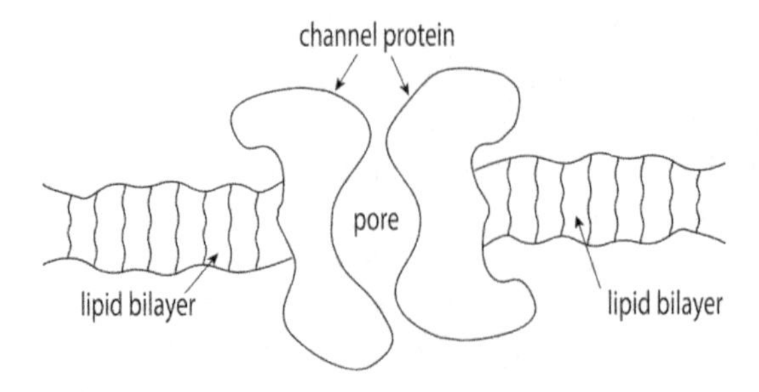

Fig. 3.6

travel through channels down gradients of electrochemical potentials. These potential gradients have two distinct components: the diffusion component due to ion concentration gradients and drift component due to the presence of electric fields (i.e. electric potential gradients). The rate of ion passage through channels is quite high and may reach about one million ions per second and higher. Nevertheless, ion currents through single channels are quite small, and they are usually on the order of picoamperes. The structures of ion channels are discussed in detail in the classical book [7] of B. Hille. It must be remarked that ion channel structures and their functioning are only partly understood. For this reason, ion channels are currently a subject of extensive research in neural science.

There exists a large variety of ion channels. Ion channels can be classified by gating, i.e. by actions responsible for opening and closing these channels. In this respect, there are voltage-gated and ligand-gated ion channels. The performance of voltage- gated channels is controlled by potential difference (voltage) across the membrane in the locations of the channels. Whereas the performance of ligand-gated channels is controlled by chemical signals produced by the binding of ligands (i.e. special stimulatory molecules) to channels.

Ion channels can also be classified by the type of ions that are allowed to selectively pass through channels. In this respect, there are four types of ion channels that are most important for the functioning of neurons. They are sodium (Na^+) channels, potassium (K^+) channels, calcium (Ca^2+) channels and chloride (Cl^-) channels. Voltage-gated sodium and potassium channels (and, to some extent, chloride channels) are instrumental in the generation, formation, and propagation of action potentials. Whereas ligand-gated channels play the central role in the formation and functioning of synaptic connections between neurons.

It must be remarked that there exists appreciable diversity within each type of channel. In this respect, potassium voltage-gated channels are most diverse. It is also important to point out that sodium and potassium voltage-gated channels pass Na^+ and K^+ ions across neuron membranes in opposite directions, respectively. Finally, sodium channels are quite fast, while potassium channels are relatively slow.

Next, we consider the principle of operation of ion channels. As discussed before, proteins are the "walls" of ion channels. Proteins usually have a very large number of metastable states corresponding to different local minima of free energy separated by some energy barriers. In biophysics and neural science, these metastable states are called conformational states. Ion channel functioning depends on these conformational states. This is because proteins assume different geometric shapes in different conformational states. In some of these conformational states, proteins may form pores that permit specific ions to pass through. Such protein metastable states can be viewed as open (conducting) conformations of ion channels. On the other hand, protein metastable states with the absence of sufficiently wide pores can be prohibitive to the passage of specific ions. Such metastable states can be viewed as closed (nonconducting) conformations of ion channels. The transition between protein metastable states and, consequently, between closed and open conformations may be triggered by changes in local membrane voltage in voltage-gated channels. This transition may also be caused by binding of special stimulating molecules in ligand-gated channels. It is quite possible that there is also another physical mechanism of switching of protein conformational states. This mechanism is related to ion flow through channels, and it was studied by V. A. Chinarov and his colleagues [8]. Indeed, the electric fields of ions at very short distances within narrow channel pore confinements may be comparable and even higher than the electric fields produced by voltage gating. Furthermore, ions traveling through channel pores may bind at some sites inside these pores. The electrostatic fields of these bound ions may also exceed the electric fields produced by voltage gating. The presented discussion suggests that ion currents through channels may result in the changes in protein conformational states leading to subsequent changes in the functioning of ion channels.

As discussed before, channel proteins have large numbers of conformational (i.e. metastable) states. For this reason, electrical properties of ion channels exhibit hysteresis. This hysteresis has been already observed experimentally and studied theoretically. Some sample publications in this area are [9]–[14], and the number of research reports related to hysteresis of ion channels is growing. The existence of hysteresis of ion channels implies that ion channels are endowed with memory. This memory is encoded in conformational states of ion channel proteins. This means that the past history of the conformational states of ion channels may effect their future functioning. As argued before, currents through ion channels may affect conformational states of their proteins and, consequently, encode new information. In other words, the past history of ion currents through channels may affect their future functioning.

Historically, ion channels were difficult to detect experimentally because of tiny currents through these channels. This difficulty was by and large removed through the development of the patch-clamp technique. This technique was introduced by Erwin Neher and Bert Sakmann in the late 1970s [15]. The patch-clamp technique made the recording of single ion channels possible, and it became one of the principal sources of information about these channels. Neher and Sakmann were awarded the Nobel Prize in 1991 for their work in this area.

In the patch-clamp technique, a hollow glass micropipette with a very narrow tip of diameter in micrometer range is pressed against a cell membrane and suction is subsequently applied to form a tight sealing around the edge of the tip. The micropipette is filled with an electrolyte solution which matches the ionic composition of the electrolyte solution in the exterior of neurons. This pipette and specially designed electronic circuitry with amplifiers are used to record ion currents. A schematic representation of such recording of ion current through a single channel is shown in Fig. 3.7.

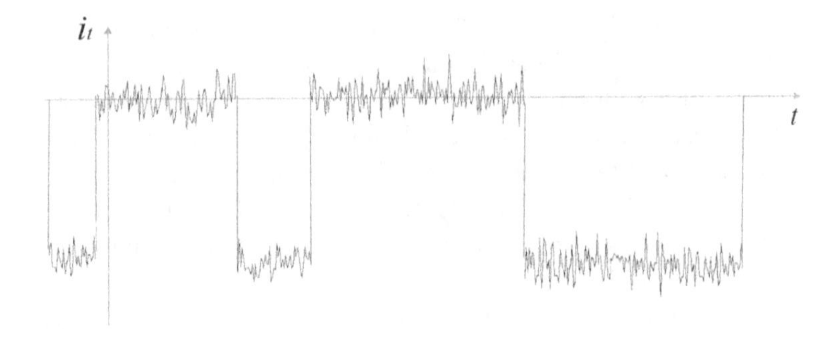

Fig. 3.7

It is apparent from the above figure that ion currents through single channels are stochastic in nature. In other words, channels randomly switch between open and closed conformations. It has been observed that random ion current recordings are modified by applied membrane voltage in the case of voltage-gated channels and by ligand bindings in the case of ligand-gated channels.

It is most likely that the randomness of channel currents is caused by thermal noise, although other sources of noise may be present as well. In the noisy environment, protein states and their geometric configurations are not static. Proteins execute random motions around their conformational configurations. These random motions occur within energy wells with energy minima corresponding to metastable (i.e. conformational) states. When sufficiently large deviations (i.e. large energy kicks) of noise are realized, they may move proteins over energy barriers into adjacent energy wells corresponding to other conformational states. This is a possible physical mechanism of random switching between protein metastable states and, consequently, between open and closed channel conformations. Small noise observed in channel current recordings during the current conduction and its absence (see Fig. 3.7) can be at least partially attributed to random protein dynamics around their conformational states. Another source of this small randomness in channel current recordings may be the electronic noise of the measuring equipment itself.

Classical kinetic theory was developed to account for random currents through ion channels. It is postulated in this theory that there are certain protein conformational states and Markov random processes are used to describe switchings between these states. These switchings are usually illustrated by kinetic diagrams with fixed switching probability rates (called kinetic constants) between conformational states. The Markov assumption in the analysis of channel switching clearly implies that this switching does not depend on the channel past history. This underlying assumption is not consistent with the hysteresis phenomena exhibited by ion channels. The presence of hysteresis implies that ion channels are endowed with memory. Furthermore, very interesting research was performed to test the validity of the Markovian condition for ion channel current recordings. The idea of testing this condition was first suggested by T. Timmer and S. Klein in [16]. This idea was further developed by A. Fulinski and his colleagues in [17]. It was demonstrated in [17] that the Markovian condition is not consistent with experimental data obtained for some potassium channels.

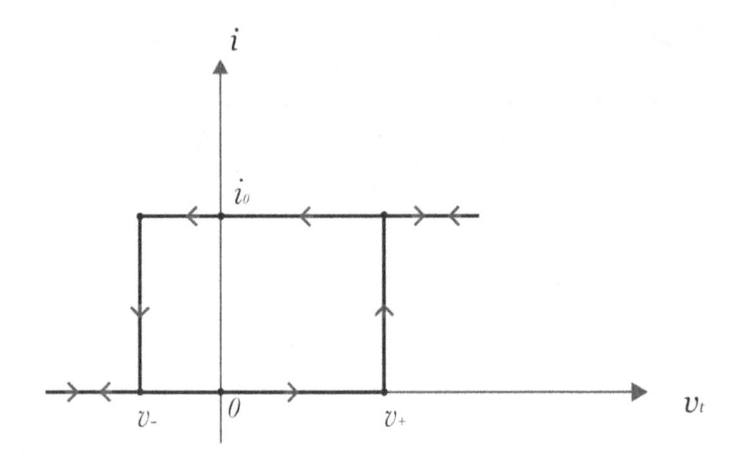

Fig. 3.8

It is therefore interesting to develop the theory of random channel currents which is free from the underlying Markovian assumption. One way of doing this is to consider the stochastic channel currents as being produced by random switching of rectangular hysteresis loops. This is illustrated by Fig. 3.8.

In this figure, the vertical axis corresponds to channel current, while random noise v_t is plotted along the horizontal axis. The choice of the rectangular loop is justified by the fact that in many single channel recordings the random ion currents are binary (as shown in Fig. 3.7). Furthermore, the switching between closed ($i = 0$) and open ($i = i_0$) conformations occurs very fast (i.e., on a very short time scale). The latter is reflected in almost vertical lines of transitions between the open and closed states in channel current recordings. Switching values v_+ and v_- depend on conformational states being switched. These states may be changed by gating, and they also may depend on the past history of channel currents.

Mathematically, the hysteresis based random switching between open and closed conformations can now be treated as an exit problem for stochastic Markov noise process v_t [18]–[19]. Indeed, when (as a result of the preceding switching), the random process v_t starts from the point v_- and then exits at the point v_+ on the semi-infinite line shown in Fig. 3.9a, switching from the closed conformations ($i = 0$) to the open conformations ($i = i_0$) occurs. Similarly, when the random noise v_t starts from the point v_+ and then exits at the point v_- on the semi-infinite line shown in Fig. 3.9b, the switching from the open conformations to the closed conformations occurs.

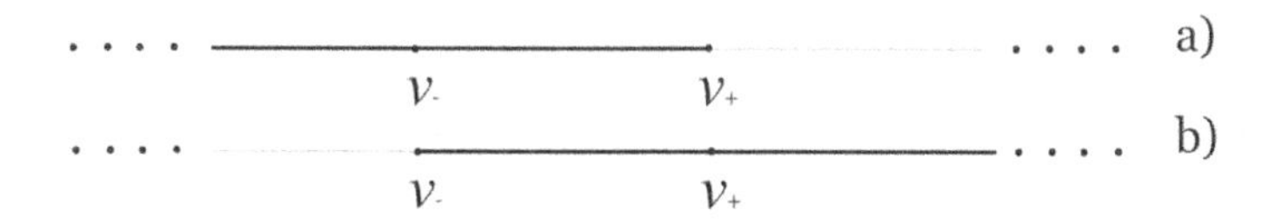

Fig. 3.9

It is apparent that these random switching times are equal to random dwell (duration) times of open and closed conformations. As far as the random process v_t is concerned, it may be natural to assume that this is a stationary Gaussian Markov process. It is shown in probability theory that the only process that satisfies these three requirements is the Ornstein-Uhlenbeck process. It must be remarked that the exit problem is one of the classical and well-studied problems in the theory of stochastic processes.

It is worthwhile to point out that the binary current i_t generated by random switching of a rectangular loop is not Markovian. However, the two-component random process $y_t = \binom{i_t}{v_t}$ is Markovian. This process is defined on a specific graph representing a rectangular loop in Fig. 3.8. The theory of Markov processes on graphs has been recently developed [20]–[22]. This theory as well as the theory of exit problems for stochastic processes will be discussed in details in the next chapter.

It is clear from Fig. 3.7 that a single protein channel randomly oscillates between open and closed conformations. These random oscillations occur regardless of whether the ion channel is gated or not. This makes the very definition of open and closed states somewhat ambiguous. It turns out that some clarity in this matter can be introduced by considering energy well structures corresponding to open and closed states of channel proteins and analyzing how these energy structures are changed by gating. In the simplest case, these energy structures are schematically shown in Fig. 3.10.

In this figure, energy minima corresponding to open and closed protein conformational configurations are marked by letters O and C, respectively, while maxima of energy barriers separating adjacent wells are marked by the letter B. It is apparent that the energy structures presented in Fig. 3.10a correspond to closed states. Indeed, for such energy structures, the energy barriers $\mathcal{E}_C$ for closed conformations are appreciably higher than the energy barriers $\mathcal{E}_O$ for open conformations. This means that on average the channel proteins spend more time fluctuating around C-conformations than around O-conformations. By gating, the energy structures may be changed to those shown in Fig. 3.10b. It is clear that such energy structures

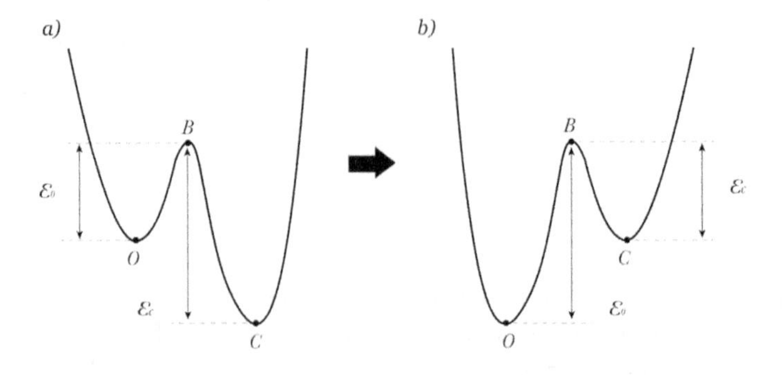

Fig. 3.10

correspond to open states. Indeed, for such energy structures energy barriers $\mathcal{E}_C$ are appreciably smaller than energy barriers $\mathcal{E}_O$. This means that on average the channel proteins spend more time fluctuating within the O-wells than within the C-wells. The presented discussion clearly reveals that switching from C-wells to O-wells and from O-wells to C-wells require different switching values of thermal noise energy to overcome different energy barriers. This is properly reflected in the different switching values v_+ and v_- of the hysteresis loop in Fig. 3.8.

We conclude the presented brief review of ion channels with the following remarks. It has been mentioned before that sodium and potassium channels are instrumental in the generation of action potentials. In contrast, calcium channels play no significant role in the formation of action potentials. Nevertheless, these channels are very important. They are crucial for neurotransmitter release, which (as discussed later) is at the very foundation of the establishing and functioning of synaptic connections. Furthermore, there are calcium activated potassium channels, which are essential for controllability of membrane potential. Finally, calcium channels are involved in regulation of many biochemical processes. The detailed account of the importance of calcium channels can be found in the book [1] of C. Koch.

As mentioned in the previous section, there are special protein channels called pumps. They are active channels in the sense that they move ions against their concentration gradients and that they require some energy for this action. The active pump transport restores the gradients of ion concentrations, which is essential for the operation of ion channels.

As discussed before, ion channels are formed by proteins. The remarkable fact is that the proteins are unstable elements. On average, they only last for a couple of days (see [23], as well as [24]), and then they are replaced by newly synthesized proteins. Thus, there exists a continuous process of protein synthesis and protein degradation. This leads to an unresolved and puzzling issue of how the integrity of neural systems and their memories remain mostly intact in the face of this volatility and fluidity.

Next, we proceed to the brief discussion of synapses. Typically, a synapse is a very complex junction between a pre-synaptic axon terminal of one neuron and a post-synaptic dendritic spine of another neuron. It is by means of such junctions that electrical and chemical signals are transmitted between neurons. In other words, synapses are structural units that are indispensable in the formation of neuronal circuits. For this reason, the importance of synapses has been recognized and greatly appreciated since the work of Ramón y Cajal, who promulgated the cellular connectionist approach in neural science at the turn of the nineteenth century. Since then, the research in the area of synapses has continued unabated.

There are two types of synapses: chemical and electrical. The latter is often referred to as a gap junction. Chemical synapses are much more common than electrical synapses, and they are immensely numerous. It is estimated that there are about 10^{15} chemical synapses in a human brain. They are also quite small with a diameter of synaptic contact being about 0.5 to 1.0 micrometers.

In the case of electrical synapses, pre- and post-synaptic membranes forming gap junctions are electrically connected by specialized ion channels that pierce through the membranes of both cells. This creates direct and high conductivity pathways for ions between adjacent neurons. The main advantage of such synapses is their speed of communication. However, no enhancement (gain) of transmitted signals is possible. In contrast, chemical synapses are much more complex. A schematic representation of such synapses is shown in Fig. 3.11.

As shown in this figure, an axon bouton and a dendritic spine are separated by a very narrow gap called synaptic cleft. There are many vesicles filled with neurotransmitters inside the axon bouton, while there are numerous receptors of these neurotransmitters on the opposite surface of the dendritic spine.

The principle of operation of chemical synapses can be briefly described as follows. When a propagating action potential reaches an axon bouton, it causes local voltage-gated calcium channels to switch to open states. This leads to an appreciable influx of calcium ions into the axon bouton, which in turn results (through some complex events) in the fusion of a certain number of synaptic vesicles with bouton membranes. As mentioned before,

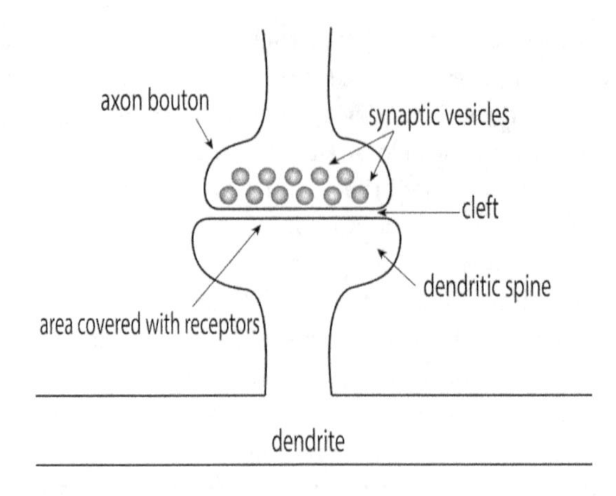

Fig. 3.11

the vesicles contain neurotransmitters, which are released into the synaptic cleft after vesicle fusion into the pre-synaptic membrane. Released neurotransmitters rapidly diffuse across the very narrow synaptic cleft and bind to post-synaptic receptors. These receptors are by and large ligand-gated ion channels. These bindings result in various intricate events, which eventually lead to increases in post-synaptic membrane potentials. In this way, electrical connections between neurons are realized by synapses. It must be pointed out that there is a great variety of neurotransmitters and post-synaptic receptors. This makes the phenomena of synaptic transmission very complex and occurring on different time and spatial scales. It is also important to note that synaptic transmission exhibits stochasticity, which is believed to be due to the probabilistic nature of neurotransmitter release.

The most remarkable phenomenon that makes synapses so vital and intriguing is their plasticity. In a nutshell, the essence of synaptic plasticity is the ability of synapses to be strengthened or weakened over time as a result of their past activity. In other words, the strength of synapses (i.e. their efficacy) is increased by their past stimulation or decreased by the lack thereof. It is apparent that the number of ion channels in post-synaptic membranes is clearly related to the strength of synapses. There exists some evidence to suggest that the density of these channels changes over time in response to synaptic activity, and this can be regarded as a molecular manifestation of synaptic plasticity.

In scientific literature, synaptic plasticity has long been regarded as a biological basis of memory formation and storage. It is usually postulated in neural science that memories are represented by interconnected networks of synapses in the brain, and synaptic plasticity is viewed as a reflection of the learning process. However, the very mechanism of synaptic growth is not fully understood yet. The clear indication of this state of affairs can be found in the review article of Eric Kandel on the biology of memory [25]. In this paper the reference is made to the classical 23 mathematical problems posed by David Hilbert in 1900 in the Second International Congress of Mathematicians in Paris, and then in a similar spirit 11 open-ended problems in the area of biological basis of memory are articulated. The first of these problems is related to synaptic growth, and it is stated as follows:

"How does synaptic growth occur, and how is signaling across the synapse coordinated to induce and maintain growth?"

There also exists the biophysical phenomenon of long-term potentiation (LTP) related to synaptic plasticity. The essence of LTP is a sustained increase in synaptic strength caused by a brief but sufficiently strong stimulus. LTP was first observed by T. V. P. Bliss and T. Lomo in 1973 [26], and since then it has been extensively studied. Nevertheless, according to C. Koch [1]:

"The field of LTP is also very controversial, so that there is only a surprisingly small number of completely accepted findings."

In particular, the issue of the location of LTP expression remains unresolved. Namely, it is not clear if the appearance of LTP is due to specific changes occurring in the pre-synaptic axon bouton or the post-synaptic dendritic spine, or in both of them.

Finally, we shall briefly mention the connection of synaptic plasticity to the phenomenological Hebbian theory. This theory can be viewed as an attempt to quantify the change in the synaptic strength W_{AB} between neurons A and B due to their simultaneous activities. In the simplest form, this change is expressed by the formula:

$$W_{AB} = \alpha V_A V_B \ , \tag{3.1}$$

where V_A and V_B are simultaneous average firing rates of neurons A and B, respectively. In a way, the last formula implies that simultaneous activation of cells is associated with appreciable increases in synaptic strength between those cells. This fact is often summarized as: "*Cells that fire together wire together.*" It is worthwhile to mention that there are mathematical modifications of the Hebb rule (3.1). However, their review is beyond the scope of our discussion.

3.3 Action Potentials

The brain and the entire nervous system function by means of generation and propagation of action potentials. These potentials are short-lasting (in time) spikes of voltages, which are generated by ion channels in neurons. This implies that the action potentials are ionic in nature.

It is the established fact that biological fluids inside and outside of neurons contain large numbers of various ions of different concentrations. In particular, the concentrations of sodium (Na^+), chloride (Cl^-), and calcium (Ca^{2+}) ions are appreciably higher outside the neurons than inside. Whereas, the concentration of potassium (K^+) ions is much higher inside rather than outside the neurons. Under unperturbed conditions, these ion concentrations result in voltages across neuron bilipid membranes, which are typically between 60 mV and 70 mV. If the potential of the exterior side of the membrane is chosen to be equal to zero, then the potential of the interior membrane side is between -70 mV and -60 mV. This potential is called the resting potential. This potential is maintained by continuous ion flow across membrane realized by ionic pumps. In this sense, the resting potential is not an equilibrium state potential. Maintaining this potential is the major energy expenditure in the nervous system.

When a neuron soma is electrically perturbed by signals coming from its dendrites or by an external stimulus, action potentials may be generated at an axon initial segment. This segment has a very high concentration of sodium and potassium ion channels, and this makes this part of the neuron very sensitive to electrical perturbations of its resting potential. In other words, the axon initial segment is a "trigger zone" that is the most excitable part of the neuron. For the action potential to be generated, the perturbed membrane potential must exceed some threshold value, which is called the threshold potential. This threshold potential is about 15 mV higher than the resting potential. As soon as the threshold potential is exceeded, a brief voltage spike is generated and starts to propagate along the axon. These spikes are peaked between $+20$ mV and $+40$mV. One typical shape of the action potential generated at the axon initial segment is schematically shown in Fig. 3.12.

It is evident from the above figure that there are three distinct phases in the time evolution of the action potential. They are the rising phase, the falling phase, and the undershoot phase. During the rising phase the membrane potential monotonically increases and changes its sign from negative to positive. That is why this phase is called the depolarization phase. The

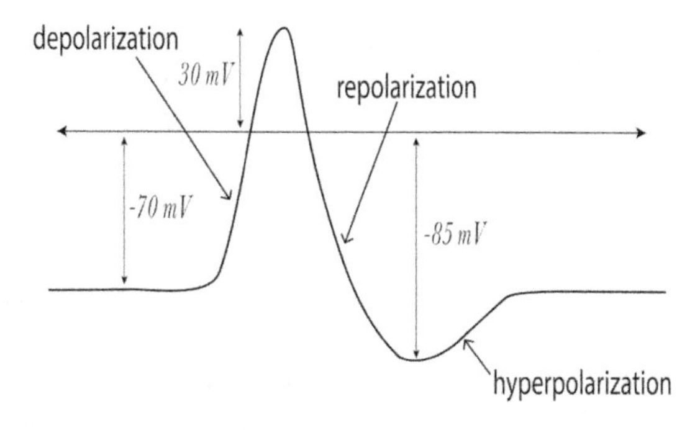

Fig. 3.12

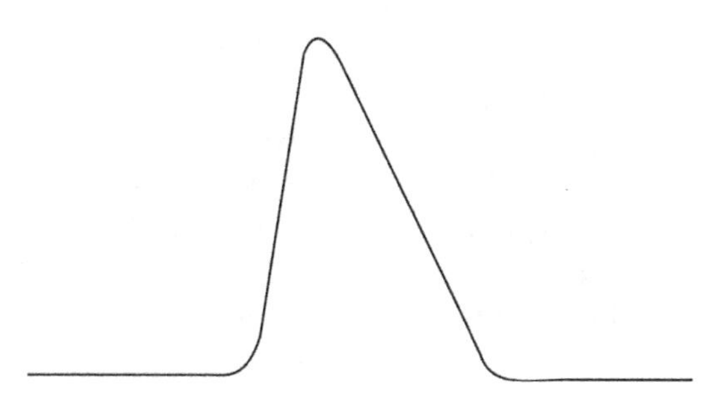

Fig. 3.13

time duration of this phase is about 1 ms. During the falling phase, the membrane potential monotonically decreases and returns to its negative value. For this reason, this phase is called repolarization phase. Its time duration is about 2 ms. During the depolarization phase, the membrane potential decreases below its resting value. For this reason, this phase is followed by the subsequent monotonic increase of membrane potential back to its resting value. This phase of restoration of the membrane potential is called hyperpolarization phase. Its time duration is about 5 ms. It is interesting to note that this hyperpolarization phase is absent for action potentials generated at Ranvier nodes of myelinated axons. A typical shape of the action potential at the node of Ranvier is schematically shown in Fig. 3.13

Typically, not a single action potential, but rather a sequence (a train) of action potentials is generated, and these potentials propagate along the axon. Remarkably, these action potentials are identical (i.e. stereotyped) in shape. Schematically, a train of such action potentials is shown in Fig. 3.14.

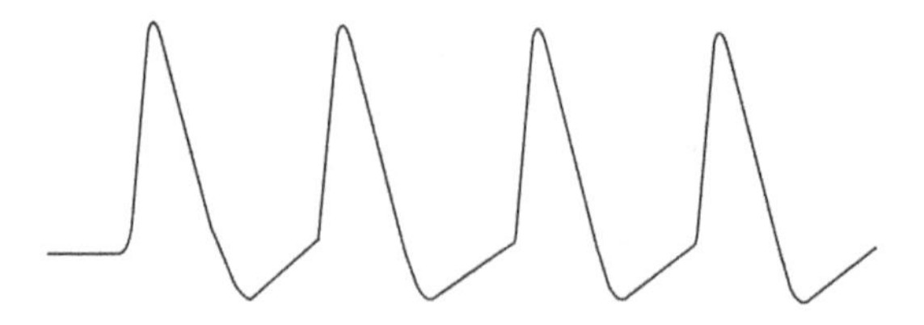

Fig. 3.14

It is evident from this figure that the voltage spikes (action potentials) have a certain separation in time, which is called the refractory period. This period can be subdivided into two distinct parts: an absolute refractory period during which no generation of action potential is possible, then followed by a relative refractory period when a stronger-than-usual stimulus is required to generate the next action potential. The physical nature of the relative refractory period is quite apparent. Indeed, if the membrane potential is below the resting potential, then a stronger stimulus is needed in order to exceed the threshold potential. On the other hand, the absolute refractory period is due to the unique feature of sodium channels, related to their inactivated state, which will be discussed later.

Next, we consider the physical mechanism of the generation of action potentials. At the very foundation of this mechanism are the properties of voltage-gated sodium and potassium channels. At the beginning of the depolarization phase when the membrane potential at a certain location exceeds the threshold potential, some voltage-gated sodium channels become open at this location. This results in the influx of positively charged sodium ions into a neuron which leads to the further increase of the membrane potential at this and adjacent locations. Consequently, new voltage-gated sodium channels get open, which brings about an additional influx of positively charged sodium ions. This further increases the local membrane potential and results again in activation of additional sodium channels. Thus, it is clear that there exists a strong positive feedback at work here, which results in a steep local increase in membrane potential. This membrane depolarization is aborted by inactivation of sodium channels resulting in some peak value of action potential. At this stage, voltage-gated potassium channels get activated, leading to the outflux of positively charged potassium ions from the neuron. This brings about the repolarization phase of membrane potential. When voltage-gated potassium channels finally close, the resting potential is then re-established during the hyperpolarization phase. There is no consensus in the literature concerning the physical mechanism of the restoration of the resting potential during the hyperpolarization phase. The most frequently expressed point of view is that this restoration occurs due to the pump (and leak) channels.

It is apparent from the above description of the action potential generation (as well as from Fig. 3.14) that as soon as the threshold membrane voltage is exceeded, the action potentials of identical (stereotyped) shape are produced. If the perturbed membrane potential is below its threshold value, then no action potential is generated. This is the essence of the **all-or-none principle**. The origin of this principle is due to the positive feedback that drives the generation of action potentials. As a result of this feedback, currents produced by the opening of voltage-gated sodium channels are much larger than stimulating currents. Consequently, if the threshold voltage is exceeded, then amplitudes and shapes of action potentials are determined by the properties of membrane channels rather than by the strength of the initial stimulus. For this reason, these shapes are stereotyped.

Next, we shall discuss two important and difficult issues related to the generation of action potentials. The first issue is related to deterministic stereotyped shapes of action potentials produced by ionic channels despite the fact that the current conduction of individual channels is stochastic in nature (as discussed in the previous section). It is intuitively clear that some averaging over large number of ionic channels is involved in the deterministic nature of the action potentials. In this sense, the deterministic action potentials can be viewed as macroscopic potentials while random characteristics of individual ion channels can be regarded as microscopic ones. The issue of how purely deterministic action potentials emerge from stochastic actions of individual channels is a very difficult one. In our discussion, this matter will be left unattended.

The second issue is related to the inactivated state of voltage-gated sodium channels. It is believed that the transition to this state occurs at (or) near peaks of action potentials and that this state persists during the repolarization phase of these potentials. In the inactivated state, the ion current flow through the sodium channel is appreciably reduced or completely stopped. For this reason, the duration of the inactivated state determines the duration of the absolute refractory period. Thus, it is clear that there are three states of voltage-gated sodium channels involved in the formation of action potentials. They are the deactivated (closed) state, activated (open) state, and inactivated state. During the action potential generation, voltage-gated sodium channels go through the following

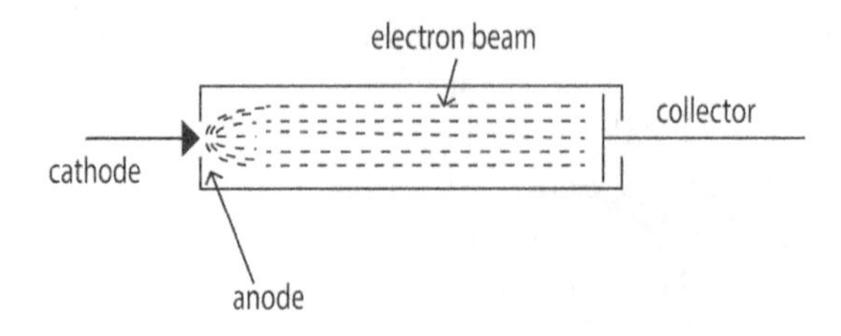

Fig. 3.15

transition cycle: deactivated → activated → inactivated → deactivated. The physical mechanism of the deactivated → activated transition is more or less clear. Namely, the applied voltage across the neuron membrane at the location of sodium channels modifies the energy well structures of open and closed conformational configurations of channel proteins by making the open conformation more probable. In contrast, the physical mechanism of the activated → inactivated transition is much less understood. Usually, it is believed that this transition is associated with the existence of the special "inactivated" gate and the efforts have been made to interpret this gate in terms of channel protein structure, as described in the work of W. A. Catterall [27]. However, there exists a fundamental difference between "deactivated → activated" and "activated → inactivated" transitions. The first transition occurs with no current through a sodium channel, while the second transition takes place when the ion flow through the sodium channel is at its peak. Since the switching to the inactivated state occurs during ion current flow, this suggests that the transition from the activated to the inactivated state cannot be explained by membrane potential control only. It is conceivable that this ion flow itself may be the cause of the transition to the inactivated state. With this point in mind, we discuss below two plausible ion current controlled mechanisms that may play key roles during the activated state and, as a result, cause the transition to the inactivated state.

It turns out that a somewhat similar phenomenon of "inactivation" has been observed for electron beams in emission diodes [28]. Such a diode is schematically shown in Fig. 3.15. Here, the emitted electrons are accelerated by the voltage applied between the cathode and the anode and propagate through the anode hole into the drift region between the anode and the collector. Such an electron beam has unique nonlinear properties. Namely, if the electron beam current I is below some critical value called the limiting current, I_L, then the electrons propagate toward the collector,

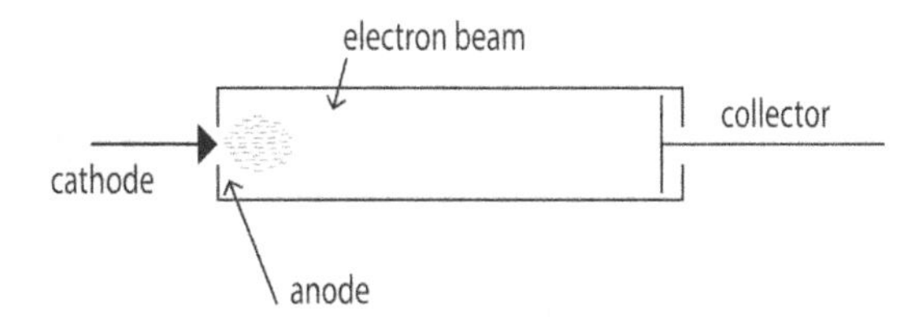

Fig. 3.16

and the full electron beam current is usually measured at the collector site. However, if the electron beam current I exceeds I_L, then an electron cloud (cluster) called a virtual cathode is formed in the close proximity to the anode as pictured in Fig. 3.16. In this situation, almost all current above the limiting value I_L is diverted to the anode. This phenomenon occurs naturally due the very strong Coulomb repulsion between similarly charged electrons.

Remarkably, the described physical phenomenon exhibits hysteresis between the injected electron beam current I and reflected electron current I_R. This hysteresis is schematically shown in Fig. 3.17. According to this figure, if the injected electron beam current I is monotonically increased, then there is no reflected current until I exceeds the threshold value I_L. After I exceeds I_L, the virtual cathode is formed and most of the injected current I is reflected. In the case of the subsequent monotonic decrease of I, this reflection persists until I is reduced below the so-called space charge limiting current I_{SC} which may be substantially smaller than I_L. Then, the virtual cathode disappears and the reflection seized to exist. The physical mechanism of the described irreversibility and hysteresis is based on the fact that in order to form the virtual cathode, an injected current I above the limiting current I_L is needed, whereas in order to maintain the virtual cathode, injection currents only above the space-charge-limited value are sufficient. In other words, when I exceeds I_L, the emission diode is switched into "inactivated" state which persists until the injection current is reduced below I_{SC}.

It is conceivable that a similar phenomenon may occur in voltage-gated sodium channels. Namely, when the ions current through the sodium channel approaches its peak, the strong repulsive Coulomb interaction between ions may lead to the formation of the ion accumulations (ion clusters) within the channels, which may result in sudden decrease and in eventual stoppage of ion currents through the channels. This is a plausible mechanism

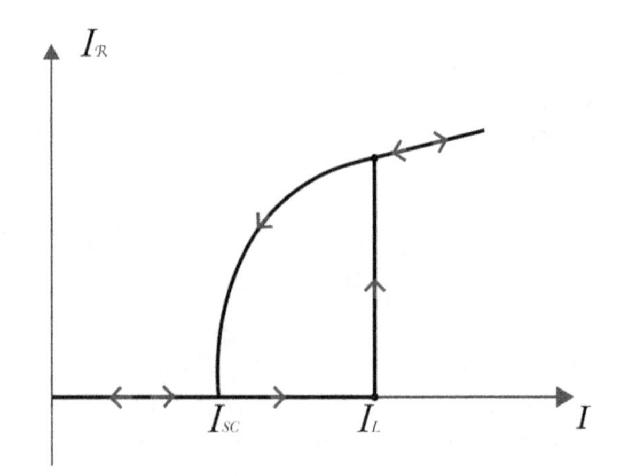

Fig. 3.17

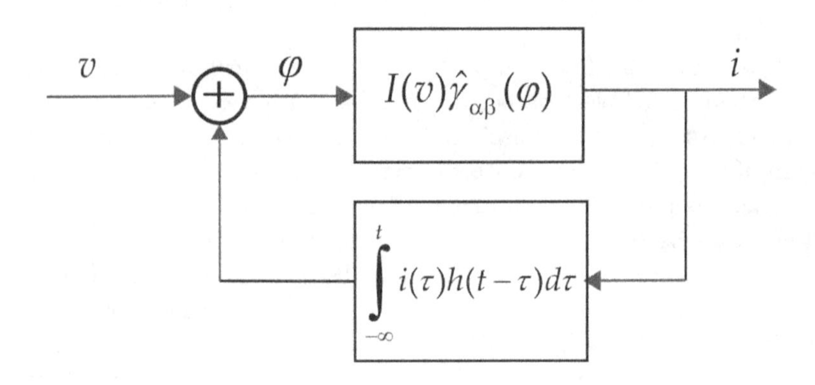

Fig. 3.18

for the activated→inactivated transition. These ion clusters may persist over time during the repolarization phase resulting in the persistence of the inactivated state. The presented idea of formation and persistence of the inactivated state merits further investigation along with the study of other affects which may be caused by ion flow through the channels.

Since the activated→inactivated sodium ion channel transition occurs during current flow, this suggests that switching between these two metastable states may be due to Coulomb interaction of channel ions in addition to the membrane potential. In order to pursue this line of reasoning further, one may consider an ion current feedback mechanism. Let us consider a sodium ion channel feedback model as shown in Fig. 3.18.

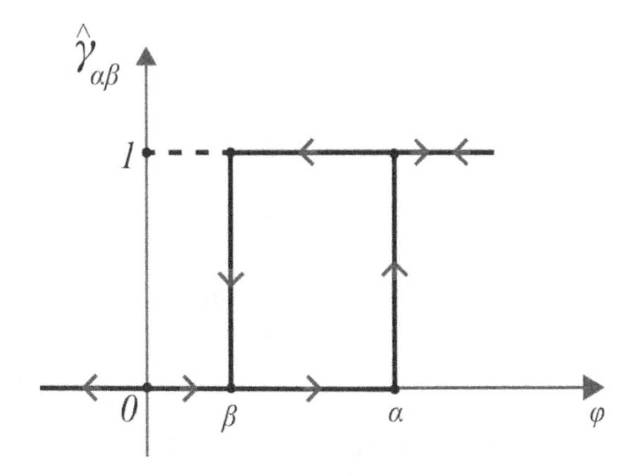

Fig. 3.19

According to this model, the ion channel is controlled by the membrane potential v and feedback of the time integral of the channel current i. Here, $I(v)$ represents the ion current when the channel is open (as measured with standard patch clamp techniques). To be consistent with standard ion channel measurements, by convention, $I(v)$ is negative in value. The binary hysteresis operator, as shown in Fig. 3.19, reflects the status of the channel where output 0 corresponds to a closed channel and output 1 corresponds to an open channel. Here, α and β denote the values of the membrane potential at which the channel is switched between the deactivated $\rightarrow$ activated and the activated$\rightarrow$ deactivated states, respectively, in the absence of ion currents.

The feedback operator represents some accumulated level of channel ion current charge and it is modeled as a time invariant linear system. It is clear that some negative feedback is needed to close the channel due to current flow. Since the channel current i is negative (by convention), the impulse response $h(t)$ should be a positive function.

Let us examine this mechanism more carefully. Consider the channel in the deactivated state and the membrane potential $v < \alpha$, where v in practice is a large negative voltage less than the resting potential. Therefore, the channel is closed and the channel current is zero. Next, the voltage is increased up to some level above the rest potential, i.e., $v > \alpha$. Now, since $v > \alpha$, the rectangular loop switches to 1, and there is sodium ion current $I(v)$. Without feedback and in the absence of noise, this current will flow indefinitely, and the channel will remain in the activated state.

However, patch clamp measurements show that this does not occur, and the current is turned off after a few milliseconds of current flow. It is worth noting here that, due to the stochastic nature of the system, the ion channel current may fluctuate between $I(v)$ and 0, corresponding to the 1 and 0 states of the rectangular hysteresis loop, respectively. Such binary step like fluctuations, commonly observed in patch clamp measurements and schematically depicted in Fig. 3.7, correspond to the transitions of the rectangular hysteresis loop as the channel stochastically opens and closes until eventually reaching the inactivated state.

Now, let us consider the simplest choice for the feedback function: a scaled unit step function, $h(t) = Ku(t)$, where $K > 0$ (Volts/Coulomb). It is clear that such a choice represents a scaled value of the cumulative ion charge flow during the activation of the ion channel. Since, by convention, the influx sodium ion current is negative, the feedback loop represents a negative feedback, $KI(v)T < 0$, where T is the total (random) time the channel stays open. Therefore, this negative feedback produces an effective input of $(v + KI(v)T)$ to the rectangular hysteresis loop. Since the membrane potential $v > \alpha$, i.e., large enough to result in the activated state, it is clear that this effective input may result in $(v + KI(v)T) < \beta$. This would clearly results in closing the channel, which the membrane potential $v > \alpha$ only cannot do in the absence of any other fluctuations.

Clearly, one may consider a wide variety of ion current feedback models, different patch clamp membrane potential protocols and, more importantly, operation of these feedback mechanism under action potentials. However, the detailed study of this feedback mechanism is left to future work, and will not be pursued further here.

Next, we proceed to the derivation of the deterministic nonlinear diffusion equation for generation and propagation of action potentials. To this end, we consider a very short (in a macroscopic sense) cylindrical region of unmyelinated axon shown in Fig. 3.20. Here x is a central point of this cylinder, while Δx is its "macroscopic" length. The latter means that the number of microscopic membrane channels along cylindrical side surface $\tilde{S}$ is very large to make their individual stochastic nature negligible.

The subsequent derivation is based on the principle of continuity of electric current, which states that the following mathematical relation is valid for any closed surface S:

$$\oiint_S \mathbf{J} \cdot d\mathbf{s} = 0 \,, \tag{3.2}$$

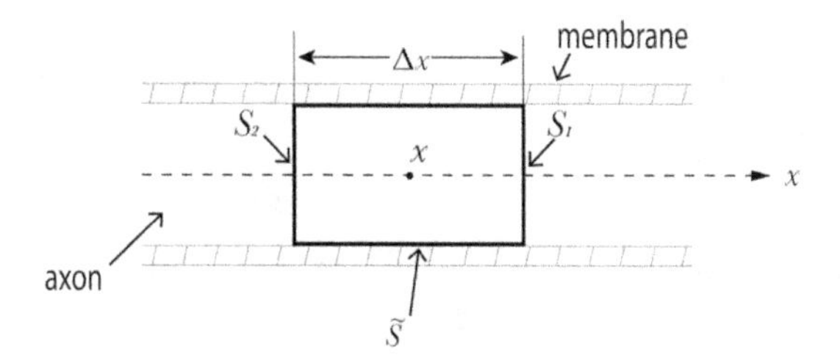

Fig. 3.20

where $\mathbf{J}$ is an electric current density, while the direction of $d\mathbf{s}$ coincides with the direction of outward normal to S.

By applying the last formula to the cylindrical surfaces shown (in bold) in Fig. 3.20, we find:

$$\iint_{\tilde{S}} \mathbf{J} \cdot d\mathbf{s} + \iint_{S_1} \mathbf{J}_a \cdot d\mathbf{s} + \iint_{S_2} \mathbf{J}_a \cdot d\mathbf{s} = 0 \,, \tag{3.3}$$

where the notation $\mathbf{J}_a$ is used for the axial (along x) component of electric current density.

The first integral in the left-hand side of formula (3.3) can be represented as follows:

$$\iint_{\tilde{S}} \mathbf{J} \cdot d\mathbf{s} = 2\pi r \Delta x J_{sides} \,, \tag{3.4}$$

where r is the axon radius, while J_{sides} is the average (over $\tilde{S}$) value of current density normal to the side surface $\tilde{S}$.

The sum of the last two integrals in the left-hand side of formula (3.3) can be written as the difference of the two axial currents $I_a\left(x + \frac{\Delta x}{2}\right)$ and $I_a\left(x - \frac{\Delta x}{2}\right)$ leaving and entering, respectively, the cylindrical axon region under consideration:

$$\iint_{S_1} \mathbf{J}_a \cdot d\mathbf{s} + \iint_{S_2} \mathbf{J}_a \cdot d\mathbf{s} = I_a\left(x + \frac{\Delta x}{2}\right) - I_a\left(x - \frac{\Delta x}{2}\right) . \tag{3.5}$$

By substituting the last two formulas into the equation (3.3), we find:

$$2\pi r J_{sides} + \frac{I_a\left(x + \frac{\Delta x}{2}\right) - I_a\left(x - \frac{\Delta x}{2}\right)}{\Delta x} = 0. \tag{3.6}$$

Since Δx is macroscopically small, the last term in the left-hand side of formula (3.6) can be replaced by the derivative, which leads to the following equation:

$$2\pi r J_{sides} + \frac{\partial I_a}{\partial x} = 0. \tag{3.7}$$

The current J_{sides} can be represented as a sum of average displacement (capacitive) current J_{dis} through $\tilde{S}$ and the average ion current $J_{ch}(\varphi)$ through membrane channels along $\tilde{S}$:

$$J_{sides} = J_{dis} + J_{ch}(\varphi). \tag{3.8}$$

The ion current through $\tilde{S}$ depends on (average) potential φ on $\tilde{S}$, which is reflected in its notation. On the other hand, the average displacement current can be written as follows:

$$J_{dis} = C\frac{\partial \varphi}{\partial t}, \tag{3.9}$$

where C is the per unit surface membrane capacitance.

In the case when an axial diffusion current of ions within the axon is a small effect in comparison with the ion drift current, then the axial current I_a is only of resistive nature and can be represented by formula:

$$I_a = -\frac{1}{R}\frac{d\varphi}{dx}, \tag{3.10}$$

where R is the per unit length resistance of the axon.

By substituting the last three formula into (3.7), we end up with the following nonlinear diffusion equation:

$$b\frac{\partial \varphi}{\partial t} - \frac{\partial^2 \varphi}{\partial x^2} + f(\varphi) = 0, \tag{3.11}$$

where

$$b = 2\pi rRC \tag{3.12}$$

and

$$f(\varphi) = 2\pi rRJ_{ch}(\varphi)\ . \tag{3.13}$$

The derived diffusion equation (3.11) is nonlinear because the term $f(\varphi)$ which is proportional to average channel current density is a nonlinear function of φ. The nonlinear diffusion equation (3.11) was (and still is) the foundation of the Hodgkin Huxley theory of the action potential generation and propagation [29]–[32]. It is worthwhile to mention that Hodgkin and Huxley developed their theory when the existence of ionic channels and their individual stochastic nature were not known. This fact once again supports the statement of J. Larmor (see Section 1.2) that "... *scientific progress, considered historically, is not a strictly logical process* ..."

Hodgkin and Huxley realized the importance of sodium and potassium ion currents through a neuron membrane for the generation and propagation of action potentials. They introduced these currents (along with small leakage currents) into a diffusion equation as nonlinear functions of some gating variables (a term not used by Hodgkin and Huxley but later adopted in the neural science literature). Furthermore, they proposed separate first order ordinary differential equations with respect to time for these variables with coefficients being nonlinear functions of potential φ. Finally, Hodgkin and Huxley used these equations to numerically study the finite speed propagation of action potentials for unmyelinated axons and compare their computations with experimental results obtained for the giant squid axon.

Below, we describe another **inverse problem** approach which reveals the hysteretic nature of macroscopic sodium and potassium ion currents. The central idea of this approach is to treat the functions $f(\varphi)$ in the nonlinear diffusion equation (3.11) as unknown and determine it from such experimental data as the measured deterministic shape of the action potential and its finite speed of propagation. It is worthwhile to mention that such a speed does not exist for linear diffusion equations, but it is quite possible for nonlinear diffusion equations. This possibility has been already discussed in Section 2.5 for type II superconductors.

To start the discussion, we assume that the solution of equation (3.11) has the form:

$$\varphi(x,t) = \varphi(vt - x) \ , \tag{3.14}$$

where function φ and speed v are known (they have been measured). We want to determine the function $f(\varphi)$ in equation (3.11) from its solution (3.14). To do this, we introduce the variable:

$$\lambda = vt - x \tag{3.15}$$

and, according to equation (3.14), we treat the electric potential as a function of this variable:

$$\varphi(x,t) = \varphi(\lambda) \ . \tag{3.16}$$

It is apparent that

$$\frac{\partial \varphi}{\partial t} = v\varphi^{'}(\lambda) \tag{3.17}$$

and

$$\frac{\partial^2 \varphi}{\partial x^2} = \varphi^{''}(\lambda) \ . \tag{3.18}$$

By substituting the last two formulas into the nonlinear differential equation (3.11), we obtain:

$$bv\varphi^{'}(\lambda) - \varphi^{''}(\lambda) + f\left(\varphi(\lambda)\right) = 0 \ , \tag{3.19}$$

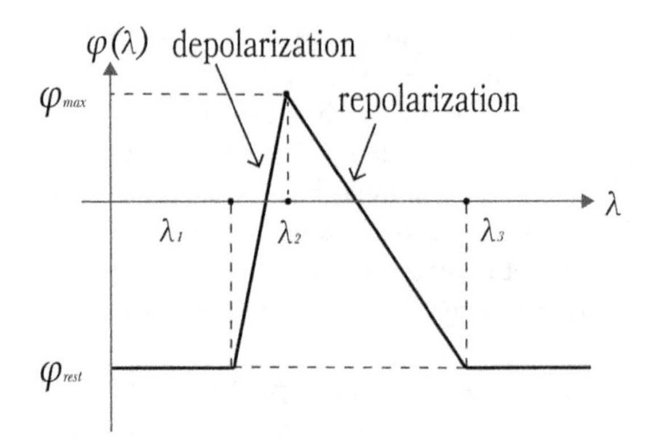

Fig. 3.21

which leads to

$$f\left(\varphi(\lambda)\right) = -bv\varphi'(\lambda) + \varphi''(\lambda)\ . \tag{3.20}$$

The last equation can be used to determine the function $f(\varphi)$. We shall demonstrate this for the simple case of the triangular shaped action potential shown in Fig. 3.21. The triangular shape can be viewed as a reasonable approximation of the actual shape of the action potential. It is also clear that the linear upstroke of triangular shape is produced by sodium ion currents, while the linear potential reversal is due to the potassium ion currents. For this reason, function $f(\varphi)$ can be split into the sum of two functions $f_{Na^+}(\varphi)$ and $f_{K^+}(\varphi)$ corresponding to sodium and potassium currents, respectively:

$$f(\varphi) = f_{Na^+}(\varphi) + f_{K^+}(\varphi)\ . \tag{3.21}$$

Now, from Fig. 3.21 and formula (3.20) we find

$$f_{Na^+}(\varphi) = \begin{cases} -vb\dfrac{\varphi_{max} - \varphi_{rest}}{\lambda_2 - \lambda_1} & ,\ \text{if}\ \lambda_1 < \lambda < \lambda_2 \\ 0 & ,\ \text{otherwise} \end{cases}\ . \tag{3.22}$$

Similarly, from Fig. 3.21 and equation (3.20), we derive

$$f_{K^+}(\varphi) = \begin{cases} vb\dfrac{\varphi_{max} - \varphi_{rest}}{\lambda_3 - \lambda_2} & ,\ \text{if}\ \lambda_2 < \lambda < \lambda_3 \\ 0 & ,\ \text{otherwise} \end{cases}\ . \tag{3.23}$$

As expected, the term $f_{Na^+}(\varphi)$, corresponding to sodium current is nonpositive because of the influx of Na^+ ions, whereas the term $f_{K^+}(\varphi)$ is nonnegative because of outward flow of K^+ ions.

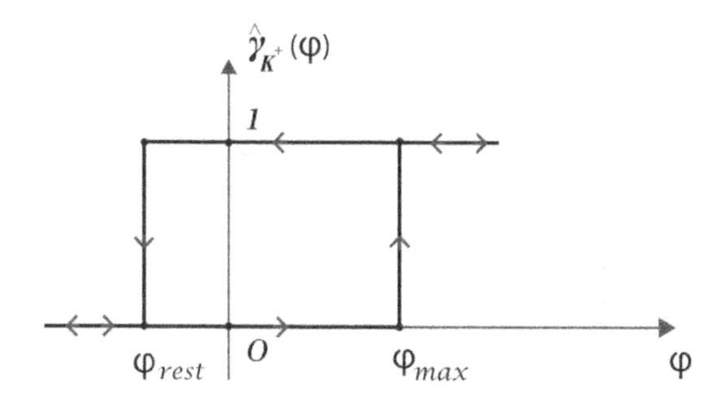

Fig. 3.22

It turns out that sodium and potassium ion current terms can be represented in terms of rectangular hysteresis loops. To demonstrate this, we start with the potassium ion current and introduce the hysteresis loop shown in Fig. 3.22.

From formula (3.23) and Fig. 3.22, it is clear that $f_{K^+}(\varphi)$ can be expressed as follows:

$$f_{K^+}(\varphi) = vb\frac{\varphi_{max} - \varphi_{rest}}{\lambda_3 - \lambda_2}\hat{\gamma}_{K^+}(\varphi) \, . \tag{3.24}$$

It is clear that the use of two-state rectangular hysteresis operators is sufficient to represent potassium currents, and this is consistent with the fact that the underlying potassium ion channels have only *two* states, i.e., deactivated and activated.

The sodium current given in (3.22) can also be expressed in terms of rectangular hysteresis loops. However, it requires one key modification because sodium channels have three distinct states, i.e., deactivated, activated and inactivated. With this in mind, it is clear that $f_{Na^+}(\varphi)$ can be expressed as follows:

$$f_{Na^+}(\varphi) = -vb\frac{\varphi_{max} - \varphi_{rest}}{\lambda_2 - \lambda_1}u(\varphi - \varphi_{rest})\hat{\gamma}_{Na^+}(\varphi) \, . \tag{3.25}$$

Here, u denotes the unit step function shown in Fig. 3.23a, and $\hat{\gamma}_{Na^+}(\varphi)$ is the rectangular hysteresis loop shown in Fig. 3.23b. According to this formula and Fig. 3.23, we can conclude that the sodium current term $f_{Na^+}(\varphi)$ is equal to zero if $\varphi < \varphi_{rest}$, then it jumps to its negative value given by the formula (3.22) as φ reaches φ_{rest}, it remains at this negative value as the potential φ is monotonically increased between φ_{rest} and φ_{max}. Finally, this current jumps back to zero as φ reaches φ_{max} and it equals to zero as the potential φ is decreased from φ_{max} to φ_{rest}, and it remains zero thereafter as $u(\varphi - \varphi_{rest})$ is zero.

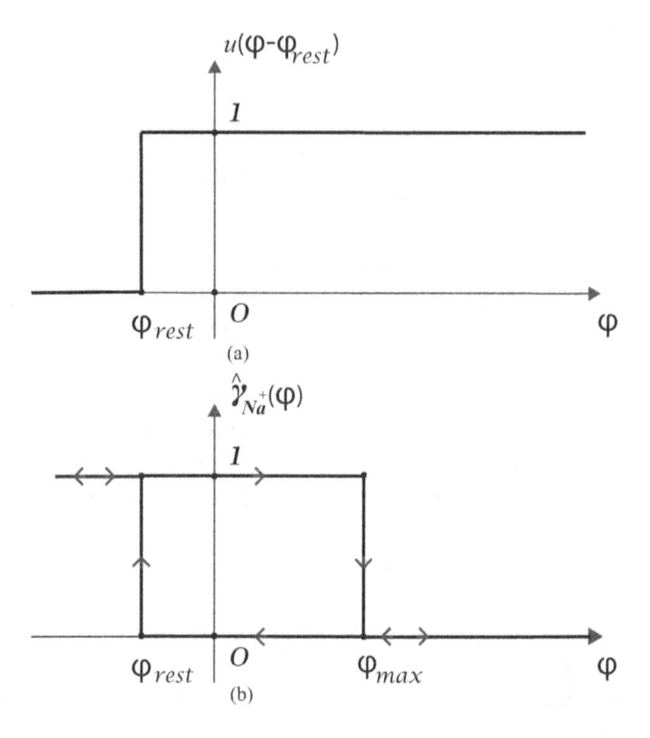

Fig. 3.23

Now, we consider regeneration of action potentials at the nodes of Ranvier of myelinated axons. These action potentials do not have the hyperpolarization phase (see Fig. 3.13) and, for this reason, they can be reasonably well approximated by a triangular shape shown in figure (see Fig. 3.24).

As discussed earlier, nodes of Ranvier are separated by myelinated segments (see Fig. 3.3), and there are no ion channels embedded in axon membranes along these segments. Whereas, there are high concentrations of ion channels at nodes of Ranvier. This implies that the electric potential along the myelinated axon membrane is described by two separate equations, which are particular cases of the diffusion equation (3.11). Namely, the electric potential φ along myelinated inter-node segments satisfies the linear diffusion equation:

$$b\frac{\partial \varphi}{\partial t} - \frac{\partial^2 \varphi}{\partial x^2} = 0 \, , \tag{3.26}$$

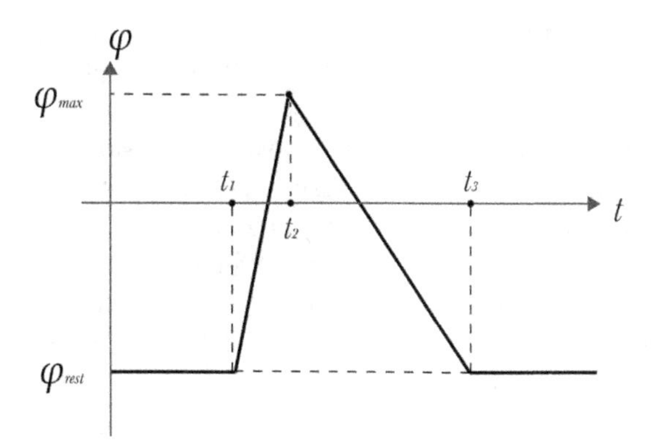

Fig. 3.24

while the regeneration of action potentials at the nodes of Ranvier is described by the following differential equation:

$$b\frac{\partial \varphi}{\partial t} + f(\varphi) = 0 \,. \tag{3.27}$$

By using the last equation and Fig. 3.24, as well as the same line of reasoning as in the derivation of formulas (3.24) and (3.25), we find the following expressions for $f(\varphi)$:

$$f(\varphi) = f_{Na^+}(\varphi) + f_{K^+}(\varphi) \,, \tag{3.28}$$

$$f_{Na^+}(\varphi) = -b\frac{\varphi_{max} - \varphi_{rest}}{t_2 - t_1} u(\varphi - \varphi_{rest})\hat{\gamma}_{Na^+}(\varphi) \,, \tag{3.29}$$

$$f_{K^+}(\varphi) = b\frac{\varphi_{max} - \varphi_{rest}}{t_3 - t_2}\hat{\gamma}_{K^+}(\varphi) \,, \tag{3.30}$$

where $\hat{\gamma}_{Na^+}(\varphi)$ and $\hat{\gamma}_{K^+}(\varphi)$ are the rectangular hysteresis loop shown in Figs. 3.23 and 3.22, respectively. It is clear that $f_{Na^+}(\varphi)$ is the component of $f(\varphi)$ representing the sodium channel currents which are responsible for a steep upstroke in the action potential, while $f_{K^+}(\varphi)$ represents the potassium channel currents responsible for the reversal branch of the action potential. It must be remarked that the nature of potassium channels at the node of Ranvier is still a matter of discussion. There exists the point of view that these are special calcium-activated potassium channels. Another point of view is that the action potential repolarization is achieved due to strong leakage channels, and this explains the absence of any hyperpolarization in action potentials at nodes of Ranvier.

Between the nodes of Ranvier, the dynamics of electric potential is described by equation (3.26). This is a linear diffusion equation. It is known that for such an equation, the speed of propagation of zero front is infinite. In this sense, it does not describe any wave propagation effects. However, it does describe fast-in-time spatial variation of the potential φ due to diffusion. It is clear from equation (3.26) that the smaller the coefficient b, the faster the process of diffusion. The smallness of b is achieved by decreasing the per unit surface capacitance C (see formula (3.12)) through the myelination of axon. This leads to the following picture of saltatory signal conduction in myelinated axons. Namely, the potential perturbations caused by the action potential at a node of Ranvier is transmitted through a fast diffusion process to another node of Ranvier where this perturbation leads to regeneration of the action potential and its further transmission to yet another node of Ranvier. In this way, the transmission of the action potential occurs through multiple repetitions of the described process of "hopping" of the action potential from node to node.

In our previous discussion, we used triangular shape approximations of action potentials, which appreciably simplified the solution of the inverse problem for determination of $f(\varphi)$. This solution clearly reveals the hysteretic nature of macroscopic sodium and potassium currents, which are expressed in terms of the rectangular loops shown in Figs. 3.23 and 3.22, respectively. Similar calculations can be performed for more realistic shapes of action potentials and they will lead to hysteresis loops with gradual (instead of vertical) transitions between two states. The possibility of such calculation is especially evident from equation (3.27) for generation of the action potential at the nodes of Ranvier. Similar calculations can also be carried out by using equation (3.20), however, they are more involved.

It must be remarked that in the case of the unmyelinated axon the use of the triangular shapes of action potentials may result in δ-function terms in ionic currents at the locations corresponding to λ_1, λ_2 and λ_3. This is due to the idealization of actual shapes of action potentials. The above issue was left unattended in our discussion because it does not exist for actual shapes of action potentials. It also does not affect the hysteretic nature of macroscopic sodium and potassium channels. This hysteretic nature is due to the fact that these channels are turned on and off at different values of membrane potential.

3.4 Hysteresis Models of Neural Memory

In this section, hysteresis modelling of neural memory is explored. The idea that the physical phenomenon of hysteresis may be related to neural memory was suggested before. As mentioned in the end of Section 1.1, the papers of B. G. Cragg and H. N. V. Temperley, "*Memory: The Analog with Ferromagnetic Hysteresis*" (Journal "Brain", 1955) [33] and A. Katchalsky and E. Neuman "*Hysteresis and Molecular Memory Record*" (International Journal of Neuroscience, 1972) [34] were probably the very first publications where this idea was discussed. In retrospect, this is not surprising because hysteresis is endowed with memory. This fact was the central point of the discussions presented in the above papers.

Naturally, the second paper was more advanced, and its conclusion was stated as follows:
"*There is accumulative evidence that the first step of the memory record is a physical process. A plausible mechanism is based on conformational changes in biopolymers, which produced long-lived metastable states. Such metastable states, incorporated in crystalline domains, can be readily detected in hysteresis phenomena.*"

It should be kept in mind that the paper of A. Katchalsky and E. Neuman was written at a time when the existence of ionic channels formed by proteins embedded in neuron membranes was not known. Furthermore, at the time of publication of the above papers, the Preisach-type models of hysteresis were not yet sufficiently developed. The purpose of this section is to demonstrate that by using Preisach-type models, the connection between neural memory and hysteresis can be further elaborated. Namely, it is shown below that memory of Preisach-type hysteresis models has many unique features, which have been observed (or suspected) for neural memory. In this sense, the Preisach-type models of neural memory are attractive, and they may eventually lead to new insights concerning the nature of actual neural memories. The interesting connections between neural memories and Preisach hysteresis models were first pointed out in the paper [35], which was subsequently reviewed by Sir John Maddox in the paper "*Is there Inanimate Memory?*" (Nature, 1986) [36].

The necessity of using the mathematical tools equipped with memory in neural science is stressed in the book of P. S. Churchland and T. J. Sejnowski [2], where it is stated (see p. 46):
"*Our understanding of the nervous system at the subcellular level is changing rapidly, and it is apparent that neurons are dynamic and complex*

entities whose computational properties cannot be approximated by memoryless response functions, a common idealization"
In this respect, the use of the Preisach model endowed with memory can be viewed as a step in the right direction.

It is important to stress here that the Preisach hysteresis models of neural memory may naturally have some limitations. These models (as any model) are products of mind, while actual neural memories are products of the evolution process. The scientific process of modelling is driven by observations, intuition, and logical reasoning. Whereas, the slow and cumbersome evolution process is driven by random mutations and survivalistic selection. As a result, the evolution process builds on what has been already there. For this reason, biology (in contrast with physics and mathematics) does not have rigid principles and laws. There are very few (if any) principles in biology and neural science, which are rigidly valid and do not allow for at least some partial exceptions. Theoretical models may only imitate certain important properties of actual neural memories, but it is doubtful that they may ever fully account for their immense complexity.

Biological memory is a very broad area of neural science research, which is being conducted at different levels. One of them is the top-down approach, which deals with the functioning and manifestations of memory, and it is characterized by such terms as declarative memory, procedural memory, short-term memory, long-term memory, memory consolidation etc. Declarative (explicit) memory is memory of facts, people, and events. In contrast, procedural (implicit) memory is memory of perceptions and motor skills. Declarative memory requires conscious recall, while procedural memory is realized without conscious recall of past events, but by means of spontaneous reflexes. Extensive research has been conducted to identify the structures of the brain associated with declarative and procedural memories. It has been established that procedural memory involves such parts of the brain as the cerebellum and the motor cortex. Declarative memory, on the other hand, involves the hippocampus and the neocortex. The most famous study revealing the separation of procedural and declarative memories was performed in the case of the unfortunate patient known as "H.M." This patient has two-thirds of his hippocampus and parts of his medial temporal lobe and amygdala removed through surgery in an attempt to cure his epilepsy. After surgery, H.M. could still form new procedural memories. However, he became unable to form new declarative memories of facts and events.

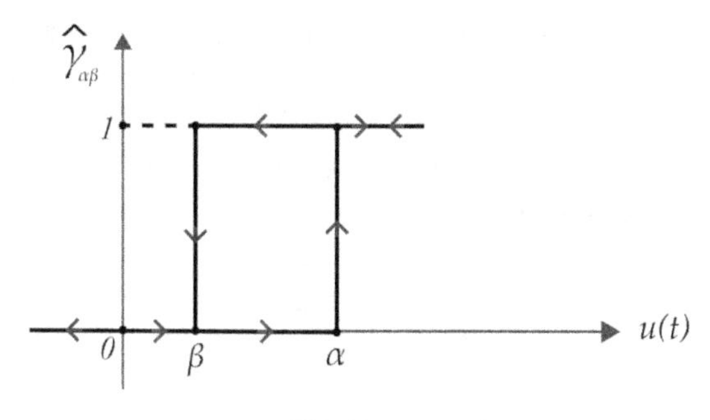

Fig. 3.25

It has been also established that the initial storage of long-term declarative memory requires the hippocampus. This stored information is thereafter transferred to the neocortex for final consolidation, and the hippocampus is not required once the consolidation of memory has been achieved. It is still enigma why the long-term declarative memory storage proceeds through these two distinct steps.

Another level of memory studies is the bottom-up approach, which is concerned with the physical molecular basis of memory storage. The central issue here is to identify specific classes of molecules as well as certain changes induced in their structures, which make the memory storage possible. Our subsequent discussion is related to this area of memory studies, and it is based on the Preisach models of hysteresis, considered in detail in the previous chapters.

As a reminder, the classical Preisach model is given by the formula:

$$f(t) = \iint\limits_{\alpha \geq \beta} \mu(\alpha, \beta) \hat{\gamma}_{\alpha,\beta} u(t) d\alpha d\beta \ , \tag{3.31}$$

where $u(t)$ is an input signal, $f(t)$ is an output signal, $\hat{\gamma}_{\alpha,\beta}$ are rectangular hysteresis loops (operators) with α and β being "up" and "down" switching thresholds, respectively (see Fig. 1.13), while $\mu(\alpha, \beta)$ is some weight function. It was mentioned in Section 1.2 that this model can be viewed as a parallel connection of rectangular loops, scaled by $\mu(\alpha, \beta)$ (see Fig. 1.14).

It is apparent from formula (3.31) that the Preisach model is of hybrid (mixed) nature. Namely, its main building blocks are binary elements $\hat{\gamma}_{\alpha,\beta}$, while its input $u(t)$ and output $f(t)$ are continuous signals of time. Previously, rectangular loops $\hat{\gamma}_{\alpha,\beta}$ with binary output values ± 1 were used in the construction of the Preisach model. However, these rectangular loops can be replaced by the loops shown in Fig. 3.25, and this replacement will not affect the properties of the Preisach model discussed in Chapter 1. The loops $\hat{\gamma}_{\alpha,\beta}$ shown in Fig. 3.25 are more convenient for their biological interpretation.

It was briefly mentioned at the end of the Section 1.3 that the Preisach model (3.31) is endowed with memory, which exhibits the properties similar to those observed in neural memories. This matter is further elaborated below. Namely, the subsequent discussion will be focused on the following issues:

- **The molecular basis of neural memory**
- **Selective memories and their extraction**
- **Distributed memories and their engrams (memory traces)**
- **Memory formation as an emerging property of sparse connectivity**
- **Memory stability with respect to protein turnover; fading memory**
- **Memory storage and plasticity**
- **Memory recall**

We start with the first issue.

- **The molecular basis of neural memory**

It is accepted by most (but not all) neuroscientists that learning and new memory formation requires synthesis of new proteins. There exists some experimental evidence for the validity of the above statement. This evidence was obtained by using protein synthesis inhibitors. These inhibitors are a special class of antibiotics, which prevent the production of new proteins. It was found that the injection of protein synthesis inhibitors in the hippocampus resulted in amnesia. Namely, the memories undergoing consolidation at the time of injection were lost. These experiments resulted in the *de novo* protein synthesis theory, which states that the formation of long-term memory requires the synthesis of new proteins.

The *de novo* theory is attractive from the purely theoretical point of view. Indeed, proteins are macromolecules with many metastable (conformational) states. For this reason, proteins exhibit hysteresis and, as a result, they are endowed with memory. This leads to the reasonable conclusion that memory may be stored in conformational states of proteins. This can be viewed as a plausible hypothesis concerning the molecular basis for memory formation.

There is a huge number of different types of proteins in neurons. The immediate question is which proteins are most likely to be involved in the memory storage process. A strong argument can be made that ionic channel proteins are best suited for this purpose. Indeed, the two most important biophysical operations, which underlie all electrical signaling in the brain, are the generation of action potentials and the signal transmission across the synaptic clefts. These operations are accomplished by the means of ionic channels. These channels may be subject to electrical sensory signals with memory data, and these signals may modify accordingly the conformational states of channel proteins. Furthermore, ion channels are electrically interconnected by conducting biofluids inside and outside the neurons. This electric connectivity may lead to the formation of hysteresis-based memory similar to the Preisach model memory.

Now, the question can be raised concerning the biological interpretation of rectangular loops $\hat{\gamma}_{\alpha,\beta}$ and function $\mu(\alpha,\beta)$ in the Preisach model (3.31). The simplest interpretation would be that the rectangular loops $\hat{\gamma}_{\alpha,\beta}$ model ionic channels. This interpretation is supported by the fact that in most single channel patch clamp recordings the ion currents are binary (as shown in Fig. 3.7). Furthermore, the random switchings between closed ($i = 0$) and open ($i = i_0$) conformations are represented in these recordings by almost vertical lines. This implies that similar random switchings would occur if rectangular loops $\hat{\gamma}_{\alpha,\beta}$ shown in Fig. 3.25 are subject to stochastic input $u(t)$. In this interpretation, the function $\mu(\alpha,\beta)$ can be viewed as an average value of random ion current of the channel represented by the loop $\hat{\gamma}_{\alpha,\beta}$ shown in Fig. 3.25. Since the number of ion channels is finite, the integral in the formula (3.31) should be replaced by the sum:

$$f(t) = \sum_{k=1}^{N} \mu(\alpha_k, \beta_k)\hat{\gamma}_{\alpha_k,\beta_k} u(t) \ , \tag{3.32}$$

where N is a very large number of channels. It can be easily shown that the discrete version (3.32) of the Preisach model (3.31) has the same properties which were established for the model (1.3) in Chapter 1.

Another (more sophisticated) approach would be to model each hysteretic ion channel by the Preisach model (3.31). Assuming that these channels are connected in parallel (that is the same input $u(t)$ is applied to them), we find:

$$f_k(t) = \iint_{\alpha \geq \beta} \mu_k(\alpha,\beta)\hat{\gamma}_{\alpha,\beta} u(t) d\alpha d\beta \tag{3.33}$$

and

$$f(t) = \sum_{k=1}^{N} f_k(t) , \tag{3.34}$$

where, as before, N is a large number of interconnected channels. From the last two formulas we obtain:

$$f(t) = \iint_{\alpha \geq \beta} \mu(\alpha, \beta) \hat{\gamma}_{\alpha,\beta} u(t) d\alpha d\beta , \tag{3.35}$$

where

$$\mu(\alpha, \beta) = \sum_{k=1}^{N} \mu_k(\alpha, \beta) . \tag{3.36}$$

Thus, a group of parallelly connected hysteretic channels can be described by the model (3.35), which is mathematically identical to the model (3.31).

Up to this point, it has been tacitly assumed that the same voltage input $u(t)$ is applied to each hysteretic ion channel. However, due to voltage changes along membranes, these channels may be subject to different voltage inputs. One simple way to account for this is to use the following individual channel inputs:

$$u_k(t) = v_k + u(t) , \tag{3.37}$$

where v_k is a voltage across the membrane at the location of the channel number k. Then, formula (3.33) should be replaced by the equation:

$$f_k(t) = \iint_{\alpha \geq \beta} \mu_k(\alpha, \beta) \hat{\gamma}_{\alpha,\beta} \big[v_k + u(t) \big] d\alpha d\beta . \tag{3.38}$$

Next, it can be shown that

$$\hat{\gamma}_{\alpha,\beta} \big[v_k + u(t) \big] = \hat{\gamma}_{\alpha - v_k, \beta - v_k} u(t) . \tag{3.39}$$

Indeed, $\hat{\gamma}_{\alpha,\beta}[v_k + u(t)]$ is switched from 0 to 1 when $u(t)$ is monotonically increased and reaches such values that

$$v_k + u(t) > \alpha , \tag{3.40}$$

which means that

$$u(t) > \alpha - v_k . \tag{3.41}$$

The last inequality implies that $\hat{\gamma}_{\alpha - v_k, \beta - v_k} u(t)$ is switched from 0 to 1. Similarly, $\hat{\gamma}_{\alpha,\beta}[v_k + u(t)]$ is switched from 1 to 0, if $u(t)$ is monotonically decreased and reaches such values that

$$v_k + u(t) < \beta , \tag{3.42}$$

which means that

$$u(t) < \beta - v_k \ . \tag{3.43}$$

The last inequality implies that $\hat{\gamma}_{\alpha-v_k,\beta-v_k}u(t)$ is switched from 1 to 0. The presented reasoning proves the validity of formula (3.39). By using this formula, equation (3.38) can be written as follows:

$$f_k(t) = \iint_{\alpha\geq\beta} \mu_k(\alpha,\beta)\hat{\gamma}_{\alpha-v_k,\beta-v_k}u(t)d\alpha d\beta \ . \tag{3.44}$$

Now, by introducing the new variables

$$\alpha' = \alpha - v_k \ , \quad \beta' = \beta - v_k \ , \tag{3.45}$$

the equation (3.44) can be modified as follows

$$f_k(t) = \iint_{\alpha'\geq\beta'} \mu_k(\alpha' + v_k, \beta' + v_k)\hat{\gamma}_{\alpha',\beta'}u(t)d\alpha' d\beta' \ . \tag{3.46}$$

Finally, by using formulas (3.34) and (3.46), we arrive at:

$$f(t) = \iint_{\alpha'\geq\beta'} \mu(\alpha',\beta')\hat{\gamma}_{\alpha',\beta'}u(t)d\alpha' d\beta' \ , \tag{3.47}$$

where

$$\mu(\alpha',\beta') = \sum_{k=1}^{N} \mu_k(\alpha' + v_k, \beta' + v_k) \ . \tag{3.48}$$

It is clear that formula (3.47)) is mathematically identical to the classical Preisach model and, consequently all the results obtained in Chapter 1 are valid.

Next, we proceed to the discussion of the following issue.

- **Selective memories and their extraction**

It is often emphasized in neural science that brains are similar to computers. The whole research area of neural networks has been developed to explore these similarities. However, as far as memory is concerned, brains are strikingly different from computers. In computers, binary storage is employed, while this is not true for brain memory storage. Furthermore, identical storage elements are used in computers, while biological diversity is probably utilized for storage purposes in brains. In computers, binary data are **assigned** for storage in addressable memory locations. In the case of brains, the stored data are not assigned, but **selectively extracted** from the incoming analog (i.e., time-continuous) sensory input. This extraction is selective. The latter means that only a few features are extracted from the incoming sensory data, while most of this data is not stored. Furthermore, the selectively extracted data stored in brains are not **immutable**. Instead, the stored data continuously evolve over time by being updated, distorted or suppressed into oblivion.

It turns out that the Preisach hysteresis model interpreted as a storage device exhibits the above-mentioned memory properties observed in brains. Indeed, the storage in the Preisach memory is accomplished by using qualitatively similar but quantitively different rectangular loop elements $\hat{\gamma}_{\alpha,\beta}$. In other words, diversity of these elements is crucial for storage. If these elements are interpreted as models for protein channels, then their diversity reflects the biological diversity of channels.

When the Preisach memory is subject to time-continuous inputs $u(t)$, then it detects and extracts from these inputs their extremum values and stores them in the memory structure. Indeed, it has been demonstrated in Section 1.3 that if input $u(t)$ is applied to the Preisach memory during the time interval $t_0 < t < t'$, then the detected, extracted and stored extremum values are specified by the following formulas:

$$M_1 = u(t_1^+) = \max_{t_0<t<t'} u(t) , \tag{3.49}$$

$$m_1 = u(t_1^-) = \min_{t_1^+<t<t'} u(t) , \tag{3.50}$$

$$M_2 = u(t_2^+) = \max_{t_1^-<t<t'} u(t) , \tag{3.51}$$

$$m_2 = u(t_2^-) = \min_{t_2^+<t<t'} u(t) , \tag{3.52}$$

$$\cdots\cdots\cdots\cdots$$

$$M_k = u(t_k^+) = \max_{t_{k-1}^-<t<t'} u(t) , \tag{3.53}$$

$$m_k = u(t_k^-) = \min_{t_k^+<t<t'} u(t) . \tag{3.54}$$

It is apparent that the storage of the extracted extremum input values in the Preisach memory is not digital but rather analog in nature. It is also clear from formulas (3.49)–(3.54) that this storage is not immutable but evolves

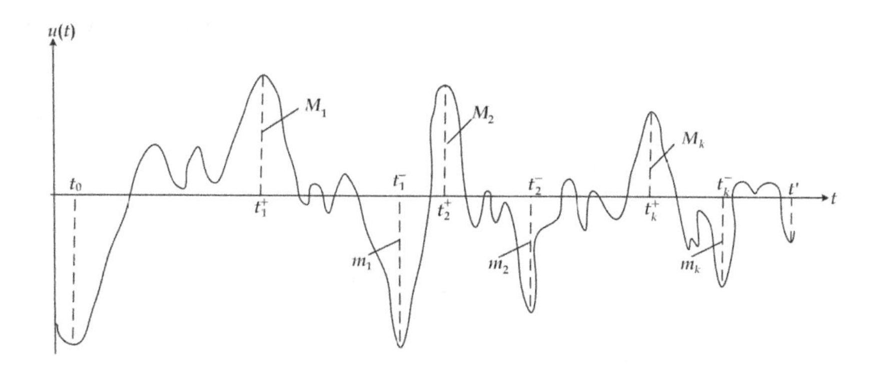

Fig. 3.26

over time. Indeed, it is clear that formulas (3.49)–(3.54) define a sequence of alternating dominant input extrema, and all intermediate input extrema are erased. The latter is illustrated by Fig. 3.26, which is similar to Fig. 1.27. This is the so-called erasure property of the Preisach memory. This erasure property implies that the most dominant input extrema may persist, while other extrema may be erased by subsequent variations of input $u(t)$. In other words, the erasure property of the Preisach memory describes data storage updating, its persistence, and its extinction. The relevant question is why the extremum values of input are selected for extraction and storage. The plausible answer is that the extremum values of continuous input are most distinct in comparison with other values. It is natural that brains are most impacted by strong impressions and feelings, which may be caused by extremum values of incoming sensory inputs. It is also natural that new stronger impressions and feelings caused by new and more dominant sensory input extrema may suppress the previous impressions stored in brains. This is fully consistent with the erasure property of the Preisach memory.

It is worthwhile to mention that some modification is possible in data extraction as a result of the processing of sensory input. Indeed, the incoming sensory input $u(t)$ may be subject to processing before it reaches the memory extraction and storage stage. Consider the simplest case when the processed input $\tilde{u}(t)$ can be represented as

$$\tilde{u}(t) = c_1 u(t) + c_2 v(t) , \tag{3.55}$$

where c_1 and c_2 are some constants, while $v(t)$ is some function produced by processing. Then, the Preisach memory will extract and store extremum values of the processed input, which may not coincide with extremum values of sensory input. Indeed, the extracted values of sensory input $u(t)$ will be its values at the time instants at which

$$c_1 \frac{du(t)}{dt} + c_2 \frac{dv(t)}{dt} = 0 \, , \tag{3.56}$$

which may be different from the time instants when

$$\frac{du(t)}{dt} = 0 \, . \tag{3.57}$$

More complicated cases of processed sensory inputs can be treated in a similar way.

Next, we proceed to the discussion of the following issue.

- **Distributed memories and their engrams (memory traces)**

It is well known that memory storage in brains is of highly distributed nature. This stands in striking contrast with computer memory, where storage of information is localized and specific storage sites for particular data can be clearly identified. The latter is not the case for distributed memory. This led to the search of memory engrams. These engrams are also called memory traces. The term "engram" was first coined in the first decade of the twentieth century by Richard Semon, a German evolutionary biologist and zoologist. This term usually refers to specific changes in brain cellular structures which underlie memory storage. These cellular changes can be viewed as imprints of memory. It is natural to assume that different memories have different engrams.

The extensive research on memory engrams was conducted by Karl Lashley, a famous professor from Harvard University. He tried to identify brain localizations of memory engrams by performing numerous experiments on rats. Ultimately his search for engrams was unsuccessful. In his paper "*In search of the engram*" (see [37]) he wrote:

"*I sometimes feel, in reviewing the evidence on the localization of the memory trace, that the necessary conclusion is that learning just is not possible. It is difficult to conceive of a mechanism which can satisfy the conditions set for it. Nevertheless, in spite of such evidence against it, learning does sometimes occur.*"

In the abstract to the above paper, Lashley expressed this fact more succinctly:

"*... there is no demonstrable localization of memory trace.*"

Nevertheless, after the work of Lashley, the pursuit of engram search has continued unabated, but it has proved to be elusive. This elusiveness is best reflected in the following statement of C. Koch in his article "*Computation and the single neuron*" [38], as well as in his book "*Biophysics of Computation*" (see [1], p. 471):

"*And what of memory? It is everywhere (but can't be randomly addressed). It resides in concentration of free calcium in dendrites and the cell body; in the density and exact voltage-dependency of the various ionic conductances; and in the density and configuration of specific proteins in the postsynaptic terminals.*"

After the cited statement, C. Koch remarked:

"*Only very little of this complexity is reflected in today's neural-network theory.*"

The Preisach hysteresis memory is also of highly distributed nature. In this sense, it mimics neural memory. As discussed in the previous section, the Preisach memory detects, extracts, and stored alternating dominant input extrema determined by formulas (3.49)–(3.54). These extrema are not stored in specific rectangular cell elements $\hat{\gamma}_{\alpha,\beta}$, but all these cell elements are involved in storage of the above extrema regardless of their values. Remarkably, in the case of the distributed storage of the Preisach hysteresis memory, the engrams (i.e. memory traces) can be clearly identified. This identification is based on the diagram technique discussed in detail in Section 1.3. Here, we briefly summarized the most relevant facts of this technique.

In the diagram technique, each rectangular cell $\hat{\gamma}_{\alpha,\beta}$ is identified with a point (α, β) of the half-plane $\alpha \geq \beta$. The function $\mu(\alpha, \beta)$ is usually defined on some triangle T of this half plane. At any instant of time this triangle is divided into two sets $S^{+}(t)$ and $S^{0}(t)$ for which $\hat{\gamma}_{\alpha,\beta}u(t) = 1$ and $\hat{\gamma}_{\alpha,\beta}u(t) = 0$, respectively. (Please note that here rectangular loops shown in Fig. 3.25 are used, instead of rectangular loops in Fig. 1.13.) This division of T on $S^{+}(t)$ and $S^{0}(t)$ is due to a staircase interface $L(t)$ with vertices whose α and β coordinates are determined by the dominant past maxima M_k and minima m_k, respectively. This is illustrated below in Figs. 3.26 and 3.27, which correspond to the cases of monotonically increasing and decreasing input $u(t)$, respectively. The final link of the interface $L(t)$ is attached to the line $\alpha = \beta$. This link is a horizontal one and it moves upward as the input $u(t)$ is monotonically increased (see Fig. 3.27). On the other hand, this link is a vertical one and it moves from right to left as the input $u(t)$ is monotonically decreased (see Fig. 3.28).

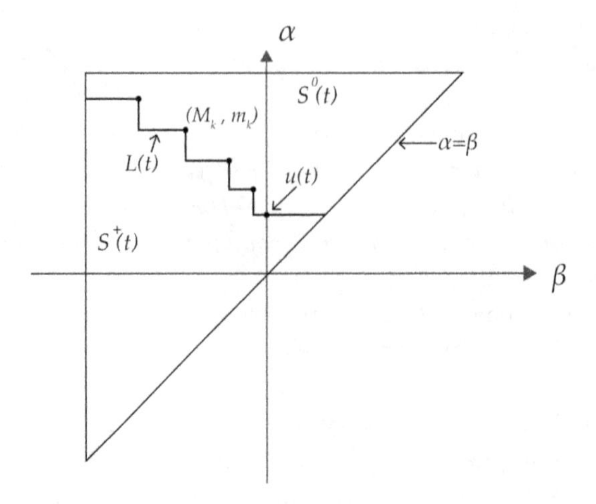

Fig. 3.27

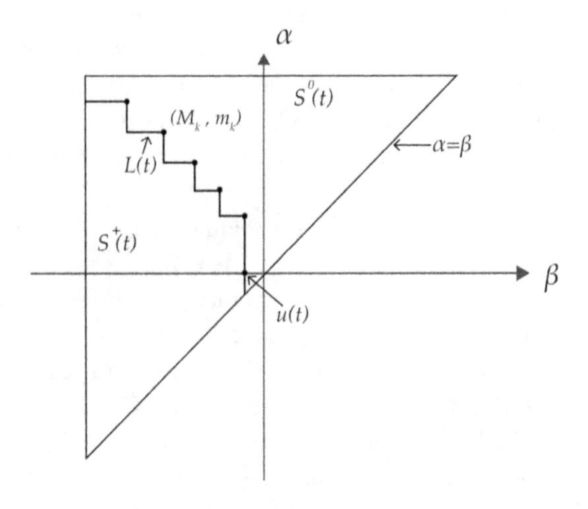

Fig. 3.28

Now, it is clear that at any instant of time t the input $f(t)$ of the Preisach model (3.31) can be computed using the formula:

$$f(t) = \iint_{S^+(t)} \mu(\alpha, \beta) d\alpha d\beta \; . \tag{3.58}$$

It is evident from the above formula that the current value of output $f(t)$ is determined by the geometry of the set $S^+(t)$, which, in turn, is completely defined by the shape of the staircase interface $L(t)$. This interface depends on stored past input extrema. Thus, the interface $L(t)$ can be viewed as an imprint of memory storage. In this sense, **the interface $L(t)$ is a memory engram (or a memory trace)**. It is also apparent that the geometric shape of engram $L(t)$ changes with time, reflecting that stored data continuously evolve over time by being updated, modified, or suppressed into oblivion.

Up to this point, our discussion has been merely theoretical and centered on the identification of engrams in the Preisach memory. Another very important issue is how these memory engrams can be experimentally revealed. It is apparent from the previous analysis that only the recall of the entire stored data may provide a complete information concerning Preisach memory engrams. The memory recall is quite problematic in its own right, and it will be discussed later in this section. Furthermore, huge numbers of $\hat{\gamma}_{\alpha,\beta}$ are involved in shaping memory engrams $L(t)$, and this involvement depends on conformational (metastable) states of proteins, which they represent. For this reason, one may say that memory engrams are **hidden in protein conformational states**. This may explain their elusiveness.

In the conclusion of our discussion of engrams, it is interesting to point out that the Preisach model can be completely defined in terms of its memory engram. Indeed, this model can be defined by formula (3.58) and by the rules for the modifications of $L(t)$ for monotonically increasing and decreasing variations of input $u(t)$. In this way, the Preisach model is defined without any reference to rectangular loops $\hat{\gamma}_{\alpha,\beta}$. Nevertheless, this definition is fully equivalent to the previous definition given by formula (3.31). It is interesting that the new definition of the Preisach model in terms of its engram opens the opportunities for further generalizations of the Preisach model. Namely, new and more general rules of the modifications of the engram $L(t)$ may be introduced. In these rules, the links of $L(t)$ may not be the segments of straight lines parallel to coordinate axes (see, for instance, Fig. 3.29). These segments may be curved lines as well. Furthermore, different functions $\mu^+(\alpha, \beta)$ and $\mu^0(\alpha, \beta)$ may be defined on $S^+(t)$ and $S^0(t)$, respectively. These generalizations may account for more complicated (rather than parallel) connectivity of $\hat{\gamma}_{\alpha,\beta}$. The above generalizations have not yet been fully explored.

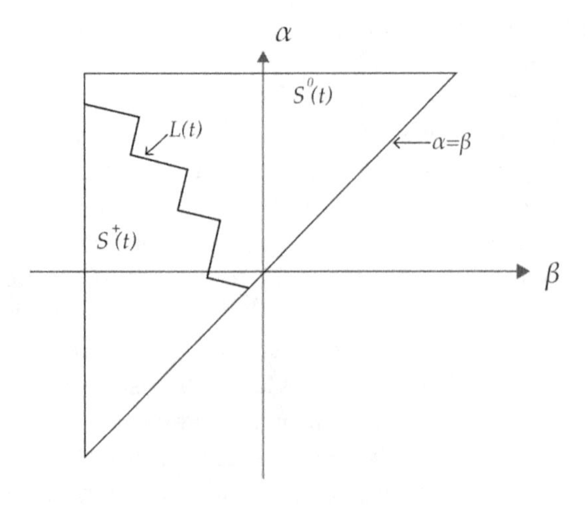

Fig. 3.29

Now, we proceed to the discussion of the following issue.

- **Memory formation as an emergent property of sparse connectivity**

The Preisach memory is a result of the parallel connectivity of rectangular hysteresis loop elements $\hat{\gamma}_{\alpha,\beta}$. This memory is an emergent property because it is not exhibited by individual elements $\hat{\gamma}_{\alpha,\beta}$. Indeed, the property of input extrema detection, their extraction and their storage is due to the parallel connectivity of the simplest hysteretic elements. It is quite remarkable that simplest parallel connectivity of the simplest rectangular hysteresis loop elements leads to the emergent phenomena when the whole seems to be much greater than the sum of the parts.

The parallel connectivity is very sparse. It is doubtful that the parallel connectivity is actually realized in neural memories. In other words, it is doubtful that this connectivity was discovered by nature as a result of the evolution process. However, there are indications that the sparse connectivity between neurons is typical in brains. In the book "*The Computational Brain*" by P. S. Churchland and T. J. Sejnowski (see [2] p. 51), the sparse connectivity is regarded as one of the most basic structural features relevant to brain functioning. Namely, it is stated there that:

"*Not everything is connected to everything else. Each cortical neuron is connected to a roughly constant number of other neurons, irrespective of brain size, namely about 3% of the neurons underlying the surrounding square millimeter of cortex,*" and then it is followed by the comment:

"*... cortical neurons are actually rather sparsely connected relative to the population of neurons in a cell's neighborhood.*"

It is possible that the sparsity of connectivity is beneficial for the formation of numerous interconnected neuron circuits. As a result, these numerous interconnected neural circuits (which may be in some sense similar to the parallel Preisach hysteresis circuit) can be used for memory storage and enhance in this way the storage capacity.

It must be remarked that experimental and theoretical study of connectivity in the brain is a very active area of research nowadays. In this research, such tools as functional magnetic resonance imaging (fMRI) and graph theory are extensively used. There are many publications in which sparse brain connectivity patterns are studied and the benefits of such connectivity are explored. The detail analysis of this matter is beyond the scope of our discussion.

Instead, we proceed to the discussion of the following issue:

- **Memory stability with respect to protein turnover; fading memory**

It was discussed in this section that it is highly plausible that proteins of ion channels form a molecular basis for brain data storage. Indeed, proteins have many conformational (metastable) states. For this reason, they exhibit hysteresis, and they are endowed with memory. However, as mentioned in Section 3.2, proteins are unstable elements, there exists a continuous process of protein degradation and synthesis. This biological phenomenon is called protein turnover. Different protein turnover rates have been observed in different tissues and different brain locations. On average, proteins last for several days. This brings the question of how stable memories, which may last for many years, can be stored by unstable elements. In other words, it is important to understand how neural systems and their memories are remained mostly intact in the face of volatility and fluidity brought about by protein turnover.

This important issue of memory stability was first raised by Francis Crick in 1984 in his paper in *Nature* [23] entitled "*Memory and molecular turnover.*" In this paper, this issue was framed as follows:

"*Time span of human memory (without obvious rehearsal) is often a matter of years, sometimes even ten years. Yet it is believed that almost all the molecules in our bodies, with the exception of DNA, turn over in a matter of days, weeks, or at the most a few months. How then is memory stored in the brain so that its trace is relatively immune to molecular turnover?"*

In the above paper, F. Crick proposed a plausible explanation for memory stability based on molecular symmetry arguments. More importantly, this paper was the starting point for the extensive research. The main results of this research, obtained after thirty years since the publication of the above paper, are summarized by R. B. Meagher in [24]. In parallel with this research, extensive studies have been conducted to understand the distributed nature of protein synthesis, which makes this synthesis possible in locations (such as synapses, for instance) that may be separated by hundreds of microns from neuron soma and its nucleus. It has been found in these studies that protein synthesis in remote locations is performed by distributed mRNA molecules [39], [40].

Next, we consider a plausible explanation for data storage stability in the face of protein turnover in the case of Preisach memory. This explanation is based on the distributed nature of data storage in the Preisach memory and its engram. In the case of the Preisach model, all elementary cells $\hat{\gamma}_{\alpha,\beta}$ are involved in the storage of data at any instant of time t. This storage is reflected in the output value of $f(t)$ given by formula (3.58). Within the Preisach approach, the protein turnover can be viewed as a removal of some terms in formula (3.36), representing the ion channels affected by protein degradation. This removal affects the values of the function $\mu(\alpha,\beta)$ in formula (3.58), but it does not affect the shape of engram $L(t)$, which is the imprint of the stored data. Thus, the protein turnover may lead to a very slow decay of $\mu(\alpha,\beta)$ which, in turn, may lead to a very slow decay of $f(t)$ representing a specific pattern of the stored memory. The slowness of the decay may be due to a very large number N in formula (3.36), which represents a very large number of interconnected protein channels. This argument is supported by the existence of a huge number of proteins resident in neurons. It is estimated that there are about 250 million various proteins in the dendrites of a single neuron and about 500 million in a neuron total [41]. Thus, the protein turnover may lead to a slow decay of memory, which is known as fading memory. This is usually the case in the absence of stored memory rehearsing.

It is important to point out that another stochastic mechanism of fading memory may also exist. In this mechanism, the stored memory is weakened by inherently present noise. Mathematically, it means that the input to the

Preisach model is a stochastic process describing this noise. In this case, formula (3.31) can be written as follows:

$$f_t = \iint\limits_{\alpha \geq \beta} \mu(\alpha, \beta) \hat{\gamma}_{\alpha,\beta} u_t d\alpha d\beta \ , \tag{3.59}$$

where f_t and u_t are typically used notations for output and input stochastic processes, respectively. Large deviations of (generally small) input noise u_t may lead to switchings of many hysteresis loop elements $\hat{\gamma}_{\alpha,\beta}$, which may result in the modification of engram $L(t)$ and slow memory decay typical for fading memory. This decay is slow because it usually takes a long time to develop large random deviations in the presence of small noise. This memory fading mechanism is mathematically studied in the next chapter.

Now, we shall proceed to the discussion of the following issue.

- **Memory storage plasticity**

As discussed in Section 3.2, the essence of synaptic plasticity is the strengthening or weakening of synapses as a result of their past activity. In modern neuroscience, synaptic plasticity is regarded as the foundation for memory formation and learning. For example, it is stated in the book of C. Koch [1] (see p. 329) that:

"*Changes in synaptic strength are widely postulated to be the primary biophysical substrate for many forms of behavioral plasticity, including learning and memory, although our understanding of the link remains far from complete.*"

It is interesting to explore how the Preisach model of neural memory may account for the phenomenon of plasticity. In the case of the classical Preisach model (3.35), the plasticity can be accounted for by using the number N of interconnected channels as a function of time, $N(t)$, or as a function of input, $N(u(t))$. Another option is to use N as a function of dominant past input extrema. In this way, the proliferation of spine ion channels or their reduction occurring as a result of synaptic plasticity can be accounted for.

Another approach is to use generalizations of the classical Preisach model discussed in the Chapter 2. For instance, the so-called "restricted" Preisach model defined by the formula:

$$f(t) = \iint\limits_{T_{M_1}} \mu(\alpha, \beta, M_1) \hat{\gamma}_{\alpha,\beta} u(t) d\alpha d\beta \ + \ C_{M_1} \tag{3.60}$$

was introduced and studied in Section 2.3.

In the last formula, M_1 is the largest past input maximum, triangle T_{M_1} is a part of triangle T defined by inequalities $\beta \leqslant \alpha \leqslant M_1$ and C_{M_1} is some constant (see formula (2.73)). The model (3.60) is called restricted, because the definition of $\mu(\alpha, \beta, M_1)$ is restricted to the triangle T_{M_1}.

It is clear from formula (3.60) that the past input variations may strengthen the memory. Indeed, if function $\mu(\alpha, \beta, M_1)$ is a monotonically increasing one with respect to M_1, then the output $f(t)$ defined by the formula:

$$f(t) = \iint_{S^+_{M_1}(t)} \mu(\alpha, \beta, M_1) d\alpha d\beta \; + \; C_{M_1} \tag{3.61}$$

will also increase with respect to M_1. In this way, the past history may enhance the future memory. This property does not exist in the classical Preisach memory model specified by formula (3.31).

The memory model (3.60) can be further generalized to account for what can be called synaptic depression. Indeed, the following Preisach model:

$$f(t) = \iint_{T_{M_1 m_1}} \mu(\alpha, \beta, M_1, m_1) \hat{\gamma}_{\alpha,\beta} u(t) d\alpha d\beta \; + \; C_{M_1 m_1} \tag{3.62}$$

was introduced in Section 2.3. Here: M_1 and m_1 are the largest and the smallest past input maximum and minimum, respectively, the triangle $T_{M_1 m_1}$ is a part of the triangle T defined by inequalities $m_1 \leq \beta \leq \alpha \leq M_1$, while $C_{M_1 m_1}$ is some constant (see formula (2.105)).

As before, the last formula can be written in the form:

$$f(t) = \iint_{S^+_{M_1 m_1}(t)} \mu(\alpha, \beta, M_1, m_1) d\alpha d\beta \; + \; C_{M_1 m_1} \; , \tag{3.63}$$

where $S^+_{M_1 m_1}(t)$ is a set of points (α, β) of the triangle $T_{M_1 m_1}$, for which $\hat{\gamma}_{\alpha,\beta} u(t) = 1$.

If function $\mu(\alpha, \beta, M_1, m_1)$ is a monotonically decreasing one with respect to m_1, then according to the formula (3.63) the output $f(t)$ will also decrease with respect to m_1. This means that the past input variations represented by M_1 and m_1 may suppress the future values of output $f(t)$ defined by the input extrema extracted and stored after M_1 and m_1 are reached. In other words, the past input history represented by M_1 and m_1 may suppress manifestations of future data storage, that is it may weaken future memories.

Finally, it is worthwhile to point out that the Preisach model (2.26) may also be useful for plasticity modelling.

In the presented discussion of the Preisach modelling of plasticity it was tacitly assumed that proteins of ionic channels in synapses form a molecular basis for memory formation. The plausibility of this assumption can be justified as follows. There are two biophysical operations that make all electrical signaling in brains possible. They are the action potential generation and the electric signal transmission across synaptic clefts. These two operations are performed by using ionic channels. As discussed in the previous section, action potentials are identical (stereotyped) in shape. This may suggest that the performance of ionic channels responsible for action potential generation is not affected by continuous process of memory acquisition and storage. The latter implies that performance of ionic channels involved in synaptic transmission may be mostly affected by the data storage process. In other words, it is plausible to conclude that synaptic channel protein may form a molecular basis for data storage.

Next, we proceed to the discussion of the issue.

- **Memory recall**

This is a very difficult issue. In the paper [42], Eric R. Kandel states:

"*Finally, we need to understand how memory is recalled. This is a deep problem whose analysis is just beginning.*"

There are at least two reasons why the memory recall problem is so difficult.

First, a special recall signal must be produced for memory retrieval. The generation of this signal may require some conscious actions. In this way, the memory recall is related to consciousness. The neuroscientific research on consciousness is currently at its initial stage. It is a great challenge to understand how an unconscious molecular basis of the brain may result in the emergence of consciousness. A very interesting framework of consciousness is proposed in the paper [43] of Francis Crick and Christof Koch. This framework is based on the notion of neural correlates of consciousness formed as a result of competition between assemblies (i.e., coalitions) of interconnected neurons.

Second, it has been found that the memory recall is detrimental to the stability of the stored memory subject to the retrieval process. This process may convert a stable (consolidated) memory into a labile state, in which it can be distorted and even erased. For this reason, it is believed that the reconsolidation of retrieved memory is needed for its preservation.

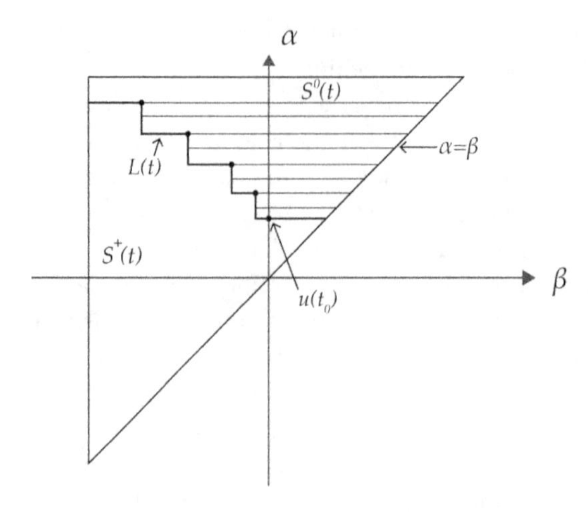

Fig. 3.30

The Preisach model of neural memory clearly mimics this second difficulty of the recall process. Indeed, the memory readback process requires such an input signal $u(t)$, which will reveal the structure of engram $L(t)$. This can be achieved by using monotonically increasing or monotonically decreasing inputs $u(t)$ as illustrated in Figs. 3.30 and 3.31, respectively. These variations of input $u(t)$ will result in modifications of geometric diagrams in Figs. 3.30 and 3.31. These modifications are marked by horizontal and vertical lines, respectively. The variations of output $f(t)$, corresponding to the above monotonic variations of input $u(t)$, will exhibit jumps in its output derivatives at instant of times when corner points of staircase line $L(t)$ are erased. These jumps and the values of input at their occurrence reveal the stored data.

It is apparent that the described recall process results in the erasure of the engram $L(t)$ and of the retrieved memory. Consequently, the recalled memory must be stored anew, which is tantamount to its reconsolidation.

In the conclusion of this section, it must be remarked that the Preisach memory has a remarkably simple structure consisting of the simplest (parallel) connectivity of the simplest (rectangular loop) memory elements $\hat{\gamma}_{\alpha,\beta}$. Nevertheless, its memory properties are quite similar to those observed in neural memory. For this reason, it is hoped that the Preisach model may provide useful insights into the nature of actual neural memory.

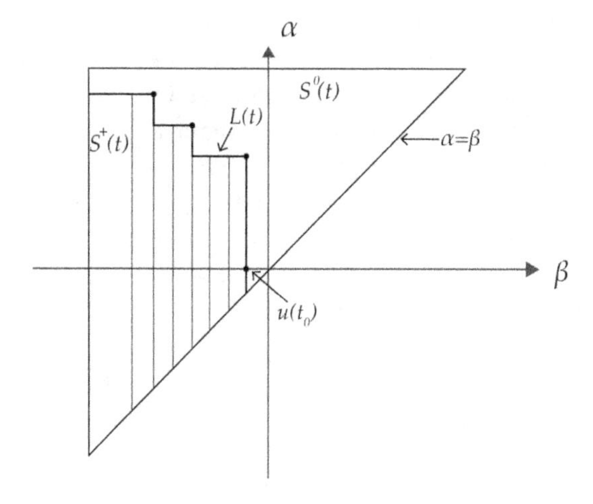

Fig. 3.31

3.5 Preisach-Based Data Storage and Global Optimizers

This short section is not related to neural memory. Its purpose is to suggest that the unique features of the Preisach model may be explored for the future development of data storage devices and hardware-type global optimizers.

The existing conventional data storage systems are based on the availability of identical microelectronic devices used for the storage of binary numbers. However, the relentless process of miniaturization has resulted in the transition of digital electronic devices from microscale to nanoscale. At the nanoscale, electronic devices are very susceptible to random dopant fluctuations which occur due to the random nature of ion implantation and diffusion. There are also random fluctuations of oxide thickness in MOSFET devices. All these random fluctuations lead to fabrication deviations that are strongly pronounced at the nanoscale and which appreciably affect the characteristics of digital semiconductor devices. This makes the fabrication of almost identical storage elements very expensive and even unattainable in the case of their further miniaturization. The nonidentical nature of digital devices is detrimental to the existing principles of computer storage. On the other hand, the nonidentical nature of storage elements is beneficial for the design of Preisach-type memory devices. Actually, it is at the very foundation of the design of such devices. For this reason, this type of devices may find some applications in future data storage systems.

One of the main difficulties in the Preisach-based data storage is that the data subject to storage must be represented as sequences of alternating maxima and minima of decreasing magnitude. Only in this case (as clear from Section 1.3), the Preisach storage without any erasure, i.e., without any information loss, can be accomplished. This requires special formatting of the data subject to storage. This formatting is discussed below.

Suppose that we have a set of numbers subject to storage. First, we subdivide this set of numbers into two subsets of positive and negative numbers, respectively. Namely, numbers

$$x_1, x_2, \ldots, x_n \tag{3.64}$$

are positive, while numbers

$$y_1, y_2, \ldots, y_m \tag{3.65}$$

are negative.

Then, we introduce the following sequence of all positive numbers:

$$x_1, x_2, \ldots, x_n, x_{n+1}, x_{n+2}, \ldots, x_N \ , \tag{3.66}$$

where

$$x_{n+1} = -y_1, \ x_{n+2} = -y_2, \ldots, x_N = -y_m \tag{3.67}$$

and

$$N = n + m \ . \tag{3.68}$$

Next, we design the following sequence of numbers X_k in the case when $N = 2i$:

$$X_{2i} = \sum_{k=1}^{2i} x_k, \ X_{2i-2} = \sum_{k=1}^{2i-2} x_k, \ldots, X_2 = \sum_{k=1}^{2} x_k \ , \tag{3.69}$$

$$X_{2i-1} = -\sum_{k=1}^{2i-1} x_k, \ X_{2i-3} = -\sum_{k=1}^{2i-3} x_k, \ldots, X_1 = -x_1 \ . \tag{3.70}$$

It is clear that

$$X_{2i} > X_{2i-2} > \cdots > X_2 \ , \tag{3.71}$$

and

$$X_{2i-1} < X_{2i-3} < \cdots < X_1 \ . \tag{3.72}$$

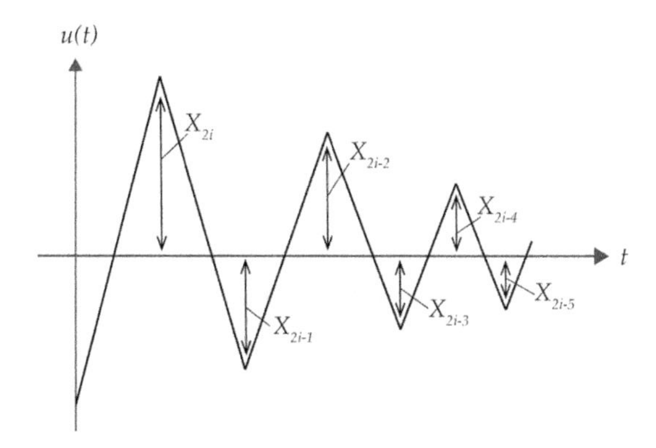

Fig. 3.32

In the case when $N = 2i + 1$, we define sequence X_k as follows:

$$X_{2i+1} = \sum_{k=1}^{2i+1} x_k,\ X_{2i-1} = \sum_{k=1}^{2i-1} x_k, \ldots, X_1 = x_1\ , \tag{3.73}$$

$$X_{2i} = -\sum_{k=1}^{2i} x_k,\ X_{2i-2} = -\sum_{k=1}^{2i-2} x_k, \ldots, X_2 = -\sum_{k=1}^{2} x_k\ . \tag{3.74}$$

It is clear that

$$X_{2i+1} > X_{2i-1} > \cdots > X_1\ , \tag{3.75}$$

while

$$X_{2i} < X_{2i-2} < \cdots < X_2\ . \tag{3.76}$$

The above defined sequences X_k can be stored in the Preisach memory devices consisting of parallel connectivity of $\hat{\gamma}_{\alpha,\beta}$ without being affected by the erasure property of the Preisach model. Indeed, by using an input shown in Fig. 3.32, we shall end up with the Preisach memory engram shown in Fig. 3.33. The last figure corresponds to the case when $N = 2i$. In this case, the last link of the engram connected to the line $\alpha = \beta$ is a vertical one. The α and β coordinates of the vertices of the protruding angles of the engram are equal to X_{2j} and X_{2j+1}, respectively.

In the case when $N = 2i + 1$, the engram will be similar to one shown in Fig. 3.33, except the last link of the engram will be a horizontal one and the α and β coordinates of the vertices of the protruding angles of the engram are equal to X_{2j+1} and X_{2j}, respectively.

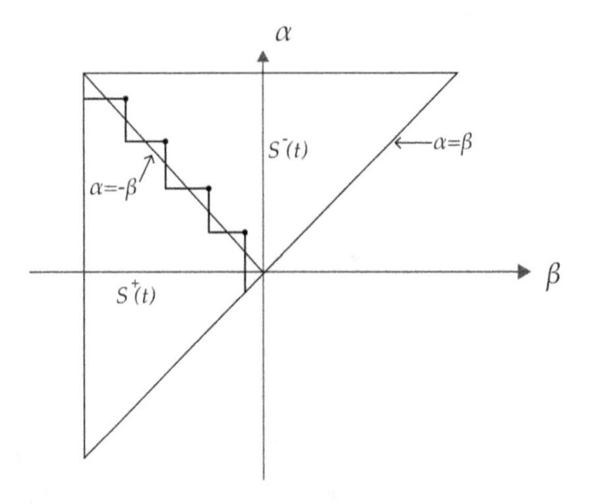

Fig. 3.33

As discussed below, the recorded data X_k can be read back by monotonically increasing the input $u(t)$ and properly analyzing the output $f(t)$. As soon as numbers X_k are read, the original numbers in formulas (3.64) and (3.65) can be recovered by using formulas (3.67), (3.69), and (3.70) in the case when $N = 2i$, and formulas (3.67), (3.73), and (3.74) in the case when $N = 2i + 1$.

It is clear from Fig. 3.33 that the Preisach memory with only symmetric ($\alpha = -\beta$) rectangular loops $\hat{\gamma}_{\alpha,\beta}$ can be used. Indeed, it is clear from formulas (3.69)–(3.70) and (3.73)–(3.74) that the vertices of the protruding angles of the engram are above the line $\alpha = -\beta$, while the vertices of other ("caving in") angles of the engram are below the line $\alpha = -\beta$. This fact follows from the inequality

$$X_{2j} > |X_{2j-1}| > X_{2j-2} \tag{3.77}$$

in the case when $N = 2i$, and the inequality

$$X_{2j+1} > |X_{2j}| > X_{2j-1} \tag{3.78}$$

in the case when $N = 2i + 1$.

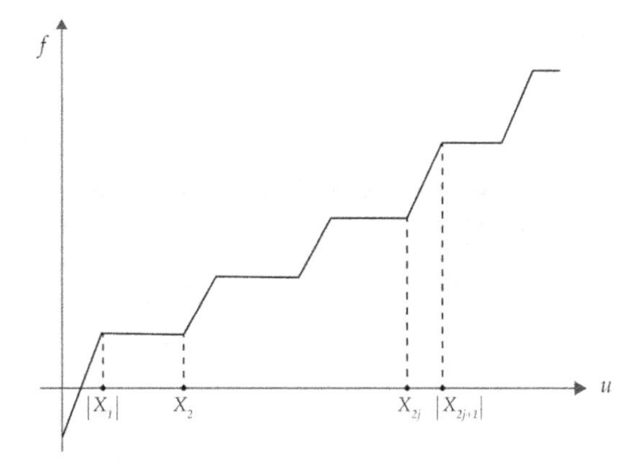

Fig. 3.34

The output of the Preisach model in the case of symmetric rectangular loops can be written as follows

$$f(t) = C \int_{\alpha} \hat{\gamma}_{\alpha,-\alpha} u(t) d\alpha \ , \tag{3.79}$$

where it is assumed (for the sake of simplicity) that $\mu(\alpha, -\alpha) = C$.

Now, it is clear that in the case of the reading back process when the input is monotonically increased, rectangular loops $\hat{\gamma}_{\alpha,-\alpha}$ corresponding to the points of the line $\alpha = -\beta$ inside $S^-(t)$ will be switched upwards. It is clear from Fig. 3.33 that the above points belong to the disjoint parts of the line $\alpha = -\beta$. When the switching of $\hat{\gamma}_{\alpha,-\alpha}$ along these parts occurs, then according to the formula (3.79) the output $f(t)$ is linearly increased as a function of input $u(t)$. Between these switchings, the output $f(t)$ remains constant. Furthermore, it is clear from Fig. 3.33, that the linear output increase starts at the input values $u(t_{2j}) = X_{2j}$ and ends at the input values $u(t_{2j+1}) = |X_{2j+1}|$. This means that the output f as the function of input u can be represented by the graph shown in Fig. 3.34.

This graph clearly reveals that the values of X_k can be retrieved by using the described read back process. In the case when $\mu(\alpha, -\alpha)$ is not constant, the parts of the graph f vs u corresponding to the monotonic increase of output will not be linear but will be curved. However, these disjoint parts will be separated by horizontal (flat) parts whose initial and end points correspond to the input values equal to $|X_{2j-1}|$ and X_{2j}, respectively. Thus, the values of X_k can still be recovered from the f vs u function.

Next, we shall discuss how the rectangular loop elements $\hat{\gamma}_{\alpha,-\alpha}$ can be physically realized. In microelectronics, this can be accomplished by using Schmitt trigger circuits with positive feedback. There are different realizations of such circuits by using BJT transistors or operational amplifiers. These realizations also require resistors. There are circuit realizations of the Schmitt trigger that can be accomplished without resistors. These are CMOS realizations, which use six MOSFETs [45]–[46]. In magnetics, rectangular loop elements $\hat{\gamma}_{\alpha,-\alpha}$ can be realized by using nanoscale single-domain thin magnetic film particles with in-plane anisotropy. For such particles, the Stoner-Wolfarth theory can be used, which predicts rectangular magnetization loops when the applied magnetic field varies along the easy anisotropy axis [47]. Finally, in optics, rectangular loop elements can be realized by using the physical phenomena of optical bistability. This phenomenon occurs in various semiconductors, and it can be also realized on a silicon chip [48] despite the relatively weak nonlinear optical properties of silicon.

The discussed Preisach-type memory is of distributed nature, and, as a result, it is not addressable. For this reason, the most probable applications of this memory will be for massive data storage when all data stored in one Preisach memory unit is retrieved. Many identical Preisach memory units can be employed for massive data storage, and these units can be addressable.

Now, we turn to the discussion of the unique properties of the Preisach model-based global optimizers. Consider first the problem of univariate global optimization. The essence of this problem is in finding the global extremum (for instance, global minimum) of a given function $\varphi(t)$ of one variable:

$$\varphi(\tilde{t}) = \min_{t \in [0,T]} \varphi(t) \; . \tag{3.80}$$

Various numerical methods have been developed for the solution of this problem. Usually, some smoothness of is assumed in these methods. One of the most commonly used assumptions is that the minimized function $\varphi(t)$ satisfies the Lipschitz condition, i.e.,

$$|\varphi(t_2) - \varphi(t_1)| \leq L|t_2 - t_1| \; , \tag{3.81}$$

where $L > 0$ is the Lipschitz constant.

The multivariate global optimization problem is substantially more difficult. It requires the finding of the global minimum of the function of many variables

$$\varphi(\vec{x^*}) = \min_{\vec{x} \in \mathcal{D}} \varphi(\vec{x}) \; , \tag{3.82}$$

where $\vec{x} = (x_1, x_2, \ldots, x_n)$ and $\mathcal{D}$ is some region (for instance) a cube, in n-dimensional space.

It is natural to apply one-dimensional global optimization techniques to the solution of multidimensional global optimization problems. One of such approaches is the nested dimension reduction scheme.

The Preisach model based devices can be viewed as hardware-type global optimizers. Indeed, if the function $\varphi(t)$ subject to minimization is used as an input ($u(t) = \varphi(t)$) to the Preisach based device, then this device will detect, extract and store the alternating sequence of dominant extrema of $\varphi(t)$. Among these extrema are the global minima and maxima of $\varphi(t)$. The Preisach device does this due to its structure and no additional computations are needed if $\varphi(t)$ is given as an analog signal. The extracted and stored extrema of $\varphi(t)$ can then be retrieved. This retrieval is especially simple in the case when the function $\mu(\alpha, \beta)$ is constant and the output of the Preisach memory is given by the formula:

$$f(t) = C \iint_{\alpha \geq \beta} \hat{\gamma}_{\alpha,\beta} u(t) d\alpha d\beta \, . \tag{3.83}$$

Indeed, by using the diagram shown in Fig. 3.35 and taking into account that the retrieval can be accomplished by using a monotonically decreasing input $u(t)$, it can be shown that the output $f(t)$ is a piece-wise linear function of $u(t)$ shown schematically in Fig. 3.36. The transition from one linear link of the function f vs u to another occurs at the input values $u = m_k$, where m_k are extracted minima of $\varphi(t)$.

The described approach can be applied to multivariate minimization. We shall illustrate this for the two-dimensional case when $\mathcal{D}$ is a rectangle shown in Fig. 3.37.

In this case, the input $u(t)$ to the Preisach minimizer coincides with $\varphi(t)$ traced upwards along the vertical line 1 during the interval $[0, T]$ then it coincides with $\varphi(t)$ traced downwards along the vertical line 2 during the interval $[T, 2T]$, and it is defined similarly for all other vertical lines. It is apparent that the Preisach circuit minimizer will detect and store the global minima at all these vertical lines. This approach is very effective when the data along these vertical lines are available in analog form. This is the case when these data are obtained as a result of measurements. The described approach can be generalized to higher dimensions, and several Preisach minimizer units can be operated in parallel. It is apparent that some smoothness of $\varphi(\vec{x})$ is tacitly assumed when minimization along discrete parallel lines is used. The same is true when finite number of $\hat{\gamma}$-elements (instead of infinite number) are used in realizations of the Preisach model (3.83).

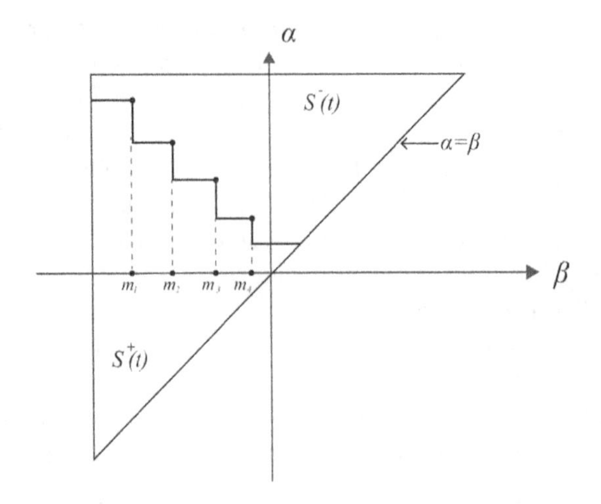

Fig. 3.35

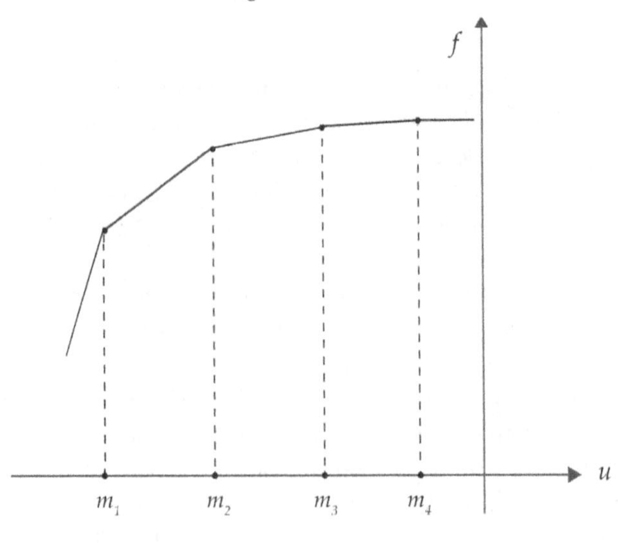

Fig. 3.36

The discussed problem of global optimization is generally regarded as a problem of high computational complexity. As a result, it has been suggested that quantum computing can be used for the solution of such problems. It is interesting to point out that the discussed Preisach based approach to the solution of global optimization problems may be realized by using classical means without resorting to quantum computing.

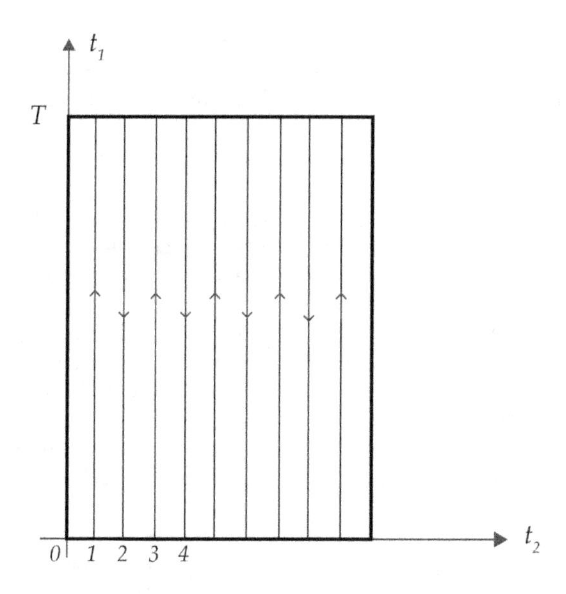

Fig. 3.37

References

[1] C. Koch, "Biophysics of Computation," Oxford University Press, 1999.
[2] P. S. Churchland and T. J. Sejnowski, "The Computational Brain," A Bradford Book, The MIT Press, 1992.
[3] P. Dayan and L. F. Abbott, "Theoretical Neuroscience," The MIT Press, 2001.
[4] C. R. Gallistel and A. P. King, "Memory and the Computational Brain," Wiley-Blackwell, 2009.
[5] H. C. Tuckwell, "Introduction to Theoretical Neurobiology," Volume 1 and Volume 2, Cambridge University Press, 1988.
[6] J. J. B. Jack, D. Noble and R. W. Tsien, "Electric Current Flow in Excitable Cells," Oxford University Press, 1983.
[7] B. Hille, "Ion Channels of Excitable Membranes," Third Edition, Sinauer Associates, Inc., 2001.
[8] V. A. Chinarov, Y. B. Gaididei, V. N. Kharkyanen and S. P. Sitko, "Ion pores in biological membranes as self-organized bistable systems," Physical Review A, Vol. 46, No. 8, pp. 5232-5241, 1992.
[9] M. A. Pustovoit, A. M. Berezhkovskii and S. M. Bezrukov, "Analytical theory of hysteresis in ion channels: two-state model," The Journal of Chemical Physics, 125(19), 194907, 2006.
[10] V. Nache, T. Eick, E. Schulz, R. Schmauder and K. Benndorf, "Hysteresis of ligand binding in CNGA2 ion channels," Nature Communications, pp. 1-9, November 29, 2013.

[11] C. Tilegenova, D. M. Cortes and L. G. Cuello, "Hysteresis of KcsA potassium channel's activation- deactivation gating is caused by structural changes at the channel's selectivity filter," PNAS, Vol. 114, No. 12, pp. 3234-3239, March 21, 2017.
[12] C. A. Villalba-Galea, "Hysteresis in voltage-gated channels," CHANNELS, Vol. 11, No. 2, pp. 140-155, 2017.
[13] H. Flyvbjerg, E. Gudowska-Nowak, P. Chrsitophersen and P. Bennekou, "Modeling Hysteresis Observed in the Human Erythrocyte Voltage-Dependent Cation Channel," Acta Physica Polonica Series B, Vol. 43, No. 11, pp. 2117-2140, November 2012.
[14] R. Männikkö, S. Pandey, H. P. Larsson and F. Elinder, "Hysteresis in the voltage dependence of HCN channels: conversion between two modes affects pacemaker properties," The Journal of General Physiology, Vol. 125, No. 3, pp. 305-326, March 2005.
[15] E. Neher and B. Sakmann, "Single-channel currents recorded from membrane of denervated frog muscle fibres," Nature, Volume 260, pp. 799-802, 29 April 1976.
[16] J. Timmer and S. Klein, "Testing the Markov condition in ion channel recordings," Physical Review E, Vol. 55, No. 3, pp. 3306-3311, 1997.
[17] A. Fulinski, Z. Grzywna, I. Mellor, Z. Siwy and P. N. R. Usherwood, "Non-Markovian character of ionic current fluctuations in membrane channels," Physical Review E, Vol. 58, No. 1, pp. 919-924, 1998.
[18] C. E. Korman and I. D. Mayergoyz, "Switching as an Exit Problem," IEEE Trans. on Magnetics, Vol. 31, No. 6, pp. 3545-3547, November, 1995.
[19] C. E. Korman and I. D. Mayergoyz, "Review of Preisach type models driven by stochastic inputs as a model for after-effect," Physica B: Condensed Matter, Vol. 233 (4), pp. 381-389, 1997.
[20] M. I. Freidlin, "Markov Processes and Differential Equations: Asymptotic Problems," Berlin: Birkhäuser-Berlin, 1996.
[21] M. E. Freidlin and A. D. Wentzell, "Diffusion Processes on Graphs and the Averaging Principle," The Annals of Probability, Vol. 21, No. 4, pp. 2215-2245, 1993.
[22] M. I. Freidlin, I. D. Mayergoyz and R. Pfeiffer, "Noise in hysteretic systems and stochastic processes on graphs," Physical Review E, Vol. 62, No. 2, pp. 1850-1855, 2000.
[23] F. Crick, "Memory and molecular turnover," Nature, Vol. 312, p. 101, 8 November 1984.
[24] R. Meagher, "'Memory and molecular turnover,' 30 years after inception," Epigenetics & Chromatin, pp. 1-9, 7(1):37, December 2014.
[25] E. R. Kandel, "The Biology of Memory: A Forty-Year Perspective," Journal of Neuroscience, Vol. 29 (41), pp. 12748-12756, 2009.
[26] T. V. P. Bliss and T. Lomo, "Long-lasting potentiation of synaptic transmission in the dentate area of the anaesthetized rabbit following stimulation of the perforant path," J. Physiol., Vol. 232 (2), pp. 331-356, 1973.
[27] W. A. Catterall, "Structure and Function of Voltage-Gated Sodium Channels at Atomic Resolution," Exp Physiol., 99(1), January 2014.

[28] I. D. Mayergoyz, W. W. Destler and F. P. Emad, "Application of intense relativistic electron beams to the switching of high currents in high power electrical networks," Journal of Applied Physics, Vol. 53, No. 11, pp. 7189-7194, 1982.
[29] A. L. Hodgkin and A. F. Huxley, "Currents Carried by Sodium and Potassium Ions Through the Membrance of the Giant Axon of Loligo," J. Physiol., Vol. 116, pp. 449-472, 1952.
[30] A. L. Hodgkin and A. F. Huxley, "The Components of Membrance Conductance in the Giant Axon of Loligo," J. Physiol., Vol. 116, pp. 473-496, 1952.
[31] A. L. Hodgkin and A. F. Huxley, "The dual effect of membrane potential on sodium conductance in the giant axon of Loligo," J. Physiol., Vol. 116 (4), pp. 497-506, 1952.
[32] A. L. Hodgkin and A. F. Huxley, "A quantitative description of membrane current and its application to conduction and excitation in nerve," J. Physiol., Vol. 117 (4), pp. 500-544, 1952.
[33] B. G. Cragg and H. N. Temperley, "Memory: The analogy with ferromagnetic hysteresis," Brain, London 78(2), pp. 304-16, 1955.
[34] A. Katchalsky and E. Neumann, "Hysteresis and Molecular Memory Record," International Journal of Neuroscience, Vol. 3, Issue 4, pp. 175-182, 1972.
[35] I. D. Mayergoyz, "Mathematical Models of Hysteresis," Phys. Rev. Lett., Vol. 56, pp. 1518-1521, 1986.
[36] J. Maddox, "Is there inanimate memory?," Nature, Vol. 321, p. 11, 1986.
[37] K. Lashley, "In search of the engram," Symposium of the Society for Experimental Biology, Vol. 4, Cambridge University Press, New York, 1950.
[38] C. Koch, "Computation and the single neuron," Nature, Vol. 385, pp. 207-210, 1997.
[39] M. A. Sutton and E. M. Schuman, "Dendritic Protein Synthesis, Synaptic Plasticity, and Memory," Cell, Vol. 127 (1), pp. 49-58, 2006.
[40] C. Hanus and E. M. Schuman, "Proteostasis in complex dendrites," Nat. Rev. Neurosci., Vol. 14, pp. 638-648, 2013.
[41] E. Schuman, "The Remarkable Neuron: Erin Schuman at TEDxCaltech," www.youtube.com.
[42] E. R. Kandel, "The molecular biology of memory: cAMP, PKA, CRE, CREB-1, CREB-2, and CPEB," Molecular Brain, Vol. 5 (14), pp. 1-12, 2012.
[43] F. Crick and C. Koch, "A framework for consciousness," Nature Neuroscience, Vol. 6 (2), pp. 119-126, 2003.
[44] I. Daubechies, "Ten Lectures on Wavelets," SIAM, 1992.
[45] I. M. Filanovsky and H. Baltes, "CMOS Schmitt trigger design," IEEE Transactions on Circuits and Systems, Vol. 41 (1), pp. 46-49, 1994.
[46] K. Madhuri, A. Srinivasulu, C. Shaker and I. Priyadarsini, "Two New CMOS Schmitt Trigger Circuits based on Current Sink and Pseudo Logic Structures," IJCA Proceedings on International Conference on Communication, Circuits and Systems, 1-24, 2013.

[47] I. D. Mayergoyz, "Mathematical Models of Hysteresis", Springer, 1991.
[48] V. R. Almeida and M. Lipson, "Optical bistability on a silicon chip," Optics Letters, Vol. 29 (20), pp. 2387-2389, 2004.

Chapter 4

Hysteresis Driven by Random Processes

4.1 Basic Facts About Stochastic Processes and Hysteresis Driven by I.I.D. Processes

It is discussed in the previous chapters that the physical origin of hysteresis is due to the multiplicity of metastable states. Under temporally constant external conditions, the presence of random (thermal) noise may cause a hysteretic system to move from one metastable state to another. This usually results in gradual (slow in time) state changes of hysteretic systems, as well as their temporal loss of memory. This phenomenon can be of practical significance in various applications where hysteresis is utilized. One important example is the magnetic data storage technology where the above phenomenon is detrimental as far as the long-time reliability of recorded information is concerned. In neural science, this phenomenon may result in gradual erasure of memory traces (memory engrams), which manifests itself as fading memory. In ion channels, the thermal noise leads to persisting temporal changes of conformational (metastable) states of channel proteins. This results in intrinsically stochastic behavior of individual channels as reflected in patch-clamp recordings of ion channel currents (see Section 3.2).

In this chapter, the effects of noise in hysteretic systems is discussed. The adopted approach is based on modelling of thermal noise as a stochastic (random) input to hysteretic systems. This approach is based on the theory of stochastic processes [1]–[2]. The very basic facts of this theory are summarized in this section without going into subtle mathematical discussions and proofs. Furthermore, the analysis of hysteresis driven by a very simple discrete-time i.i.d (independent identically distributed) random process is presented in this section as well [4]–[6].

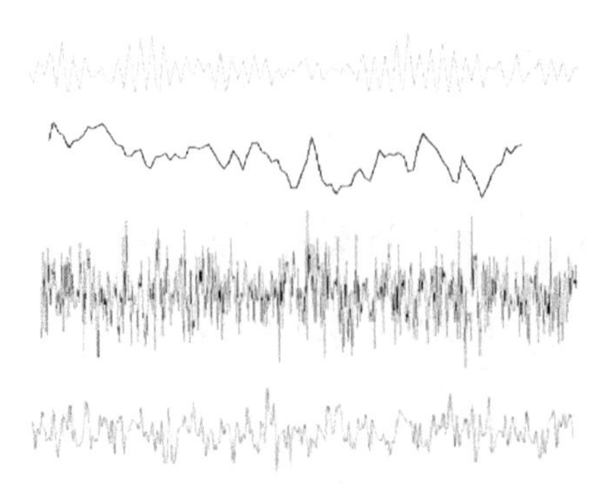

Fig. 4.1

We begin with the stochastic process definition. A stochastic process is an infinite collection (set) of random variables indexed by time (or an integer). This implies that stochastic processes describe systems, which evolve probabilistically in time and are described by random functions of time. The notation x_t is often used for these functions to distinguish them from deterministic functions. There are infinite number of random realizations (random samples) of stochastic processes. Some of these realizations in the case of time-continuous process are schematically shown in Fig. 4.1. Since these realizations are random, this implies that a probability measure can be introduced on this set of continuous functions to compute the probabilities of various subsets of realizations of random process x_t. The given descriptive (not mathematically rigorous) definition suggests that a stochastic process is a set of functions (i.e., realizations) with a probabilistic measure on them.

Another way to describe stochastic processes is by using joint probability densities. Namely, consider random variables $x_1, x_2, \cdots, x_n$ which are random values of x_t at time instants $t_1, t_2, \cdots, t_n$, respectively. Then, the joint probability density

$$\rho\big(x_1, t_1; x_2, t_2; \cdots x_n, t_n\big) \tag{4.1}$$

can be introduced. In this way, stochastic processes can be characterized by a set of joint probability densities constructed for different times $t_1, t_2, \cdots, t_n$ and different n. A very simple case of stochastic processes is when random variables $x_1, x_2, \cdots, x_n$ are independent. In this case, we find that

$$\rho(x_1, t_1; x_2, t_2; \cdots x_n, t_n) = \prod_k \rho(x_k, t_k) . \tag{4.2}$$

A more complicated case is the Markov stochastic process. To define this process, we introduce the time instants

$$t_1 > t_2 > \cdots > t_n > \tilde{t}_1 > \tilde{t}_2 > \cdots > \tilde{t}_m \tag{4.3}$$

and the conditional probability density

$$\rho(x_1, t_1; x_2, t_2; \cdots x_n, t_n | \tilde{x}_1, \tilde{t}_1; \tilde{x}_2, \tilde{t}_2; \cdots \tilde{x}_m, \tilde{t}_m) . \tag{4.4}$$

For Markov processes, the following property is valid:

$$\begin{aligned} &\rho(x_1, t_1; x_2, t_2; \cdots x_n, t_n | \tilde{x}_1, \tilde{t}_1; \tilde{x}_2, \tilde{t}_2; \cdots \tilde{x}_m, \tilde{t}_m) \\ &\qquad = \rho(x_1, t_1; x_2, t_2; \cdots x_n, t_n | \tilde{x}_1, \tilde{t}_1) . \end{aligned} \tag{4.5}$$

This property reveals that Markov processes have a short memory. Namely, only the last past measurement of $\tilde{x}_1$ at $\tilde{t}_1$ affects the conditional probability density of future measurements $x_1, x_2, \cdots, x_n$ at time instants $t_1, t_2, \cdots, t_n$, respectively. By using property (4.5), it can be proven that

$$\begin{aligned} &\rho(x_1, t_1; x_2, t_2; \cdots x_n, t_n) = \\ &\quad = \rho(x_1, t_1 | x_2, t_2) \rho(x_2, t_2 | x_3, t_3) \cdots \rho(x_{n-1}, t_{n-1} | x_n, t_n) \rho(x_n, t_n) . \end{aligned} \tag{4.6}$$

This means that the transition probability density $\rho(x, t | y, \tau)$ completely defines a Markov process.

We next consider Markov processes with continuous in time samples (realizations). The simplest and most studied example of such processes is the Wiener process W_t. This is the stochastic process with independent increments which are Gaussian random variables. More precisely, the following properties define the Wiener process:

a)

$$W_0 = 0 ; \tag{4.7}$$

b) independent (uncorrelated) increments:

$$E\Big[(W_{t_1} - W_{t_2})(W_{t_3} - W_{t_4})\Big] = 0 , \tag{4.8}$$

where $t_4 < t_3 < t_2 < t_1$ and $E[\,]$ is the notation for the expected (mean) value;

c) $W_{t_1} - W_{t_2}$ (with $t_1 > t_2 \geq 0$) is a Gaussian random variable with zero mean:

$$E\Big[W_{t_1} - W_{t_2}\Big] = 0 \tag{4.9}$$

and variance:

$$E\Big[\big(W_{t_1} - W_{t_2}\big)^2\Big] = t_1 - t_2 \ . \tag{4.10}$$

It can be shown that the Wiener process has continuous in time samples which are not differentiable at any instant of time t. Furthermore, it can also be shown that the realizations of the Wiener process satisfy with probability one the following Hölder condition:

$$\big|W_t - W_s\big| < C\big|t - s\big|^{\alpha} \ , \tag{4.11}$$

where

$$0 \leq \alpha \leq 0.5 \ . \tag{4.12}$$

The last fact is consistent with the property (see (4.10)):

$$E\Big[dW_t^2\Big] = dt \ , \tag{4.13}$$

which implies that the differential dW_t is not proportional to dt.

By using the Wiener process W_t, the broad class of Markov processes can be studied by using the stochastic differential equations:

$$\frac{dx_t}{dt} = b\big(x_t, t\big) + \sigma\big(x_t, t\big)\frac{dW_t}{dt} \ . \tag{4.14}$$

These are processes with continuous time samples and they are called diffusion processes. The term $b(x_t, t)$ in the last equation describes the drift phenomenon, while the term $\sigma(x_t, t)dW_t/dt$ describes random diffusion. The last equation is often written in the form:

$$dx_t = b\big(x_t, t\big)dt + \sigma\big(x_t, t\big)dW_t \ . \tag{4.15}$$

There are technical difficulties related to the mathematical interpretation of equation (4.14). These difficulties are related to the meaning of the derivative dW_t/dt in view of the fact that samples of the Wiener process W_t are not differentiable. These difficulties are circumvented by reducing the stochastic differential equation (4.14) to the following integral equation:

$$x_{t+s} - x_t = \int_t^{t+s} b\big(x_\lambda, \lambda\big)d\lambda + \int_t^{t+s} \sigma\big(x_\lambda, \lambda\big)dW_\lambda \ , \tag{4.16}$$

and by defining the solution of equation (4.14) as the solution of the above integral equation.

The second integral in equation (4.16) is called a stochastic integral. It can be approximated by an integral sum and defined as a limit of this sum:

$$\int_{t}^{t+s} \sigma(x_\lambda, \lambda) dW_\lambda = \lim_{n\to\infty} \sum_{k=1}^{n} \sigma(x_{\tilde{\lambda}_k}, \tilde{\lambda}_k)(W_{\lambda_{k+1}} - W_{\lambda_k}) . \quad (4.17)$$

It turns out that this limit depends on the choice of $\tilde{\lambda}_k$. The simplest choice is when $\tilde{\lambda}_k = \lambda_k$ because for this choice $\sigma(x_{\tilde{\lambda}_k}, \tilde{\lambda}_k)$ is uncorrelated with the Wiener process increment $W_{\lambda_{k+1}} - W_{\lambda_k}$. This choice leads to the Itô stochastic integral and the Itô solution of equation (4.14). Another choice is $\tilde{\lambda}_k = (\lambda_{k+1} + \lambda_k)/2$, and it leads to the Stratonovich solution of stochastic differential equation (4.14). The detailed discussion of these issues can be found in books with mathematically rigorous expositions of the stochastic process theory. This discussion is beyond the scope of this brief review. We shall only mention that the Itô solution can be reduced to the Stratonovich solution by appropriately modifying the drift term in stochastic differential equation (4.14). In the discussion below, it is assumed that the solution of equation (4.14) is defined in the Itô sense.

The Markov process defined by equation (4.14) can be also characterized by the transition probability density $\rho(x, t|y, \tau)$. It can be shown that this transition probability density satisfies the following partial differential equation:

$$\frac{\partial}{\partial t}\rho(x, t|y, \tau) = -\frac{\partial}{\partial x}\Big[b(x, t)\rho(x, t|y, \tau)\Big] + \frac{1}{2}\frac{\partial^2}{\partial x^2}\Big[\sigma^2(x, t)\rho(x, t|y, \tau)\Big] . \quad (4.18)$$

This is the equation with respect to so-called "forward" variables x and t of the transition probability density. It is often called the forward Kolmogorov equation. It turns out that there is also the partial differential equation with respect to the backward coordinates y and τ. This equation can be written as follows.

$$\frac{\partial}{\partial \tau}\rho(x, t|y, \tau) = -b(x, t)\frac{\partial}{\partial y}\rho(x, t|y, \tau) + \frac{1}{2}\sigma^2(x, t)\frac{\partial^2}{\partial y^2}\rho(x, t|y, \tau) . \quad (4.19)$$

The last equation is often called the backward Kolmogorov equation.

It is clear from the presented discussion that stochastic processes can be studied on two equivalent levels. They can be studied on the level of random realizations (samples) by solving the **nonlinear stochastic** ordinary differential equation (4.14). This is typically done by using Monte Carlo simulations. The stochastic processes can also be studied on the level of transition probability density $\rho(x, t|y, \tau)$. This requires the solution of

linear and **deterministic** equations (4.18) or (4.19). However, these are partial differential equations. Our subsequent analysis will be by and large carried out in terms of transition probability density.

In mathematics, the Wiener process and its time derivative (i.e., white noise) are used to generate a class of diffusion processes described by stochastic differential equation (4.14). In physics, the last term in equation (4.14) is used for the description of thermal noise, and the equation of the similar type as (4.14) is usually called the Langevin equation. The corresponding equation (4.18) for the transition probability density is known in physics as the Fokker-Planck equation.

Next, we consider one special diffusion process that can also be used for the modelling of realistic noise. This is the Ornstein-Uhlenbeck process. This is the stationary Gaussian Markov process. The term stationary means that all properties of the process are invariant with respect to time translations.

The Ornstein-Uhlenbeck process is described by the following stochastic differential equation:

$$dx_t = -kx_t dt + \sigma dW_t \ , \tag{4.20}$$

where k and σ are some constants. In terms of the transition probability density, the Ornstein-Uhlenbeck process is described by the following partial differential equation:

$$\frac{\partial \rho}{\partial t} = \frac{\partial}{\partial x}(kx\rho) + \frac{\sigma^2}{2}\frac{\partial^2 \rho}{\partial x^2} \ . \tag{4.21}$$

Next, we shall find the stationary distribution $\rho_{st}(x)$ of this process. For this distribution

$$\frac{\partial \rho_{st}}{\partial t} = 0 \tag{4.22}$$

and equation (4.21) is reduced to the ordinary differential equation

$$\frac{d}{dx}\left[kx\rho_{st} + \frac{\sigma^2}{2}\frac{d\rho_{st}}{dx}\right] = 0 \ , \tag{4.23}$$

which leads to

$$kx\rho_{st} + \frac{\sigma^2}{2}\frac{d\rho_{st}}{dx} = 0 \ . \tag{4.24}$$

The right-hand side of equation (4.24) is chosen to be zero instead of some constant because it is consistent with thermal equilibrium. As a result, the last equation can be written as:

$$d(\ln \rho_{st}) = -\frac{k}{\sigma^2} d(x^2) \ . \tag{4.25}$$

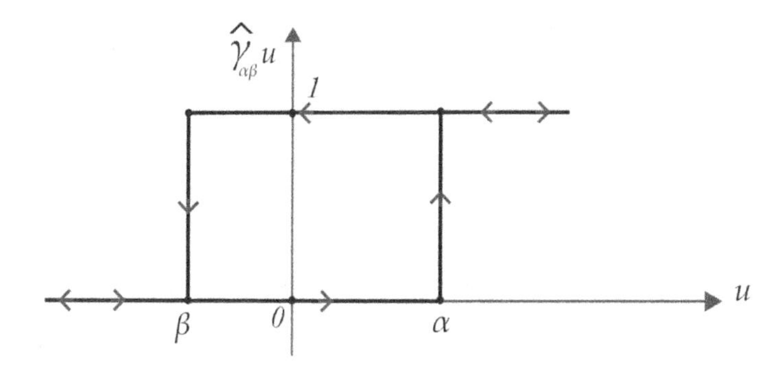

Fig. 4.2

By integrating and using the proper normalization for ρ_{st}, we finally obtain the following Gaussian stationary distribution:

$$\rho_{st}(x) = \sqrt{\frac{k}{\pi\sigma^2}} \exp\left(-\frac{kx^2}{\sigma^2} \right) . \tag{4.26}$$

In the previous discussion, we dealt with time-continuous Markov processes with continuous in time samples. There are also jump-noise type Markov processes whose samples are discontinuous functions of time. The simplest example of such processes is the discrete time i.i.d processes X_n with the property that for different n random variables X_n are independent and identically distributed. The latter means that they have the same probability density function. The analysis of hysteresis driven by the i.i.d process is relatively simple and presented below.

We begin with the case of rectangular hysteresis loop shown in Fig. 4.2. We consider this loop driven by the stochastic process

$$x_n = u + X_n . \tag{4.27}$$

It will be assumed that

$$\bar{X}_n = 0 , \tag{4.28}$$

where $\bar{X}_n$ stands for the expected value of X_n. Consequently,

$$\bar{x}_n = u , \tag{4.29}$$

where u is a constant in time value of deterministic input. If $\bar{X}_n \neq 0$, then the value $\bar{X}_n$ can be accounted for in the value of u.

We shall first introduce the notation:

$$q_{\alpha\beta}(n) = P\big(\hat{\gamma}_{\alpha\beta} x_n = 1\big) , \tag{4.30}$$

where the symbol P stands for probability. It is clear that

$$P\big(\hat{\gamma}_{\alpha\beta}x_n = 1\big) + P\big(\hat{\gamma}_{\alpha\beta}x_n = 0\big) = 1 \ . \tag{4.31}$$

Consequently,

$$P\big(\hat{\gamma}_{\alpha\beta}x_n = 0\big) = 1 - q_{\alpha\beta}(n) \ . \tag{4.32}$$

It is also clear that

$$E\big(\hat{\gamma}_{\alpha\beta}x_n\big) = P\big(\hat{\gamma}_{\alpha\beta}x_n = 1\big) = q_{\alpha\beta}(n) \ . \tag{4.33}$$

Our goal is to derive the analytical expression for $q_{\alpha\beta}(n)$. To do this, we shall first derive the finite difference equation for $q_{\alpha\beta}(n)$. This derivation is based on the following total probability relation:

$$\begin{aligned} P\big(\hat{\gamma}_{\alpha\beta}x_{n+1} = 1\big) = P\big(\hat{\gamma}_{\alpha\beta}x_{n+1} = 1 \big| \hat{\gamma}_{\alpha\beta}x_n = 1\big) P\big(\hat{\gamma}_{\alpha\beta}x_n = 1\big) \\ + P\big(\hat{\gamma}_{\alpha\beta}x_{n+1} = 1 \big| \hat{\gamma}_{\alpha\beta}x_n = 0\big) P\big(\hat{\gamma}_{\alpha\beta}x_n = 0\big) \ . \end{aligned} \tag{4.34}$$

We now introduce the following switching probabilities

$$P^{++}_{\alpha\beta}(n) = P\big(\hat{\gamma}_{\alpha\beta}x_{n+1} = 1 \big| \hat{\gamma}_{\alpha\beta}x_n = 1\big) \ , \tag{4.35}$$

$$P^{+0}_{\alpha\beta}(n) = P\big(\hat{\gamma}_{\alpha\beta}x_{n+1} = 0 \big| \hat{\gamma}_{\alpha\beta}x_n = 1\big) \ . \tag{4.36}$$

It is apparent that

$$P^{++}_{\alpha\beta}(n) + P^{+0}_{\alpha\beta}(n) = 1 \ . \tag{4.37}$$

Similarly,

$$P^{0+}_{\alpha\beta}(n) = P\big(\hat{\gamma}_{\alpha\beta}x_{n+1} = 1 \big| \hat{\gamma}_{\alpha\beta}x_n = 0\big) \ , \tag{4.38}$$

$$P^{00}_{\alpha\beta}(n) = P\big(\hat{\gamma}_{\alpha\beta}x_{n+1} = 0 \big| \hat{\gamma}_{\alpha\beta}x_n = 0\big) \ , \tag{4.39}$$

and

$$P^{0+}_{\alpha\beta}(n) + P^{00}_{\alpha\beta}(n) = 1 \ . \tag{4.40}$$

By using formulas (4.30) and (4.32) as well as the above definitions of the switching probabilities, the formula (4.34) can be written as follows

$$q_{\alpha\beta}(n+1) = P^{++}_{\alpha\beta}(n) q_{\alpha\beta}(n) + P^{0+}_{\alpha\beta}(n) \Big[1 - q_{\alpha\beta}(n)\Big] \ , \tag{4.41}$$

which can be further transformed as follows:

$$q_{\alpha\beta}(n+1) = q_{\alpha\beta}(n) \Big[P^{++}_{\alpha\beta}(n) + P^{0+}_{\alpha\beta}(n)\Big] + P^{0+}_{\alpha\beta}(n) \ . \tag{4.42}$$

Now, by using the identity (4.37), the last equation can be written as:

$$q_{\alpha\beta}(n+1) = q_{\alpha\beta}(n) \Big[1 - \big(P^{+0}_{\alpha\beta}(n) + P^{0+}_{\alpha\beta}(n)\big)\Big] + P^{0+}_{\alpha\beta}(n) \ . \tag{4.43}$$

According to the definitions of switching probabilities and Fig. 4.2, we find:

$$P^{0+}_{\alpha\beta}(n) = P\big(x_{n+1} > \alpha\big|\hat{\gamma}_{\alpha\beta}x_n = 0\big) \ , \tag{4.44}$$

$$P^{+0}_{\alpha\beta}(n) = P\big(x_{n+1} < \beta\big|\hat{\gamma}_{\alpha\beta}x_n = 1\big) \ . \tag{4.45}$$

Now, by taking into account that x_n is related to X_n by formula (4.27), we conclude that x_n are independent random variables with the common probability function $\rho(x)$. Consequently, formulas (4.44) and (4.45) can be respectively represented as follows:

$$P^{0+}_{\alpha\beta}(n) = P\big(x_{n+1} > \alpha\big) = \int_{\alpha}^{\infty} \rho(x)dx \ , \tag{4.46}$$

$$P^{+0}_{\alpha\beta}(n) = P\big(x_{n+1} < \beta\big) = \int_{-\infty}^{\beta} \rho(x)dx \ . \tag{4.47}$$

We shall next introduce the notation:

$$r_{\alpha\beta} = 1 - \left[P^{0+}_{\alpha\beta}(n) + P^{+0}_{\alpha\beta}(n)\right] \ . \tag{4.48}$$

According to the normalization condition

$$\int_{-\infty}^{\infty} \rho(x)dx = 1 \tag{4.49}$$

and formulas (4.46), (4.47) and (4.48), we find that

$$r_{\alpha\beta} = \int_{\beta}^{\alpha} \rho(x)dx \tag{4.50}$$

and

$$0 < r_{\alpha\beta} < 1 \ . \tag{4.51}$$

We shall also introduce the notation

$$d_{\alpha} = P^{0+}_{\alpha\beta}(n) < 1 \ . \tag{4.52}$$

Now, formula (4.43) can be written as follows:

$$q_{\alpha\beta}\big(n+1\big) = r_{\alpha\beta}q_{\alpha\beta}\big(n\big) + d_{\alpha} \ . \tag{4.53}$$

This is the linear finite difference equation for $q_{\alpha\beta}(n)$ with constant (i.e., independent of n) coefficients. It is clear that the latter is due to the i.i.d nature of the noise process X_n.

A general solution of the last equation has the form:

$$q_{\alpha\beta}\big(n\big) = A_{\alpha\beta}r^{n}_{\alpha\beta} + B_{\alpha\beta} \ . \tag{4.54}$$

By substituting the last formula into equation (4.53), we find:

$$A_{\alpha\beta} r_{\alpha\beta}^{n+1} + B_{\alpha\beta} = A_{\alpha\beta} r_{\alpha\beta}^{n+1} + B_{\alpha\beta} r_{\alpha\beta} + d_\alpha \ , \tag{4.55}$$

which leads to

$$B_{\alpha\beta} = \frac{d_\alpha}{1 - r_{\alpha\beta}} \ . \tag{4.56}$$

The last formula can also be written in the following two equivalent forms:

$$B_{\alpha\beta} = \frac{\int_\alpha^\infty \rho(x)dx}{1 - \int_\beta^\alpha \rho(x)dx} \ , \tag{4.57}$$

$$B_{\alpha\beta} = \frac{P_{\alpha\beta}^{0+}}{P_{\alpha\beta}^{0+} + P_{\alpha\beta}^{+0}} \ . \tag{4.58}$$

The value of $A_{\alpha\beta}$ in formula (4.54) can be determined from the initial condition

$$q_{\alpha\beta}(0) = A_{\alpha\beta} + B_{\alpha\beta} \ , \tag{4.59}$$

where

$$q_{\alpha\beta}(0) = \begin{cases} 1, & \text{if } \hat{\gamma}_{\alpha\beta} x_0 = 1 \\ 0, & \text{if } \hat{\gamma}_{\alpha\beta} x_0 = 0 \end{cases} \ . \tag{4.60}$$

From formulas (4.54) and (4.59) follows that

$$E(\hat{\gamma}_{\alpha\beta} x_n) = q_{\alpha\beta}(n) = \left[q_{\alpha\beta}(0) - B_{\alpha\beta} \right] r_{\alpha\beta}^n + B_{\alpha\beta} \ . \tag{4.61}$$

It is clear from the last equation that

$$q_{\alpha\beta}(\infty) = B_{\alpha\beta} \ , \tag{4.62}$$

which, according to formula (4.57), can be written as follows

$$\lim_{n\to\infty} E(\hat{\gamma}_{\alpha\beta} x_n) = \frac{\int_\alpha^\infty \rho(x)dx}{1 - \int_\beta^\alpha \rho(x)dx} \ . \tag{4.63}$$

Up to this point, we have discussed the case of the rectangular loop (see Fig. 4.2) driven by the i.i.d process. The obtained results can be extended to the case of the Preisach model constructed by using such loops and driven by the i.i.d process:

$$f_n = \iint_{\alpha \geq \beta} \mu(\alpha, \beta) \hat{\gamma}_{\alpha,\beta} x_n d\alpha d\beta \ . \tag{4.64}$$

Since integration is a linear operation, from the last formula we derive:

$$\bar{f}_n = \iint\limits_{\alpha \geq \beta} \mu(\alpha, \beta) E\big(\hat{\gamma}_{\alpha\beta} x_n\big) d\alpha d\beta \ . \tag{4.65}$$

Recalling the notation (4.33), the last formula can be written as follows:

$$\bar{f}_n = \iint\limits_{\alpha \geq \beta} \mu(\alpha, \beta) q_{\alpha\beta}\big(n\big) d\alpha d\beta \ . \tag{4.66}$$

From the last formula and equation (4.62), we find

$$\bar{f}_\infty = \lim_{n \to \infty} \bar{f}_n = \iint\limits_{\alpha \geq \beta} \mu(\alpha, \beta) B_{\alpha\beta} d\alpha d\beta \ . \tag{4.67}$$

Finally, from formulas (4.61), (4.66) and (4.67), we obtain

$$\bar{f}_n = \bar{f}_\infty + \iint\limits_{\alpha \geq \beta} \mu(\alpha, \beta) \Big[q_{\alpha\beta}\big(0\big) - B_{\alpha\beta} \Big] r^n_{\alpha\beta} d\alpha d\beta \ . \tag{4.68}$$

4.2 Hysteresis Driven by a Continuous-Time Noise Process

In the previous section, hysteresis driven by the discrete-time i.i.d random process was discussed. However, actual thermal noise is better described as a continuous-time random process. Mathematical analysis of hysteresis driven by a such process is a difficult problem. It is argued below that these difficulties can be mostly overcome by using the mathematical machinery of exit problems for stochastic processes [4], [7]–[10].

We start with the case of rectangular loop shown in Fig. 4.2 and assume that its driven by the stochastic process defined as

$$x_t = u_0 + X_t \ , \tag{4.69}$$

where u_0 is the initial value of the input to the hysteresis loop, while X_t is a stationary diffusion process specified by the stochastic differential equation

$$dX_t = b\big(X_t\big) dt + \sigma\big(X_t\big) dW_t \ . \tag{4.70}$$

A random output i_t of a stochastically driven rectangular loop can be written as

$$i_t = \hat{\gamma}_{\alpha\beta} x_t \ . \tag{4.71}$$

This output is a random binary process schematically shown in Fig. 4.3. Our goal is to completely mathematically describe this random non-Markovian process i_t, which is generated as a result of random switching

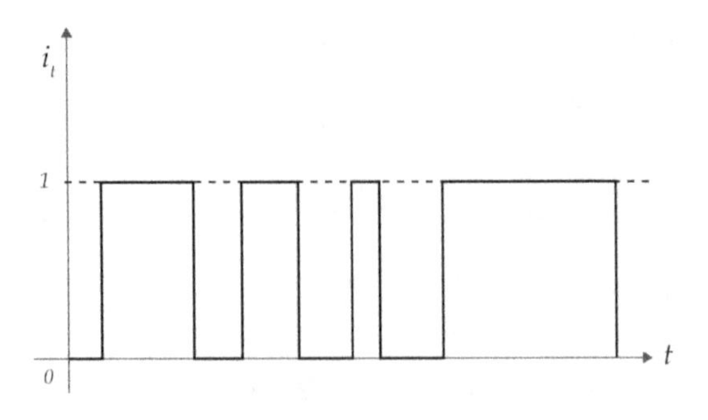

Fig. 4.3

of rectangular loop $\hat{\gamma}_{\alpha\beta}$. This will be accomplished by treating random switching as a set of exit problems for the random process X_t. Indeed, consider the case when the initial value of input and output are as follows:

$$u_0 < \alpha \quad \text{and} \quad i_0 = 0 \, . \tag{4.72}$$

Then, it is clear that the random upward switching of the rectangular loop $\hat{\gamma}_{\alpha\beta}$ occurs when the stochastic process X_t starting from the point $X_0 = 0$ exits **for the first time** the bold semi-infinite line shown in Fig. 4.4a at the point $\alpha - u_0$. Subsequently, the process switches to the branch $\hat{\gamma}_{\alpha\beta} x_t = 1$. The second random switching (downward) of the rectangular loop $\hat{\gamma}_{\alpha\beta}$ occurs when the stochastic process X_t starting from the point $\alpha - u_0$ exits the bold semi-infinite line shown in Fig. 4.4b at the point $\beta - u_0$, and the process switches back to the branch $\hat{\gamma}_{\alpha\beta} x_t = 0$. The third random switching (upward) of the rectangular loop $\hat{\gamma}_{\alpha\beta}$ occurs when the stochastic process X_t starting from the point $\beta - u_0$ exits the bold semi-infinite line shown in Fig. 4.4c at the point $\alpha - u_0$. It is clear that all subsequent even switchings occur in the same way as the second switching, while all subsequent odd switchings occur in the same manner as the third switching. Thus, it can be concluded that the random switchings of rectangular loop $\hat{\gamma}_{\alpha\beta}$ can be mathematically framed as the aforementioned sequence of exit problems for the stochastic process X_t.

The described exit problems are characterized by three random exit times:

$$\tau_0^+, \quad \tau_{\alpha - u_0}^0, \quad \tau_{\beta - u_0}^+ \, , \tag{4.73}$$

where subscripts correspond to the starting points, while superscripts indicate upward and downward switching caused by the exits of the stochastic process. It is apparent that random time $\tau_{\alpha-u_0}^0$ determines the random

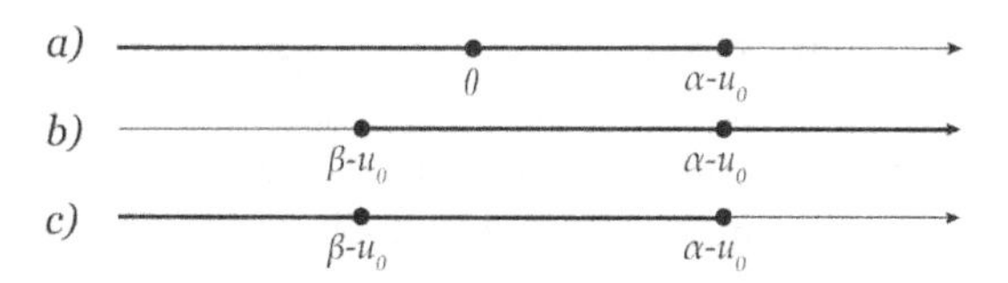

Fig. 4.4

width of rectangular pulses in Fig. 4.3, while random time $\tau^+_{\beta-u_0}$ determines the random time separation between rectangular pulses. For this reason, the statistics of random exit times τ^+_0, $\tau^0_{\alpha-u_0}$ and $\tau^+_{\beta-u_0}$ completely characterize the random binary process shown in Fig. 4.3.

Next, we shall describe the mathematical technique for the determination of these statistics. To this end, we first introduce the functions

$$v^+(x,t) = P\big(\tau^+_x \geq t\big) \tag{4.74}$$

and

$$V^+(x,t) = e(t) - v^+(x,t) \ , \tag{4.75}$$

where $e(t)$ is the unit step function. It is clear from the last two formulas that

$$V^+(x,t) = P\big(\tau^+_x < t\big) \ , \tag{4.76}$$

which means that $V^+(x,t)$ has the meaning of the probability distribution function of random exit time τ^+_x. Thus, if the function $v^+(x,t)$ is found, then the statistics of random time τ^+_x is known.

The function $v^+(x,t)$ can also be defined as

$$v^+(x,t) = P\big(X_s < \alpha - u_0, \quad 0 \leq s \leq t\big) \ , \tag{4.77}$$

which is consistent with the previous definition (4.74).

The last formula can be used to derive the initial-boundary value problem for the function $v^+(x,t)$. The derivation proceeds as follows. Let $\rho(\tilde{x},t|x,0)$ be the transition probability density for the process X_t inside the semi-infinite interval $(-\infty, \alpha - u_0]$. Then, according to the formula (4.77), we find

$$v^+(x,t) = \int_{-\infty}^{\alpha-u_0} \rho(\tilde{x},t|x,0)d\tilde{x} \ , \tag{4.78}$$

where $\rho(\tilde{x}, t|x, 0)$ is zero (absorbing boundary condition) at $\alpha - u_0$, indicating the exit of the process from the branch $\hat{\gamma}_{\alpha\beta}x_t = 0$. Since the process X_t is stationary, the transition probability density $\rho(\tilde{x}, t|x, 0)$ is invariant with respect to the translation of time. This implies that

$$\rho(\tilde{x}, t|x, 0) = \rho(\tilde{x}, 0|x, -t) . \tag{4.79}$$

By using the last identity, formula (4.78) can be written as follows:

$$v^+(x, t) = \int_{-\infty}^{\alpha - u_0} \rho(\tilde{x}, 0|x, -t)d\tilde{x} . \tag{4.80}$$

Next, we shall use the following backward Kolmogorov (Fokker-Planck) equation for $\rho(\tilde{x}, 0|x, -t)$:

$$\frac{\partial \rho(\tilde{x}, 0|x, -t)}{\partial t} = b(x)\frac{\partial}{\partial x}\rho(\tilde{x}, 0|x, -t) + \frac{\sigma^2(x)}{2}\frac{\partial^2}{\partial x^2}\rho(\tilde{x}, 0|x, -t) . \tag{4.81}$$

It is also clear that the transition probability density $\rho(\tilde{x}, 0|x, -t)$ satisfies the following initial condition:

$$\rho(\tilde{x}, 0|x, 0) = \delta(x - \tilde{x}) . \tag{4.82}$$

By integrating the last two equations with respect to $\tilde{x}$ from $-\infty$ to $\alpha - u_0$ and taking into account the formula (4.80), we respectively derive that

$$\frac{\partial v^+(x, t)}{\partial t} = b(x)\frac{\partial v^+(x, t)}{\partial x} + \frac{\sigma^2(x)}{2}\frac{\partial^2 v^+(x, t)}{\partial x^2} , \tag{4.83}$$

$$v^+(x, 0) = 1 . \tag{4.84}$$

It is also clear that, according to the definition of $v^+(x, t)$ and $\rho(\tilde{x}, t|x, 0)$, the following (absorbing) boundary condition is valid:

$$v^+(\alpha - u_0, t) = 0 . \tag{4.85}$$

Thus, the problem of calculation of function $v^+(x, t)$ is reduced to the solution of the initial boundary value problem (4.83), (4.84), and (4.85). If this problem is solved, the probability distribution function $V^0(x, t)$ for the random exit time τ_x^0 can be found in a similar way by introducing the functions

$$v^0(x, t) = P(\tau_x^0 \geq t) , \tag{4.86}$$

$$V^0(x, t) = e(t) - v^0(x, t) . \tag{4.87}$$

The above functions have the following equivalent definitions, respectively,

$$v^0(x, t) = P(X_s > \beta - u_0, \ \ 0 \leq s \leq t) , \tag{4.88}$$

$$V^0(x,t) = P(\tau_x^0 < t) \ . \tag{4.89}$$

Furthermore, the following formula is valid for $v^0(x,t)$:

$$v^0(x,t) = \int_{\beta - u_0}^{\infty} \rho(\tilde{x}, t|x, 0) d\tilde{x} \ . \tag{4.90}$$

Here, $\rho(\tilde{x}, t|x, 0)$ is the transition probability density function of the process X_t defined on the semi-infinite interval $[\beta - u_0, \infty)$ with zero (absorbing boundary condition) at $\beta - u_0$, reflecting the exit of the process from the branch $\hat{\gamma}_{\alpha\beta} x_t = 1$. Now, by almost literally repeating the same line of reasoning that was used for the function $v^+(x,t)$, we derive the following initial-boundary value problem for $v^0(x,t)$:

$$\frac{\partial v^0(x,t)}{\partial t} = b(x)\frac{\partial v^0(x,t)}{\partial x} + \frac{\sigma^2(x)}{2}\frac{\partial^2 v^0(x,t)}{\partial x^2} \ , \tag{4.91}$$

$$v^0(x,0) = 1 \ , \tag{4.92}$$

$$v^0(\beta - u_0, t) = 0 \ . \tag{4.93}$$

By solving the last problem and finding the function $v^0(x,t)$, the probability distribution function $V^0(x,t)$, for the random exit time τ_x^0 can be found by using formula (4.87).

Equations (4.83) and (4.91) are partial differential equations with variable coefficients with respect to x. Such equations are difficult to solve. However, in a special case when X_t is the Ornstein-Uhlenbeck process, some analytical results are possible. The Ornstein-Uhlenbeck process is the stationary Gaussian Markov process. This makes it very attractive as a model of thermal noise. As discussed in the previous section, the following formulas are valid for the Ornstein-Uhlenbeck process:

$$b(x) = -bx, \quad b > 0 \tag{4.94}$$

$$\sigma(x) = \sigma = \text{ const} \tag{4.95}$$

and the equations (4.83) and (4.91) are reduced to:

$$\frac{\partial v^{\binom{+}{0}}(x,t)}{\partial t} = -bx\frac{\partial v^{\binom{+}{0}}(x,t)}{\partial x} + \frac{\sigma^2}{2}\frac{\partial^2 v^{\binom{+}{0}}(x,t)}{\partial x^2} \ . \tag{4.96}$$

By applying the Laplace transform

$$\tilde{v}^{\binom{+}{0}}(x,s) = \int_0^{\infty} v^{\binom{+}{0}}(x,t) e^{-st} dt, \quad (\Re e(s) \geq 0) \ , \tag{4.97}$$

the initial-boundary problems (4.83), (4.84), (4.85) and (4.91), (4.92), (4.93) can be reduced to the following boundary value problem for the ordinary differential equation

$$\frac{\sigma^2}{2}\frac{d^2\tilde{v}^{\binom{+}{0}}(x,s)}{dx^2} - bx\frac{d\tilde{v}^{\binom{+}{0}}(x,s)}{dx} - s\tilde{v}^{\binom{+}{0}}(x,s) = -1 , \tag{4.98}$$

$$\tilde{v}^{\binom{+}{0}}\left(c^{\binom{+}{0}}, s\right) = 0 , \tag{4.99}$$

$$\lim_{|x|\to\infty} \tilde{v}^{\binom{+}{0}}(x,s) = \frac{1}{s} , \tag{4.100}$$

where

$$c^+ = \alpha - u_0 \quad \text{and} \quad c^0 = \beta - u_0 . \tag{4.101}$$

It turns out that the analytical solutions to the boundary value problems (4.98)–(4.101) can be found in terms of parabolic cylinder functions. Namely,

$$\tilde{v}^{\binom{+}{0}}(x,s) = \frac{1}{s}\left[1 - \exp\left(\frac{x^2 - \left(c^{\binom{+}{0}}\right)^2}{4\lambda^2}\right)\frac{\mathcal{D}_{-s/b}\left(\frac{x}{\lambda}\right)}{\mathcal{D}_{-s/b}\left(\frac{c^{\binom{+}{0}}}{\lambda}\right)}\right] , \tag{4.102}$$

where

$$\lambda = \sigma/\sqrt{2b} \tag{4.103}$$

and $\mathcal{D}_{-s/b}$ are parabolic cylinder functions which are special functions and are extensively studied in mathematics [1]. Next, we introduce the probability density functions

$$g^+(x,t) = \frac{dV^+(x,t)}{dt} \tag{4.104}$$

and

$$g^0(x,t) = \frac{dV^0(x,t)}{dt} \tag{4.105}$$

for the random times τ_x^+ and τ_x^0, respectively. From formulas (4.75), (4.87), (4.104) and (4.105) we find that

$$\tilde{g}^{\binom{+}{0}}(x,s) = s\tilde{V}^{\binom{+}{0}}(x,s) = 1 - s\tilde{v}^{\binom{+}{0}}(x,s) , \tag{4.106}$$

which, according to equation (4.102), leads to:

$$\tilde{g}^{\binom{+}{0}}(x,s) = \exp\left(\frac{x^2 - \left(c^{\binom{+}{0}}\right)^2}{4\lambda^2}\right)\frac{\mathcal{D}_{-s/b}\left(\frac{x}{\lambda}\right)}{\mathcal{D}_{-s/b}\left(\frac{\tilde{c}^{\binom{+}{0}}}{\lambda}\right)} . \tag{4.107}$$

Some sample computational results of the probability density functions (pdf) of the exit times by using formula (4.107) and one-sided Fourier transform ($\Re e(s) \geq 0$) can be found in publications [9], [10].

As discussed in the previous chapter, the binary random process (see Fig. 4.3) generated by random switching of a rectangular hysteresis loop $\hat{\gamma}_{\alpha\beta}$ can be useful for the modelling of binary random channel currents observed by using the patch-clamp technique. Switching values α and β of hysteresis loop $\hat{\gamma}_{\alpha\beta}$ depend on energy barriers separating adjacent energy wells corresponding to open and closed conformational states of channel proteins. The height of the loop $\hat{\gamma}_{\alpha\beta}$ can be adjusted to reflect the actual current i_0 through the ion channels in open conformations.

The discussed problem of random switchings of a rectangular loop can be also useful for generation of random binary numbers. This is especially attractive in the emerging area of spintronics where very small and sensitive to thermal noise magnetic elements (particles) with rectangular hysteresis loops can be used for random binary number generation. The presented analysis can be of help in determining the statistical properties of such random binary numbers.

Up to this point, we have discussed the case of rectangular loops driven by stochastic processes. The obtained results can be extended to the case of the Preisach model driven by stochastic process.

$$f_t = \iint\limits_{\alpha \geq \beta} \mu(\alpha,\beta)\hat{\gamma}_{\alpha,\beta}x_t d\alpha d\beta \ . \tag{4.108}$$

We would like to compute the expected value $\bar{f}_t$ of the random output. This expected value is given by the formula:

$$\bar{f}_t = \iint\limits_{\alpha \geq \beta} \mu(\alpha,\beta) E\left(\hat{\gamma}_{\alpha,\beta}x_t\right) d\alpha d\beta \ . \tag{4.109}$$

It is clear that in the case of rectangular loops shown in Fig. 4.2, we have:

$$E\left(\hat{\gamma}_{\alpha,\beta}x_t\right) = q_{\alpha\beta}(t) \ , \tag{4.110}$$

where

$$q_{\alpha\beta}(t) = P\left(\hat{\gamma}_{\alpha,\beta}x_t = 1\right) \ . \tag{4.111}$$

Consequently, formula (4.109) can be written as

$$\bar{f}_t = \iint\limits_{\alpha \geq \beta} \mu(\alpha,\beta) q_{\alpha\beta}(t) d\alpha d\beta \ . \tag{4.112}$$

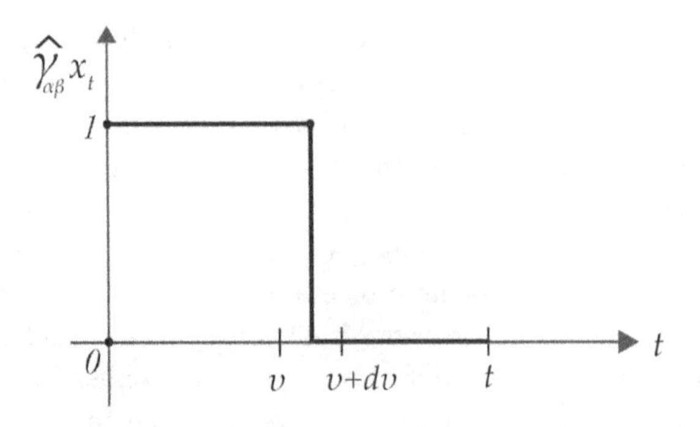

Fig. 4.5

Thus, the problem is reduced to the calculation of $q_{\alpha\beta}(t)$. The latter can be expressed in terms of switching probabilities $P_k^+(t)$ and $P_k^0(t)$, which are defined as follows:

$$P_k^+(t) = P\Big(k \text{ switchings during } (0,t)\Big|\hat{\gamma}_{\alpha,\beta}x_0 = 1\Big) , \tag{4.113}$$

$$P_k^0(t) = P\Big(k \text{ switchings during } (0,t)\Big|\hat{\gamma}_{\alpha,\beta}x_0 = 0\Big) . \tag{4.114}$$

It is clear that

$$q_{\alpha\beta}(t) = \sum_{k=0}^{\infty} P_{2k}^+(t), \text{ if } \hat{\gamma}_{\alpha,\beta}x_0 = 1 \tag{4.115}$$

and

$$q_{\alpha\beta}(t) = \sum_{k=0}^{\infty} P_{2k+1}^0(t), \text{ if } \hat{\gamma}_{\alpha,\beta}x_0 = 0 . \tag{4.116}$$

Consider first the case when $\hat{\gamma}_{\alpha,\beta}x_0 = 1$. It is clear from the definition of $\upsilon^+(x,t)$ that

$$P_0^+(t) = \upsilon^+(0,t) . \tag{4.117}$$

It is apparent from Fig. 4.5, that the occurrence of exactly one downward switching is the union of the following disjoint elementary events: downward switching occurrence in the time interval $(\nu, \nu + d\nu)$ and then no upward switching occurrence up to the time t. The probability of this elementary event, $\rho_1^+ d\nu$, is given by the formula:

$$\rho_1^+ d\nu = g^0(0,\nu)\upsilon^+(\beta - u_0, t-\nu)d\nu . \tag{4.118}$$

Now, the probability of exactly one downward switching during the time interval $(0, t)$ can be found by integrating the last formula from 0 to t:

$$P_1^+(t) = \int_0^t \rho_1^+ d\nu \ . \tag{4.119}$$

This leads to

$$P_1^+(t) = \int_0^t g^0(0, \nu) v^+(\beta - u_0, t - \nu) d\nu \ . \tag{4.120}$$

It is clear that $P_1^+(t)$ is the convolution of $g^0(0, t)$ and $v^+(\beta - u_0, t)$. Consequently, it can be written in a more concise form as

$$P_1^+(t) = g^0(0, t) * v^+(\beta - u_0, t) \ . \tag{4.121}$$

For the case when $\hat{\gamma}_{\alpha,\beta} x_0 = 0$, by using the same line of reasoning, we derive

$$P_0^0(t) = v^0(0, t) \tag{4.122}$$

and

$$P_1^0(t) = g^+(0, t) * v^0(\alpha - u_0, t) \ . \tag{4.123}$$

Next, consider the probability $P_2^+(t)$ of occurrence of exactly two switching starting from the initial state $\hat{\gamma}_{\alpha,\beta} x_0 = 1$. According to Fig. 4.6, this occurrence can be viewed as the union of the following disjoint elementary events: downward switching occurrence in the time interval $(\nu, \nu + d\nu)$ and then exactly one upward switching occurrence up to the time t. The probability of such elementary events, $\rho_2^0 d\nu$, is given by the formula:

$$\rho_2^0 d\nu = g^0(0, \nu) P_1^0(t - \nu) d\nu \ . \tag{4.124}$$

Now, the probability of exactly two switchings can be found in terms of the following convolution:

$$P_2^+(t) = \int_0^t g^0(0, \nu) P_1^0(t - \nu) d\nu \ , \tag{4.125}$$

which can also be written in the following concise form

$$P_2^+(t) = g^0(0, t) * P_1^0(t) \ . \tag{4.126}$$

By using formula (4.123), the last equation can be represented as:

$$P_2^+(t) = g^0(0, t) * g^+(\beta - u_0, t) * v^0(\alpha - u_0, t) \ . \tag{4.127}$$

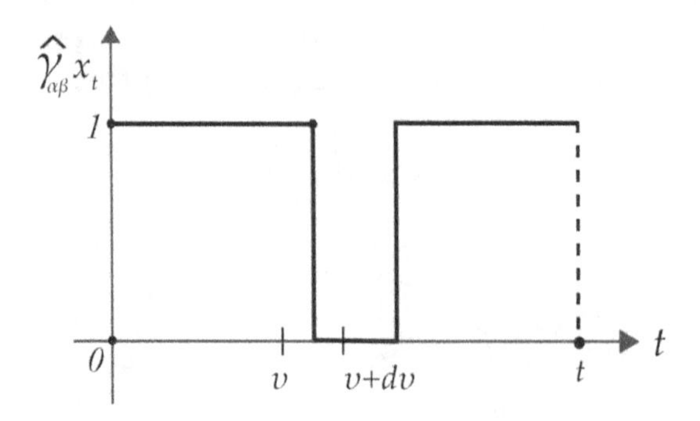

Fig. 4.6

For the sake of conciseness, we introduce the notations:

$$g^+(0,t) = g^+(t), \quad g^0(0,t) = g^0(t) \ , \tag{4.128}$$

$$g^+(\beta - u_0, t) = g^+(t), \quad g^0(\alpha - u_0, t) = g^0(t) \ , \tag{4.129}$$

$$v^+(0,t) = v_0^+(t), \quad v^0(0,t) = v_0^0(t) \ , \tag{4.130}$$

$$v^+(\beta - u_0, t) = v^+(t), \quad v^0(\alpha - u_0, t) = v^0(t) \ . \tag{4.131}$$

Now, by using the induction argument and the same line of reasoning as before, it easy to demonstrate the validity of the following formula:

$$P_{2k}^+(t) = g^0(t) * g^+(t) * \overbrace{g^0(t) * g^+(t) * \cdots * g^0(t) * g^+(t)}^{(2k-2)\ \text{terms}} * v^0(t) \ . \tag{4.132}$$

Next, we introduce the Laplace transforms:

$$\tilde{g}^+(s) = \int_0^\infty g^+(t) e^{-st} dt \ , \tag{4.133}$$

$$\tilde{g}^0(s) = \int_0^\infty g^0(t) e^{-st} dt \ , \tag{4.134}$$

$$\tilde{v}^0(s) = \int_0^\infty v^0(t) e^{-st} dt \ , \tag{4.135}$$

$$\tilde{v}^+(s) = \int_0^\infty v^+(t) e^{-st} dt \ . \tag{4.136}$$

According to formulas (4.115), (4.117), and (4.132) we have, respectively,

$$\tilde{q}_{\alpha\beta}(s) = \sum_{k=0}^{\infty} \tilde{P}_{2k}^{+}(s), \quad \text{if } \hat{\gamma}_{\alpha,\beta}x_0 = 1 \ , \tag{4.137}$$

$$\tilde{P}_0^{+}(s) = \tilde{v}_0^{+}(s) \ , \tag{4.138}$$

$$\tilde{P}_{2k}^{+}(s) = \tilde{g}^0(s)\tilde{g}^{+}(s)\tilde{v}^0(s)\left[\tilde{g}^0(s)\tilde{g}^{+}(s)\right]^{k-1} . \tag{4.139}$$

It can be proven that

$$\left|\tilde{g}^0(s)\right| < 1, \quad \left|\tilde{g}^{+}(s)\right| < 1 \ . \tag{4.140}$$

Indeed, according to equation (4.104), we have

$$\tilde{g}^{+}(s) = \int_0^{\infty} \frac{dV^{+}(x,t)}{dt} e^{-st} dt \ . \tag{4.141}$$

By taking into account that

$$\frac{dV^{+}(x,t)}{dt} \geq 0 \tag{4.142}$$

and that

$$\left|e^{-st}\right| = e^{-at}, \quad (a = \Re e(s)) \ , \tag{4.143}$$

from formula (4.141) we derive:

$$\left|\tilde{g}^{+}(s)\right| < \int_0^{\infty} \frac{dV^{+}(x,t)}{dt} e^{-at} dt < \int_0^{\infty} \frac{dV^{+}(x,t)}{dt} dt = 1 \ . \tag{4.144}$$

The inequality $|\tilde{g}^0(s)| < 1$ is similarly established.

By substituting formulas (4.138) and (4.139) into equation (4.137), we obtain:

$$\tilde{q}_{\alpha\beta}(s) = \tilde{v}_0^{+}(s) + \tilde{g}^0(s)\tilde{g}^{+}(s)\tilde{v}^0(s) \sum_{k=1}^{\infty} \left[\tilde{g}^0(s)\tilde{g}^{+}(s)\right]^{k-1} . \tag{4.145}$$

It is clear from inequalities (4.140) that the infinite sum in formula (4.145) is a converging geometric series. Consequently,

$$\tilde{q}_{\alpha\beta}(s) = \tilde{v}_0^{+}(s) + \frac{\tilde{g}^0(s)\tilde{g}^{+}(s)\tilde{v}^0(s)}{1 - \tilde{g}^0(s)\tilde{g}^{+}(s)} \ , \quad \text{if } \hat{\gamma}_{\alpha,\beta}x_0 = 1 \ . \tag{4.146}$$

Similar mathematical expression can be derived for $\tilde{q}_{\alpha\beta}(s)$ if $\hat{\gamma}_{\alpha,\beta}x_0 = 0$. These expressions along with formulas (4.102) and (4.107) can be used for calculations of $\tilde{q}_{\alpha\beta}(s)$. By performing the inverse Laplace transform $q_{\alpha\beta}(t)$ can be found. It is apparent that the described approach is very computationally expensive. For this reason, in the next section another approach is explored by using stochastic processes on graphs.

4.3 Noise in Hysteretic Systems and Stochastic Processes on Graphs

In the previous section, hysteresis driven by a continuous time and continuous sample diffusion process is discussed. The mathematical treatment of this problem is reduced to the so-called "exit problem" for diffusion processes. Although the concept of random switching as an exit problem is quite transparent from the physical point of view, its mathematical implementation is somewhat complicated. It turns out that the mathematical treatment can be simplified by using an entirely different approach based on theory of stochastic processes on graphs. This theory has recently been developed and applied to the study of random perturbations of Hamiltonian dynamical systems [11]. The main purpose of this section is to demonstrate that the mathematical machinery of this theory is naturally suitable for the analysis of random output processes of hysteretic systems. The discussion presented below closely follows the paper [12].

This discussion is based on the following simple fact. The output of the rectangular hysteresis loop $i_t = \hat{\gamma}_{\alpha\beta}\ x_t$ is a random binary process. This process is not Markovian. However, the two-component process $\vec{y}_t = \binom{i_t}{x_t}$ is Markovian. This is because the rectangular loop operators describe hysteresis with local memory. This means that joint specifications of current values of input and output uniquely define the states of this hysteresis. The two-component process $\vec{y}_t$ is defined on the four-edge graph shown in Fig. 4.7, which corresponds to rectangular loop $\hat{\gamma}_{\alpha\beta}$ with output values of ± 1. The binary process i_t presumes constant values on each edge I_k, $(k = 1, 2, 3, 4)$ of this graph.

In this section, we consider symmetric rectangular loops with output values ± 1, because this simplifies the mathematical treatment of the problem. However, the presented analysis can be used for nonsymmetric rectangular loops shown in Fig. 4.2. This is because the latter rectangular loop can be obtained from the symmetric loop by shifting its output by one half and subsequently scaling it by two.

The two component Markovian process $\vec{y}_t$ can be characterized by the transition probability density:

$$\rho(\vec{y}, t|\vec{y}_0, t_0) \tag{4.147}$$

defined on all edges of the above graph. This justifies the following equations:

$$\rho(\vec{y}, t|\vec{y}_0, t_0)\big|_{\vec{y}\in I_k} = \rho^{(k)}(x, t|\vec{y}_0, t_0)\ . \tag{4.148}$$

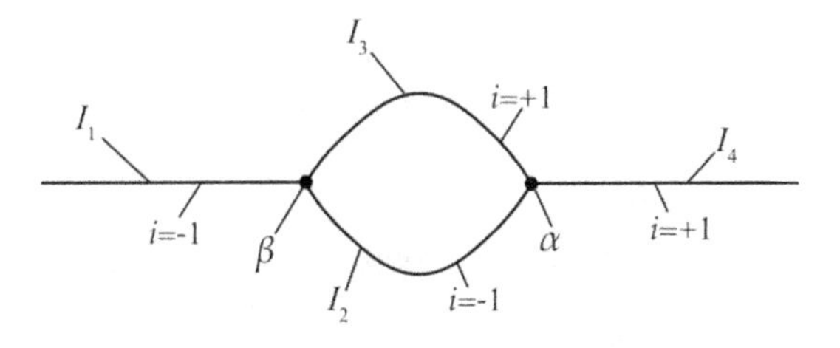

Fig. 4.7

It is apparent that

$$\rho^{(1)} = \rho, \text{ for } x \leq \beta , \tag{4.149}$$

$$\rho^{(4)} = \rho, \text{ for } x \geq \alpha , \tag{4.150}$$

and

$$\rho^{(2)} + \rho^{(3)} = \rho, \text{ for } \beta \leq x \leq \alpha , \tag{4.151}$$

where ρ is the transition probability density of the process $\vec{y}_t$, which is assumed to be known. It is also clear that on each edge of the graph the following forward Kolmogorov equation is valid

$$\frac{\partial \rho^{(k)}}{\partial t} = \frac{1}{2}\frac{\partial^2}{\partial x^2}\left[\sigma^2(x)\rho^{(k)}\right] - \frac{\partial}{\partial x}\left[b(x)\rho^{(k)}\right] . \tag{4.152}$$

Furthermore, the Markovian nature of the process $\vec{y}_t$ on the entire graph implies certain boundary conditions for $\rho^{(k)}$ at graph vertices [11]. It can be shown that these vertex boundary conditions impose continuity of transition probability density when the transition through a vertex from one graph edge to another occurs without rectangular loop switching, and zero boundary condition is imposed on the third graph edge connected to this vertex. Namely, for edge I_3 we have:

$$\rho^{(3)}\Big|_{x=\beta} = 0 , \tag{4.153}$$

while

$$\rho^{(3)}\Big|_{x=\alpha} = \rho\Big|_{x=\alpha} . \tag{4.154}$$

Similarly, for edge I_2 we find:

$$\rho^{(2)}\Big|_{x=\beta} = \rho\Big|_{x=\beta} , \tag{4.155}$$

while

$$\rho^{(2)}\Big|_{x=\alpha} = 0 . \tag{4.156}$$

In addition, the so-called probability current

$$J_k(x) = -\frac{\sigma^2(x)}{2}\frac{\partial \rho^{(k)}}{\partial x} + b(x)\rho^{(k)}(x) \tag{4.157}$$

must be conserved at each vertex. According to formulas (4.153)–(4.157), this implies the following boundary conditions:

$$\frac{\partial \rho}{\partial x}\Big|_{x=\beta} = \frac{\partial \rho^{(2)}}{\partial x}\Big|_{x=\beta} + \frac{\partial \rho^{(3)}}{\partial x}\Big|_{x=\beta}, \tag{4.158}$$

$$\frac{\partial \rho}{\partial x}\Big|_{x=\alpha} = \frac{\partial \rho^{(2)}}{\partial x}\Big|_{x=\alpha} + \frac{\partial \rho^{(3)}}{\partial x}\Big|_{x=\alpha}. \tag{4.159}$$

Furthermore, the following initial condition is valid

$$\rho(x, 0|x', 0) = \delta_{kk'}\delta(x - x'). \tag{4.160}$$

Equations (4.152) along with boundary conditions (4.153)–(4.156) and (4.158)–(4.159) as well as initial condition (4.160) completely define the dynamics of the transitional probability density for the two component Markovian process $\vec{y}_t$ on the graph shown in Fig. 4.7. The solutions to the above initial-boundary value problem can be found in terms of parabolic cylinder functions and their Laplace transforms in the case when x_t is the Ornstein-Uhlenbeck. It turns out that simple analytical results can be obtained for stationary densities $\rho_{\text{st}}^{(3)}$ and $\rho_{\text{st}}^{(2)}$. In this case, we have to deal with the following boundary value problem for ordinary differential equations: find the solution of equation

$$\frac{1}{2}\frac{d^2}{dx^2}\left[\sigma^2(x)\rho_{\text{st}}^{(3)}(x)\right] - \frac{d}{dx}\left[b(x)\rho_{\text{st}}^{(3)}(x)\right] = 0 \tag{4.161}$$

subject to the boundary conditions

$$\rho_{\text{st}}^{(3)}(\beta) = 0, \tag{4.162}$$

while

$$\rho_{\text{st}}^{(3)}(\alpha) = \rho_{\text{st}}(\alpha). \tag{4.163}$$

The above boundary conditions follow from formulas (4.153) and (4.154).

Having solved the boundary value problem (4.161)–(4.163) for $\rho_{\text{st}}^{(3)}$, $\rho_{\text{st}}^{(2)}$ can be found from formula (4.151) as

$$\rho_{\text{st}}^{(2)}(x) = \rho_{\text{st}}(x) - \rho_{\text{st}}^{(3)}(x). \tag{4.164}$$

The last equation implies that the boundary conditions (4.158) and (4.159) will be satisfied. The analytical solution to the boundary value problem (4.161)–(4.163) can be found for any stationary diffusion process x_t.

However, below we present this solution only for the important case of the Ornstien-Uhlenbeck process. By integrating equation (4.161) for this process, we find:

$$\frac{\sigma^2}{2}\frac{d\rho_{\rm st}^{(3)}}{dx} + kx\rho_{\rm st}^{(3)}(x) = C = \text{const.} \; . \tag{4.165}$$

We look for the solution of equation (4.165) in the form

$$\rho_{\rm st}^{(3)}(x) = \rho_{\rm st}(x)\varphi(x) \; , \tag{4.166}$$

where $\rho_{\rm st}(x)$ is the Gaussian stationary distribution of the Ornstein-Uhlenbeck process (see Section 4.1), while $\varphi(x)$ must be determined. By substituting formula (4.166) into equation (4.165), we find:

$$\frac{\sigma^2}{2}\rho_{\rm st}(x)\frac{d\varphi(x)}{dx} + \varphi(x)\left[\frac{\sigma^2}{2}\frac{d\rho_{\rm st}(x)}{dx} + kx\rho_{\rm st}(x)\right] = C \; . \tag{4.167}$$

For the stationary Ornstein-Uhlenbeck process, the probability current (4.157) is equal to zero, which means that

$$\frac{\sigma^2}{2}\frac{d\rho_{\rm st}(x)}{dx} + kx\rho_{\rm st}(x) = 0 \; . \tag{4.168}$$

From the last two equations, we find

$$\frac{\sigma^2}{2}\rho_{\rm st}(x)\frac{d\varphi(x)}{dx} = C \; . \tag{4.169}$$

By integrating equation (4.169) and taking into account boundary condition (4.162) and formula (4.166), we obtain:

$$\varphi(x) = \frac{2C}{\sigma^2}\int_\beta^x \frac{dy}{\rho_{\rm st}(y)} \; . \tag{4.170}$$

From boundary condition (4.163) and formula (4.166), it follows that

$$\varphi(\alpha) = 1 \; . \tag{4.171}$$

From equations (4.170) and (4.171), we find:

$$1 = \frac{2C}{\sigma^2}\int_\beta^\alpha \frac{dy}{\rho_{\rm st}(y)} \; , \tag{4.172}$$

and

$$\frac{2C}{\sigma^2} = \frac{1}{\displaystyle\int_\beta^\alpha \frac{dy}{\rho_{\rm st}(y)}} \; . \tag{4.173}$$

Now, by recalling formula (4.170), we derive

$$\varphi(x) = \frac{\displaystyle\int_\beta^x \frac{dy}{\rho_{\rm st}(y)}}{\displaystyle\int_\beta^\alpha \frac{dy}{\rho_{\rm st}(y)}} \,, \tag{4.174}$$

which according to equation (4.166) leads to

$$\rho_{\rm st}^{(3)}(x) = \rho_{\rm st}(x) \frac{\displaystyle\int_\beta^x \frac{dy}{\rho_{\rm st}(y)}}{\displaystyle\int_\beta^\alpha \frac{dy}{\rho_{\rm st}(y)}} \,, \tag{4.175}$$

where the analytical expression for $\rho_{\rm st}(x)$ is given by formula (4.26).

By using the last formula, the stationary expected value of the random binary process $i_t = \hat{\gamma}_{\alpha\beta}\, x_t$ and its variance $\sigma^2_{i_t}$ can be computed. Indeed, it is clear that

$$\bar{i_t} = E_{\rm st}\{\hat{\gamma}_{\alpha\beta}\, x_t\} = P_{\rm st}\{i_t = 1\} - P_{\rm st}\{i_t = -1\} \,. \tag{4.176}$$

Since

$$P_{\rm st}\{i_t = 1\} + P_{\rm st}\{i_t = -1\} = 1 \,, \tag{4.177}$$

we find

$$\bar{i_t} = 2P_{\rm st}\{i_t = 1\} - 1 \,. \tag{4.178}$$

On the other hand,

$$P_{\rm st}\{i_t = 1\} = \int_\beta^\alpha \rho_{\rm st}^{(3)}(x)dx + \int_\alpha^\infty \rho_{\rm st}(x)dx \,. \tag{4.179}$$

Consequently,

$$\bar{i_t} = 2\left[\int_\beta^\alpha \rho_{\rm st}^{(3)}(x)dx + \int_\alpha^\infty \rho_{\rm st}(x)dx\right] - 1 \,. \tag{4.180}$$

As soon as $\bar{i_t}$ is computed by using formulas (4.175) and (4.180), variance $\sigma^2_{i_t}$ can be calculated as well. Indeed, by using the well-known relation

$$\sigma^2_{i_t} = \bar{i^2_t} - \left(\bar{i_t}\right)^2 \tag{4.181}$$

and the fact that

$$i_t^2 = 1 \,, \tag{4.182}$$

we derive

$$\sigma^2_{i_t} = 1 - \left(\bar{i_t}\right)^2 \,. \tag{4.183}$$

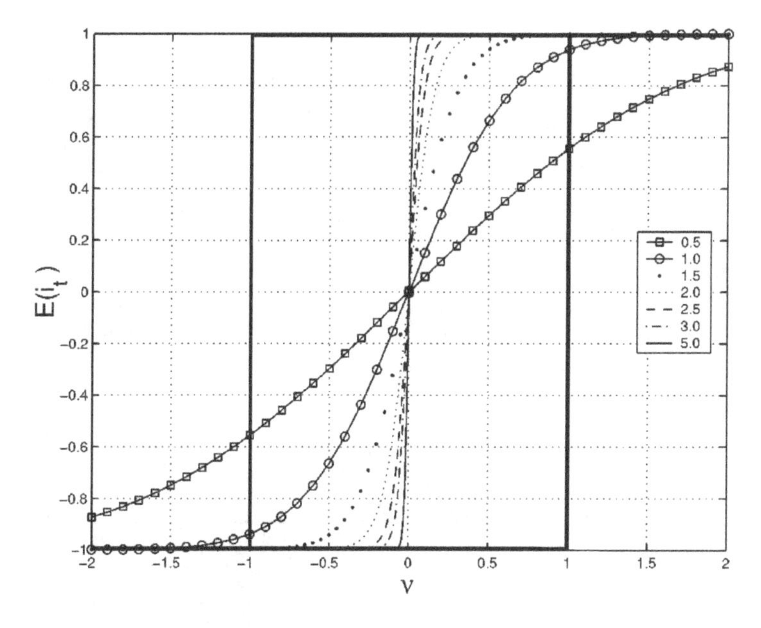

Fig. 4.8

The last formula along with equation (4.180) can be used for computations of variance $\sigma^2_{i_t}$. These computations are facilitated by the observation that

$$\int_0^x e^{y^2} dy = \frac{\sqrt{\pi}}{2} \operatorname{erfi}(x) \tag{4.184}$$

and

$$\int e^{-x^2} \operatorname{erfi}(x) dx = \frac{x^2}{\pi} \, {}_2F_2\left(1, 1; \frac{3}{2}, 2; -x^2\right) , \tag{4.185}$$

where erfi(x) and ${}_2F_2$ are the "imaginary error function" and the "generalized hypergeometric function," respectively.

By using formulas (4.175), (4.180), and (4.183), the stationary expected value $\bar{i}_t$ and variance $\sigma^2_{i_t}$ have been computed as functions of the expected ('bias') value x_0 of the input Ornstein-Uhlenbeck process x_t for symmetric rectangular loops $\hat{\gamma}_{\alpha,-\alpha} = \hat{\gamma}_\alpha$. The results of computations are presented in Figs. 4.8 and 4.9, respectively. These results are plotted for normalized x_0-values $\nu = x_0/\alpha$ and normalized values of switching thresholds $\tilde{\alpha} = \alpha/\lambda$, where $\lambda^2 = \sigma^2/b$ is the variance of the stationary distribution of Ornstein-Uhlenbeck process x_t.

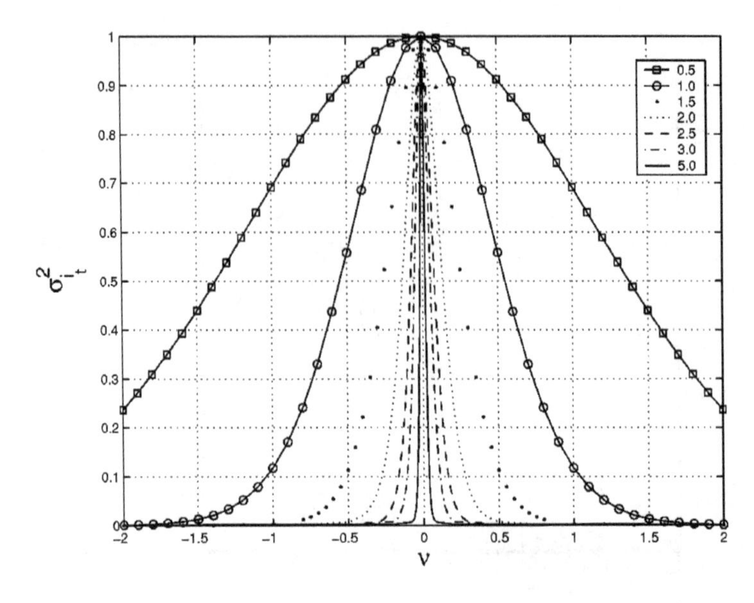

Fig. 4.9

The results obtained for the binary process $i_t = \hat{\gamma}_{\alpha\beta}$ can be used to compute the stationary characteristics of the output random process f_t of the Preisach model driven by the stochastic process x_t. Indeed, it is clear that

$$\bar{f}_t^{\text{st}} = \iint\limits_{\alpha \geq \beta} \mu(\alpha, \beta) E_{\text{st}} \left(\hat{\gamma}_{\alpha,\beta} x_t \right) d\alpha d\beta \ , \tag{4.186}$$

where $E_{\text{st}}(\hat{\gamma}_{\alpha,\beta} x_t)$ can be evaluated by using formula (4.180).

It turns out that the stationary values of the second moment $E_{\text{st}}(f_t^2)$ and the variance of f_t can be also computed by using the mathematical machinery of stochastic processes on graphs. The computations are based on the following formula:

$$E_{\text{st}} \left(f_t^2 \right) = \iint\limits_{\alpha_1 \geq \beta_1} \iint\limits_{\alpha_2 \geq \beta_2} E_{\text{st}} \left(i_t^{(1)} i_t^{(2)} \right) \mu(\alpha_1, \beta_1) \mu(\alpha_2, \beta_2) d\alpha_1 d\beta_1 d\alpha_2 d\beta_2 \ , \tag{4.187}$$

where

$$i_t^{(1)} = \hat{\gamma}_{\alpha_1, \beta_1} x_t \ , \tag{4.188}$$

$$i_t^{(2)} = \hat{\gamma}_{\alpha_2, \beta_2} x_t \ . \tag{4.189}$$

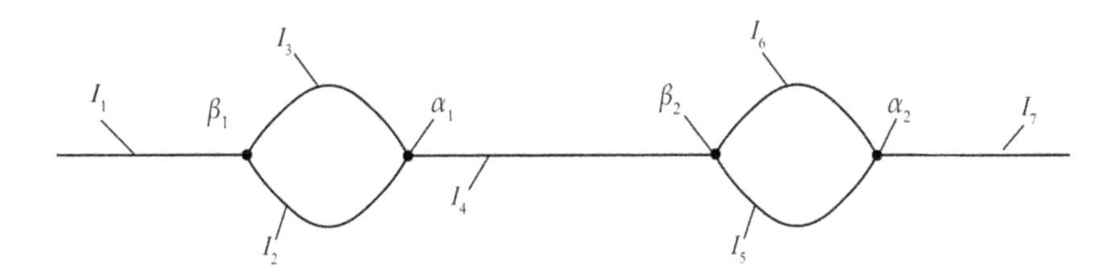

Fig. 4.10

To evaluate the quantity $E_{\rm st}(i_t^{(1)} i_t^{(2)})$, we introduce the three component Markov process $\vec{z}_t$ defined by the formula

$$\vec{z}_t = \begin{bmatrix} i_t^{(1)} \\ i_t^{(2)} \\ x_t \end{bmatrix} . \tag{4.190}$$

The process is defined on graphs whose structures depend on relations between $\alpha_1, \alpha_2, \beta_1, \beta_2$. Here, there are three distinct cases. The first is defined by inequalities

$$\beta_1 < \alpha_1 < \beta_2 < \alpha_2 \tag{4.191}$$

and it is realized when the rectangular loops $\hat{\gamma}_{\alpha_1,\beta_1}$ and $\hat{\gamma}_{\alpha_2,\beta_2}$ do not overlap. In this case, the three component Markov process $\vec{z}_t$ is defined on the graph shown in Fig. 4.10.

As before, we introduce the notations

$$\rho_{\rm st}\left(\vec{z}_t\right)\Big|_{I_k} = \rho_{\rm st}^{(k)}(x) . \tag{4.192}$$

It is clear from Fig. 4.10 that

$$\rho_{\rm st}^{(k)}(x) = \rho_{\rm st}(x) \quad \text{for} \quad k = 1, 4, 7, \tag{4.193}$$

while

$$\rho_{\rm st}^{(3)}(x) = \rho_{\rm st}(x)\varphi_3(x) , \tag{4.194}$$

$$\rho_{\rm st}^{(2)}(x) = \rho_{\rm st}(x) - \rho_{\rm st}^{(3)}(x) , \tag{4.195}$$

$$\rho_{\rm st}^{(6)}(x) = \rho_{\rm st}(x)\varphi_6(x) , \tag{4.196}$$

$$\rho_{\rm st}^{(5)}(x) = \rho_{\rm st}(x) - \rho_{\rm st}^{(6)}(x) . \tag{4.197}$$

It can be shown as before that $\varphi_3(x)$ and $\varphi_6(x)$ can be determined by using formula (4.174) by replacing α and β by α_2 and β_2 and α_1 and β_1, respectively.

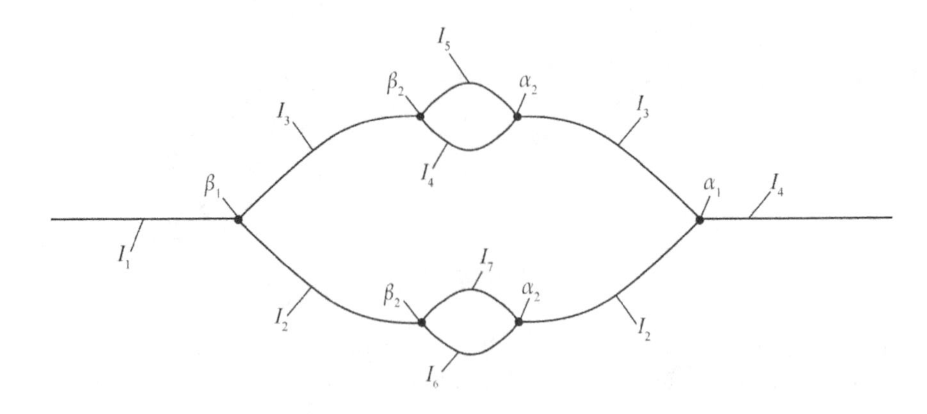

Fig. 4.11

The second case is specified by inequalities

$$\beta_1 < \beta_2 < \alpha_2 < \alpha_1 \tag{4.198}$$

and it is realized when rectangular loops $\hat{\gamma}_{\alpha_1,\beta_1}$ and $\hat{\gamma}_{\alpha_2,\beta_2}$ completely overlap. In this case, the three component Markov process $\vec{z}_t$ is defined on the graph shown in Fig. 4.11.
From this figure we find that

$$\rho_{\text{st}}^{(k)}(x) = \rho_{\text{st}}(x) \quad \text{for} \quad k = 1, 4 \,, \tag{4.199}$$

while

$$\rho_{\text{st}}^{(3)}(x) = \rho_{\text{st}}(x)\varphi_3(x) \,, \tag{4.200}$$

$$\rho_{\text{st}}^{(2)}(x) = \rho_{\text{st}}(x) - \rho_{\text{st}}^{(3)}(x) \,, \tag{4.201}$$

$$\rho_{\text{st}}^{(5)}(x) = \rho_{\text{st}}^{(3)}(x)\varphi_5(x) \,, \tag{4.202}$$

$$\rho_{\text{st}}^{(4)}(x) = \rho_{\text{st}}^{(3)}(x) - \rho_{\text{st}}^{(5)}(x) \,, \tag{4.203}$$

$$\rho_{\text{st}}^{(7)}(x) = \rho_{\text{st}}^{(2)}(x)\varphi_7(x) \,, \tag{4.204}$$

$$\rho_{\text{st}}^{(6)}(x) = \rho_{\text{st}}^{(2)}(x) - \rho_{\text{st}}^{(7)}(x) \,. \tag{4.205}$$

In the above relations, functions $\varphi_3(x)$, $\varphi_5(x)$ and $\varphi_7(x)$ are determined by formulas similar to formula (4.174).

Finally, the third case is specified by inequalities

$$\beta_1 < \beta_2 < \alpha_1 < \alpha_2 \tag{4.206}$$

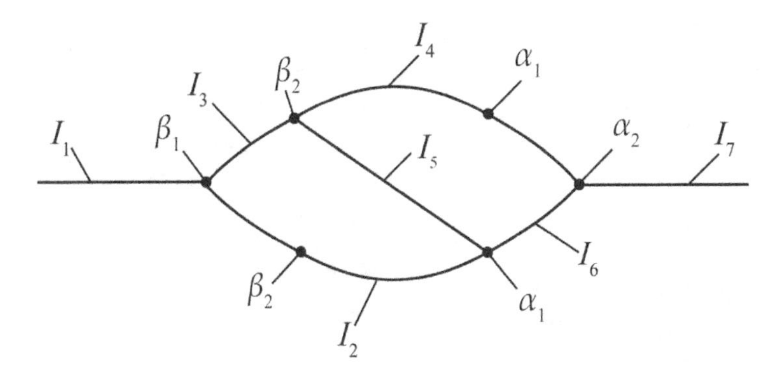

Fig. 4.12

and it is realized when rectangular loops $\hat{\gamma}_{\alpha_1,\beta_1}$ and $\hat{\gamma}_{\alpha_2,\beta_2}$ partially overlap. In this case, the three component process $\vec{z}_t$ is defined on the graph shown in Fig. 4.12. It is worthwhile to point out that in this case there is no graph edge corresponding to $i_t^{(1)} = 1$ and $i_t^{(2)} = -1$ because these simultaneous values of $i_t^{(1)}$ and $i_t^{(2)}$ are not consistent with the definition of rectangular loops $\hat{\gamma}_{\alpha_1,\beta_1}$ and $\hat{\gamma}_{\alpha_2,\beta_2}$.
It is apparent from Fig. 4.12 that

$$\rho_{\text{st}}^{(k)}(x) = \rho_{\text{st}}(x) \quad \text{for} \quad k = 1, 7 \;, \tag{4.207}$$

while

$$\rho_{\text{st}}^{(2)}(x) = \rho_{\text{st}}(x)\varphi_2(x) \;, \tag{4.208}$$

$$\rho_{\text{st}}^{(3)}(x) = \rho_{\text{st}}(x) - \rho_{\text{st}}^{(2)}(x) \;, \tag{4.209}$$

$$\rho_{\text{st}}^{(4)}(x) = \rho_{\text{st}}(x)\varphi_4(x) \;, \tag{4.210}$$

$$\rho_{\text{st}}^{(6)}(x) = \rho_{\text{st}}(x) - \rho_{\text{st}}^{(4)}(x) \;, \tag{4.211}$$

$$\rho_{\text{st}}^{(5)}(x) = \rho_{\text{st}}(x) - \rho_{\text{st}}^{(2)}(x) - \rho_{\text{st}}^{(4)}(x) \;. \tag{4.212}$$

In the above formulas, functions $\varphi_2(x)$ and $\varphi_1(x)$ can be determined in the same way as previously discussed in this section.

The calculations of $E_{\text{st}}(f_t^2)$ are considerably simplified in the particular (but important) case of the Preisach model containing only symmetric loops $\hat{\gamma}_{\alpha,-\alpha} = \hat{\gamma}_\alpha$. In this case, we have

$$f_t = \int_0^{\alpha_0} \mu(\alpha)\hat{\gamma}_\alpha x_t d\alpha \;, \tag{4.213}$$

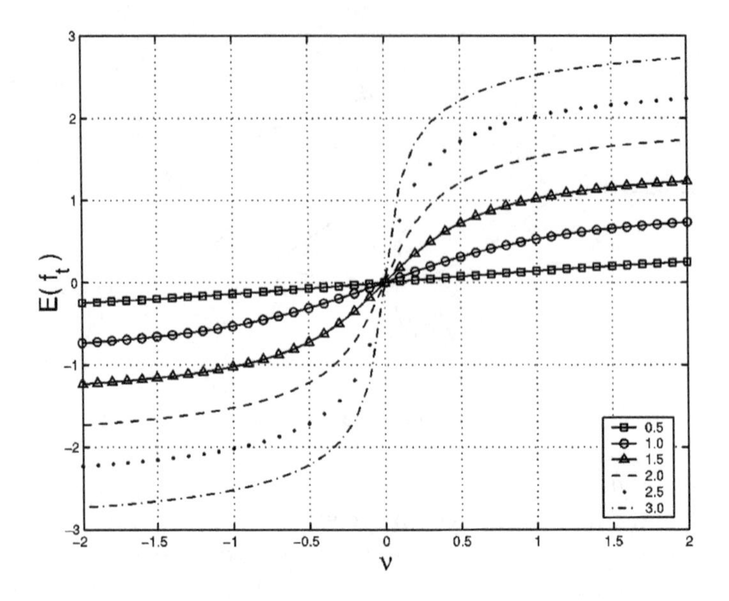

Fig. 4.13

where α_0 is the maximum value of α for rectangular loop operators $\hat{\gamma}_\alpha$. Consequently,

$$\bar{f}_t^{\text{st}} = \int_0^{\alpha_0} \mu(\alpha) E_{\text{st}}\left(\hat{\gamma}_\alpha x_t\right) d\alpha \tag{4.214}$$

and

$$E_{\text{st}}\left(f_t^2\right) = \int_0^{\alpha_0} \mu(\alpha) \left(\int_0^{\alpha_0} \mu(\alpha') E_{\text{st}}\left(\hat{\gamma}_\alpha x_t \hat{\gamma}_{\alpha'} x_t\right) d\alpha' \right) d\alpha \,. \tag{4.215}$$

The value of $E_{\text{st}}\left(\hat{\gamma}_\alpha x_t\right)$ can be evaluated in the same way as in the case of formula (4.186). The value of $E_{\text{st}}\left(\hat{\gamma}_\alpha x_t \hat{\gamma}_{\alpha'} x_t\right)$ can be evaluated by using the graph shown in Fig. 4.11 and the following formula

$$E_{\text{st}}\left(\hat{\gamma}_\alpha x_t \hat{\gamma}_{\alpha'} x_t\right) = 2P\left(\hat{\gamma}_\alpha x_t \hat{\gamma}_{\alpha'} x_t\right) - 1 \,, \tag{4.216}$$

which leads to

$$E_{\text{st}}\left(\hat{\gamma}_\alpha x_t \hat{\gamma}_{\alpha'} x_t\right) = 2\Bigg[\int_{-\alpha}^{\alpha'} \rho_{\text{st}}^{(5)}(x) dx + \int_{\alpha'}^{\alpha} \rho_{\text{st}}^{(3)}(x) dx + \int_{\alpha}^{\infty} \rho_{\text{st}}(x) dx + \\ + \int_{-\alpha'}^{\alpha} \rho_{\text{st}}^{(6)}(x) dx + \int_{-\alpha}^{-\alpha'} \rho_{\text{st}}^{(2)}(x) dx + \int_{-\infty}^{\alpha'} \rho_{\text{st}}(x) dx \Bigg] - 1 \,. \tag{4.217}$$

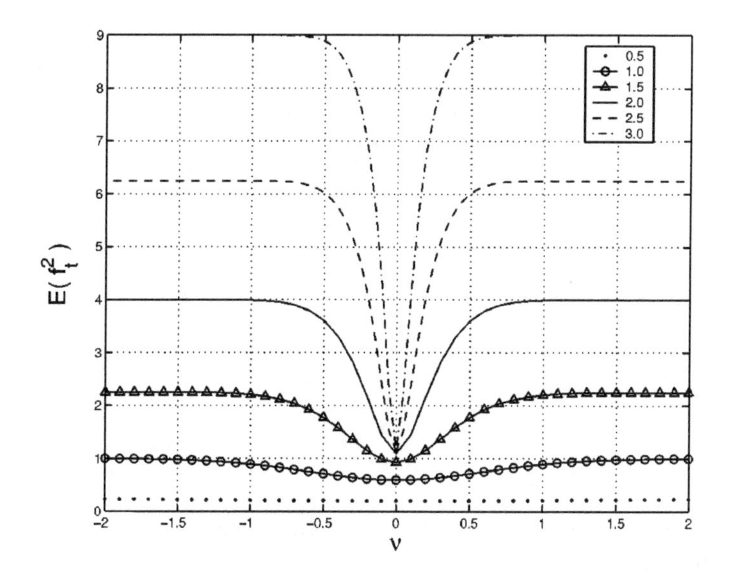

Fig. 4.14

Some sample results of calculations are shown in Figs. 4.13 and 4.14 for $\bar{f}_t^{\text{st}}$ and $E_{\text{st}}(f_t^2)$, respectively. It was assumed in these calculations that $\mu(\alpha) = 1$, and $\bar{f}_t^{\text{st}}$ and $E_{\text{st}}(f_t^2)$ were computed as functions of $\nu = x_0/\alpha_0$ for various values of $\tilde{\alpha}_0 = \alpha_0/\lambda$, where as before λ^2 is the variance of the stationary distribution of Ornstein-Uhlenbeck process. Furthermore, the values of $\bar{f}_t^{\text{st}}$ and $E_{\text{st}}(f_t^2)$ have been normalized by λ and λ^2, respectively.

The technique of stochastic processes on graphs can be further extended to compute higher order moments of the random output process f_t. This extension is more or less straightforward in the case of hysteresis model (4.212). In this case, the relevant multicomponent Markovian processes are defined on the graphs schematically shown in Fig. 4.15.

Indeed, by using the same line of reasoning as before, the following explicit expressions $\rho_{\text{st}}^{(2k+1)}$ for edges I_{2k+1} can be derived:

$$\rho_{\text{st}}^{(2k+1)}(x) = \rho_{\text{st}}(x) \prod_{j=1}^{k} \varphi_{2j+1}(x) \, . \tag{4.218}$$

Similar expressions can be derived for other graph edges.

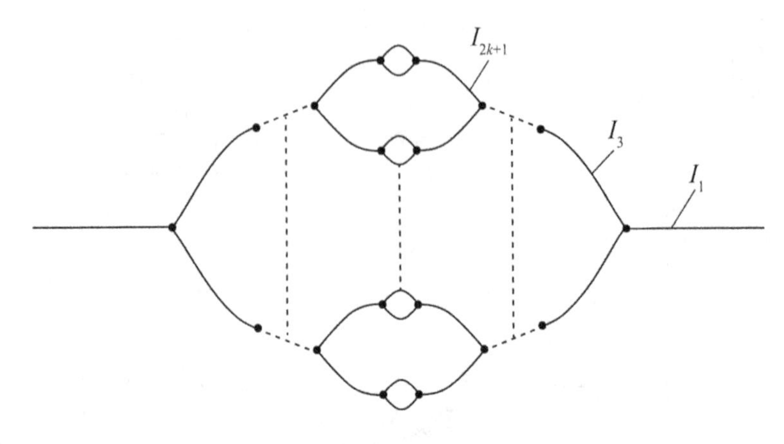

Fig. 4.15

4.4 Spectral Density of Outputs of Hysteretic Systems Driven by Noise

Spectral density functions are widely used for the characterization of stationary random processes. The spectral density is introduced as the power content of a random process versus frequency. For this reason, it is also called the power spectral density. The most known result in the area of power spectral density is established for linear time-invariant systems. This result is presented by the following formula

$$S_i(\omega) = |H(\omega)|^2 \, S_x(\omega) \ , \tag{4.219}$$

where $S_i(\omega)$ is the power spectral density of the output random process i_t, $S_x(\omega)$ is the power spectral density of the input random process x_t, while $H(\omega)$ is the transfer function of linear time-invariant system.

In this section, a method for the calculation of spectral density of random outputs of hysteretic systems driven by stationary stochastic processes is presented. The discussion is started with the case of a rectangular hysteresis loop $\hat{\gamma}_{\alpha,\beta}$ driven by a diffusion process. The problem of calculation of the spectral density of the output stochastic process i_t, defined as

$$i_t = \hat{\gamma}_{\alpha,\beta} x_t \ , \tag{4.220}$$

is of considerable mathematical difficulty for the following two reasons. The first reason is that the process i_t is not Markovian. This difficulty is overcome by using the mathematical machinery of stochastic processes on graphs discussed in the previous section. The second reason is that hysteresis loop transformation of stochastic process x_t is nonlinear in nature. This difficulty is overcome by studying process i_t in terms of its transition probability density which is described by the linear Kolmogorov (Fokker Planck) equation. Furthermore, the so-called "effective" distribution function is introduced that appreciably simplifies the calculation of spectral density. A similar approach was first developed in [13] for the analysis of spectral density in the case of semiclassical transport in semiconductors, and then it was extended in [14] and [15] to the calculation of spectral density of noise-driven hysteretic systems.

To start the discussion, consider as before the two component Markovian process $\vec{y}_t$:

$$\vec{y}_t = \begin{bmatrix} i_t \\ x_t \end{bmatrix} \tag{4.221}$$

defined on the four-edge graph shown in Fig. 4.7.

Next, we shall define the autocovariance matrix for $\vec{y}_t$. To do this, consider two random vectors

$$\vec{y} \equiv \vec{y}_\tau = \begin{bmatrix} i \\ x \end{bmatrix} \tag{4.222}$$

and

$$\vec{y}^{\,'} \equiv \vec{y}_0 = \begin{bmatrix} i^{'} \\ x^{'} \end{bmatrix} \tag{4.223}$$

generated by the process $\vec{y}_t$ at times $t = \tau$ and $t = 0$, respectively. Then, the autocovariance matrix $\hat{C}(\tau)$ can be defined as follows:

$$\hat{C}(\tau) = \left\langle \left(\vec{y} - \langle \vec{y} \rangle\right) \left(\vec{y}^{\,'} - \langle \vec{y}^{\,'} \rangle\right)^T \right\rangle , \tag{4.224}$$

where the symbol "$\langle\ \rangle$" is used for the notation of average value, while the superscript "T" denotes a transposed vector.

By using the joint probability function $\rho(i, x, \tau; i^{'}, x^{'}, 0)$ and stationary distribution function $\rho_{\mathrm{st}}(i, x)$ of the process $\vec{y}_t$, the autocovariance matrix can be represented as follows:

$$\begin{aligned} \hat{C}(\tau) = &\int\!\!\int \sum_i \sum_{i'} \vec{y} \left(\vec{y}^{\,'}\right)^T \rho(i, x, \tau; i^{'}, x^{'}, 0) dx dx^{'} \\ &- \left(\int \sum_i \vec{y} \rho_{\mathrm{st}}(i, x) dx \right) \left(\int \sum_{i'} \vec{y}^{\,'} \rho_{\mathrm{st}}(i^{'}, x^{'}) dx^{'} \right) . \end{aligned} \tag{4.225}$$

Since the process $\vec{y}_t$ is Markovian, its joint probability function can be represented as the product of the transition probability function $\rho(i, x, \tau | i^{'}, x^{'}, 0)$

and the stationary probability function. This leads to the following simplification of formula (4.225):

$$\hat{C}(\tau) = \int\int\sum_i\sum_{i'}\vec{y}\left(\vec{y'}\right)^T\left[\rho(i,x,\tau|i',x',0) - \rho_{\rm st}(i,x)\right]\rho_{\rm st}(i',x')dxdx' . \tag{4.226}$$

To further simplify the calculations, the following two-component "effective" distribution function is introduced:

$$\begin{aligned}\vec{g}(i,x,\tau) &= \begin{bmatrix} g_1(i,x,\tau) \\ g_2(i,x,\tau)\end{bmatrix} \\ &= \int\sum_{i'}\vec{y'}\left[\rho(i,x,\tau|i',x',0) - \rho_{\rm st}(i,x)\right]\rho_{\rm st}(i',x')dx' .\end{aligned} \tag{4.227}$$

If this "effective" distribution function is somehow found, then the autocovariance matrix can be computed as follows:

$$\hat{C}(\tau) = \int\sum_i \vec{y}\vec{g}^T(i,x,\tau)dx . \tag{4.228}$$

Next, we shall derive the initial-boundary value problem for $\vec{g}(i,x,\tau)$ on the graph shown in Fig. 4.7. On each edge of this graph, the transition probability density function satisfies the forward Kolmogorov equation

$$\frac{\partial\rho(i,x,\tau|i',x',0)}{\partial\tau} + \hat{\mathcal{L}}_x\rho(i,x,\tau|i',x',0) = 0 , \tag{4.229}$$

where $\hat{\mathcal{L}}_x$ is the second-order differential operator identical to the one in the right-hand side of equation (4.152). The transition probability density function satisfies the obvious initial condition

$$\rho\left(i,x,\tau|i',x',0\right) = \delta_{ii'}\delta(x-x') \tag{4.230}$$

and certain boundary conditions at graph vertices $x = \alpha$ and $x = \beta$. These "vertex" boundary conditions are discussed in the previous section and they express the continuity of the transition probability function when the transition from one graph edge to another through a vertex occurs without switching of the rectangular loop $\hat{\gamma}_{\alpha\beta}$, and zero boundary condition is imposed on the third graph edge connected to this vertex. In addition, the probability current is conserved at each vertex.

The stationary probability function satisfies the equation

$$\hat{\mathcal{L}}_x\rho_{\rm st}(i,x) = 0 \tag{4.231}$$

on each edge of the graph and the "vertex" boundary conditions. By using the formulas (4.229)–(4.231) and the definition (4.227) of $\vec{g}(i,x,\tau)$, the following initial-boundary-value problem on the graph can be derived for the "effective" distribution function: $\vec{g}(i,x,\tau)$ satisfies the equation

$$\frac{\partial \vec{g}(i,x,\tau)}{\partial \tau} + \hat{\mathcal{L}}_x \vec{g}(i,x,\tau) = 0 \tag{4.232}$$

on each graph edge, the following initial condition

$$\vec{g}(i,x,\tau)\Big|_{\tau=0} = \Big(\vec{y} - \langle \vec{y} \rangle\Big) \rho_{\mathrm{st}}(i,x) \tag{4.233}$$

and the "vertex" boundary conditions.

It is well-known that the matrix of spectral density is related to the autocovariance matrix through the Fourier transform:

$$\hat{S}(\omega) = \int\limits_{-\infty}^{\infty} \hat{C}(\tau) e^{-j\omega\tau} d\tau \ . \tag{4.234}$$

The element $S_{11}(\omega)$ of the matrix $\hat{S}(\omega)$ can be construed as the spectral density of the output process i_t. By introducing the Fourier transform of the "effective" distribution function

$$\vec{G}(i,x,\omega) = \begin{bmatrix} G_1(i,x,\omega) \\ G_2(i,x,\omega) \end{bmatrix} = \int\limits_{0}^{\infty} \vec{g}(i,x,\omega) e^{-j\omega\tau} d\tau \ , \tag{4.235}$$

and using formulas (4.228) and (4.234), we find:

$$S_i(\omega) = S_{11}(\omega) = 2\Re e \left(\int \sum_i i G_1(i,x,\omega) dx \right) \ . \tag{4.236}$$

Thus, if $G_1(i,x,\omega)$, is found, then the spectral density of the process i_t can be computed. To find $G_1(i,x,\omega)$, we perform Fourier transformation of the initial-boundary-value problem (4.232)–(4.233). As a result, we arrive at the following boundary-value problem for $G_1(i,x,\omega)$: it satisfies the following equation

$$j\omega G_1(i,x,\omega) + \hat{\mathcal{L}}_x G_1(i,x,\omega) = (i - \langle i \rangle)\, \rho_{\mathrm{st}}(i,x) \tag{4.237}$$

on each graph edge and the "vertex" boundary conditions. Thus, by solving this boundary value problem for equation (4.237) and by using formula (4.236) the spectral density of the output process i_t can be computed for any input process x_t. Analytical results can be obtained when x_t is the Ornstein-Uhlenbeck process. This process is very appealing as a noise model because of its stationary and Gaussian nature. In the case of Ornstein-Uhlenbeck process the operator $\hat{\mathcal{L}}_x$ has the form:

$$\hat{\mathcal{L}}_x G_1(i,x,\omega) = -\frac{\sigma^2}{2}\frac{d^2 G_1(i,x,\omega)}{dx^2} + b\frac{d}{dx}\left[(x-x_0)G_1(i,x,\omega)\right] , \quad (4.238)$$

where x_0 is the expected value of x_t. Formulas (4.237)–(4.238) lead to a linear second-order, inhomogeneous differential equation whose solution has two distinct components: particular solution of the inhomogeneous equation and general solution of the homogeneous equation:

$$j\omega G_1^0 - \frac{\sigma^2}{2}\frac{d^2 G_1^0}{dx^2} + b\frac{d}{dx}\left[(x-x_0)G_1^0\right] = 0 . \quad (4.239)$$

It is apparent from formula (4.231) that the particular solution of the inhomogeneous equation has the form $-\frac{j}{\omega}(i - \langle i\rangle)\rho_{\text{st}}(i,x)$. Because the particular solution is purely imaginary, it does not contribute to the spectral density computed in accordance with formula (4.236). Thus, G_1 in formula (4.236) can be replaced by G_1^0 that satisfies the equation (4.239) and can be expressed as follows:

$$G_1^0 = -\frac{j}{\omega}\left[\frac{\sigma^2}{2}\frac{d^2 G_1^0}{dx^2} - b\frac{d}{dx}\left((x-x_0)G_1^0\right)\right] . \quad (4.240)$$

By substituting expression (4.240) into formula (4.236), performing integration and using the “vertex” boundary condition, the following formula can be derived for the spectral density:

$$S_i(\omega) = -\frac{2\sigma^2}{\omega}\Im m\left[\frac{dG_1^0}{dx}(1,\alpha^+,\omega) - \frac{dG_1^0}{dx}(1,-\alpha^-,\omega) + \frac{dG_1^0}{dx}(1,\beta^+,\omega)\right] , \quad (4.241)$$

where α^+ and β^+ denote the limiting values of these respective variables from the positive direction, and α^- denotes the limiting value of this variable from the negative direction.

The solution of equation (4.239) can be expressed in terms of parabolic cylinder functions. This fact along with formula (4.241) leads to the following analytical expression for the spectral density

$$S_i(\omega) = -\frac{2\sigma^2}{\omega}\Im m\left[\sum_{k=1}^{2}\left(b_k(\omega)\frac{dz_k}{dx}(\alpha,\omega) + c_k(\omega)\frac{dz_k}{dx}(\beta,\omega)\right)\right] , \quad (4.242)$$

where functions $z_k(x,\omega)$ are related to the parabolic cylinder functions $\mathcal{D}_k(x,\omega)$ by the formula:

$$z_k(x,\omega) = \mathcal{D}_k\left(\sqrt{\frac{2b}{\sigma^2}}(x-x_0)\omega\right)\exp\left(-\frac{b}{2\sigma^2}(x-x_0)^2\right) \quad (4.243)$$

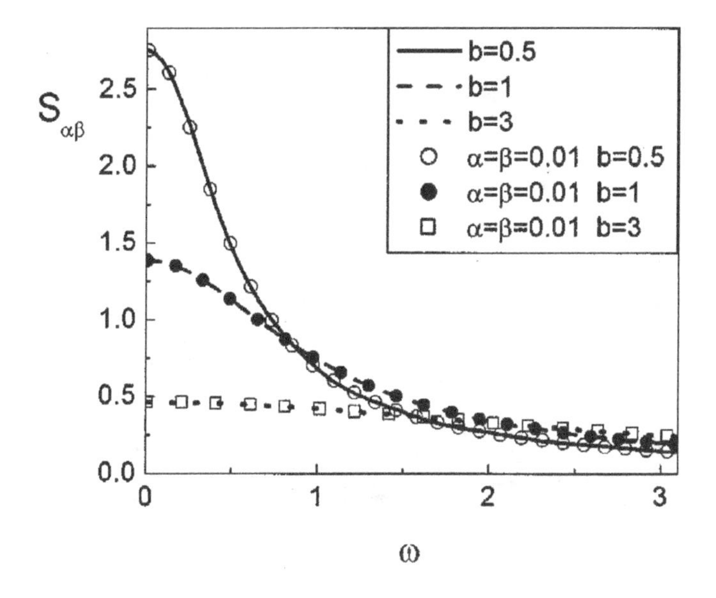

Fig. 4.16

and coefficients b_k and c_k are found from the "vertex" boundary conditions. The functions $\mathcal{D}_1$ and $\mathcal{D}_2$ are the parabolic cylinder functions that vanish at $+\infty$ and $-\infty$, respectively.

The presented technique of computing the power spectral density of the random output of rectangular loop driven by the Ornstein-Uhlenbeck process can be extended to the calculation of the spectral density of the random output of the Preisach model. For the sake of simplicity, we consider below the case of the Preisach model constructed as a superposition of only symmetric loops $\hat{\gamma}_{\alpha,-\alpha} = \hat{\gamma}_\alpha$:

$$f_t = \int_0^{\alpha_0} \mu(\alpha)\hat{\gamma}_\alpha x_t d\alpha \ . \tag{4.244}$$

The autocorrelation function of the output random process f_t is

$$C_f(\tau) = \langle f_\tau f_0 \rangle \ . \tag{4.245}$$

By using formulas (4.244) and (4.245), we find

$$C_f(\tau) = \int_0^{\alpha_0} \int_0^{\alpha_0} \langle i_\tau^\beta i_0^\alpha \rangle \mu(\alpha)\mu(\beta) d\beta d\alpha \ , \tag{4.246}$$

where

$$i_\tau^\beta = \hat{\gamma}_\beta x_\tau \tag{4.247}$$

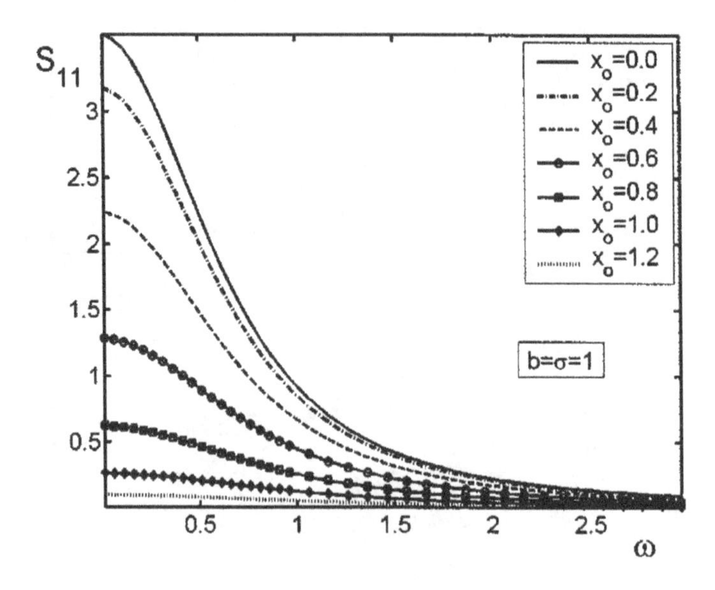

Fig. 4.17

and

$$i_0^{\alpha} = \hat{\gamma}_{\alpha} x_0 \; . \tag{4.248}$$

Since $C_f(\tau)$ is an even function of τ, the power spectral density is given by the formula:

$$S_f(\omega) = 2\Re e\left[\int_0^{\infty} C_f(\tau) e^{-j\omega\tau} d\tau\right] \; . \tag{4.249}$$

By substituting formula (4.246) into equation (4.249), we derive:

$$S_f(\omega) = \int_0^{\alpha_0} \int_0^{\alpha_0} S_{\alpha\beta}(\omega) \mu(\alpha) \mu(\beta) d\beta d\alpha \; , \tag{4.250}$$

where

$$S_{\alpha\beta}(\omega) = 2\Re e\left[\int_0^{\infty} \langle i_{\tau}^{\beta} i_0^{\alpha} \rangle e^{-j\omega\tau} d\tau\right] \; . \tag{4.251}$$

Thus, the problem of computing the power spectral density $S_f(\omega)$ is reduced to the problem of computing the "cross-spectral density" $S_{\alpha\beta}(\omega)$ defined by formula (4.251). The latter problem can be handled in the way conceptually

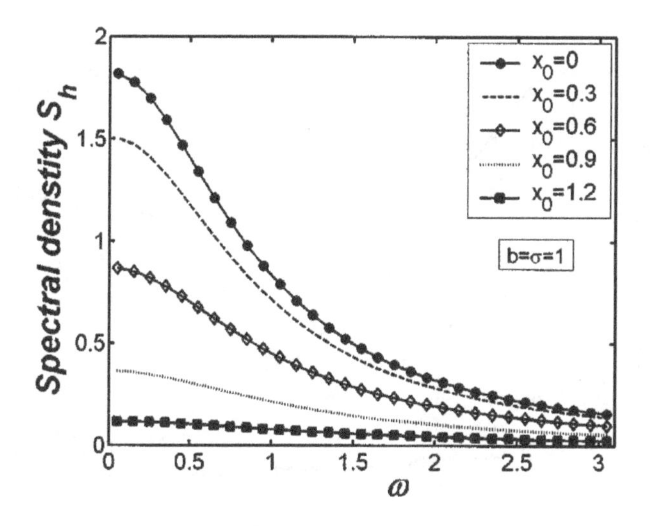

Fig. 4.18

similar to the calculation of $S_i(\omega)$ discussed above. Namely, we introduce the three component Markovian process

$$\vec{y}_t = \begin{bmatrix} i_t^\beta \\ i_t^\alpha \\ x_t \end{bmatrix} , \tag{4.252}$$

defined on the graph shown in Fig. 4.11. Furthermore, we introduce the "effective" distribution function $g(\vec{y}, \tau)$, which on each edge of the above graph satisfies the partial differential equation

$$\frac{\partial g(\vec{y}, \tau)}{\partial \tau} + \hat{\mathcal{L}}_x g(\vec{y}, \tau) = 0 \tag{4.253}$$

and initial condition

$$g(\vec{y}, 0) = i_0^\alpha \rho_{\text{st}}(\vec{y}) \tag{4.254}$$

as well as the vertex boundary conditions. It can be shown that by using the Fourier transform of $g(\vec{y}, \tau)$

$$G(\vec{y}, \omega) = \int_0^\infty g(\vec{y}, \tau) e^{-j\omega\tau} d\tau , \tag{4.255}$$

the cross-sectional density $S_{\alpha\beta}(\omega)$ can be represented as

$$S_{\alpha\beta}(\omega) = 2\Re e \left[\int_0^\infty \sum_{i^\alpha i^\beta} i^\alpha i^\beta G(\vec{y}, \omega) dx \right] . \tag{4.256}$$

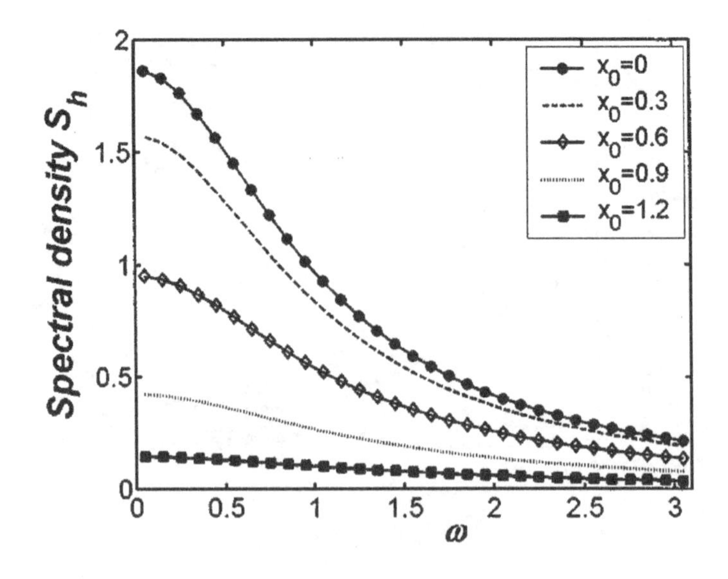

Fig. 4.19

In the above formula, the sum is taken over all graph edge values of i^β and i^α.

By performing the Fourier transform of the initial boundary value problem (4.253)–(4.254), we arrive at the following boundary value problem for $G(\vec{y}, \omega)$:

$$j\omega G(\vec{y}, \omega) + \hat{\mathcal{L}}_x G(\vec{y}, \omega) = i^\alpha \rho_{\text{st}}(\vec{y}) \tag{4.257}$$

with vertex boundary conditions. Now, it is apparent that power spectral density $S_f(\omega)$ can be computed by using formulas (4.250), (4.256), and (4.257).

In our discussion of the computation of $S_f(\omega)$ some mathematical details were omitted. These details can be found in paper [15].

We conclude this section by illustrating the presented technique with some sample computations. As a test of our technique, we compare the computational results for $S_i(\omega)$ in the case of symmetric rectangular loop $\alpha = \beta$ with the computational results for a hard limiter system. The latter system is the limiting case of the rectangular loop when its width is reduced to zero. It can be shown that the autocorrelation of the output i_t of the hard limiter is related to the autocorrelation of stochastic input x_t by the "arcsine law":

$$C_i(\tau) = \frac{2}{\tau} \arcsin \frac{C_x(\tau)}{C_i(0)} \,. \tag{4.258}$$

In the case where x_t is the Ornstein-Uhlenbeck process, from the last formula we find

$$S_i(\omega) = \frac{4}{\pi} \int_0^\infty \arcsin\left(e^{-b\tau}\right) \cos(\omega\tau) d\tau \ . \tag{4.259}$$

In Fig. 4.16, the results of computations of the power spectral density $S_i(\omega)$ for the hard limiter (shown by lines) and the rectangular symmetric loop $\hat{\gamma}_{\alpha,-\alpha}$ with $\alpha = 0.01$ are compared for different values of b. In Fig. 4.17, the results of computations of $S_i(\omega)$ for rectangular loop $\hat{\gamma}_{\alpha,-\alpha} = \hat{\gamma}_\alpha$ and different values of x_0 are presented.

Finally, Figs. 4.18 and 4.19 represent the result of calculations of $S_f(\omega)$ for the Preisach model (4.244) for the cases when $\mu(\alpha) = 1$ and $\mu(\alpha)$ is a Gaussian distribution, respectively.

In conclusion of this section, we want to mention that interesting results on the analysis of power spectral density of the random output of the Preisach model driven by stochastic processes are obtained in publications [16]–[19].

4.5 Functional (Path) Integration Models of Hysteresis

The Preisach model is designed as a continuous superposition of the simplest rectangular loop operators $\hat{\gamma}_{\alpha\beta}$. These operators can be construed as elementary building blocks of the Preisach model. A natural way to generalize the Preisach model is to consider more sophisticated elementary hysteresis operators and to design hysteresis models as continuous superpositions of such elementary operators. In this section we pursue this approach and consider functional (path) integration models of hysteresis that are designed as superpositions of elementary hysteresis operators generated by continuous functions. A physical interpretation of the path integration models as well as their various connections with the classical Preisach model are presented. The discussion in this section follows (to a certain extent) the paper [20].

Consider a continuous function $g(x)$ on some closed interval $[x_-, x_+]$ that satisfies the condition

$$u_- = g(x_-) \leq g(x) \leq g(x_+) = u_+ \ . \tag{4.260}$$

Such a function will be called a generating function, while x_- and x_+ can be termed as lower and upper saturation values, respectively.

An elementary hysteresis operator $\hat{\gamma}_g u(t)$ can be associated with each generating function by traversing its upper or lower envelopes (see Fig. 4.20). This can be done as follows. Suppose that at time t_0 the input $u(t)$ assumes some extremum value u_0 and

$$u_0 = g(x_0) \ . \tag{4.261}$$

If u_0 is some minimum value, then for the subsequent monotonic increase of input the upper envelope

$$g^+_{u_0}(x) = \max_{[x_0,x]} g(x) \tag{4.262}$$

is traversed. On the other hand, if u_0 is some maximum value, then for the subsequent monotonic decrease of the input the lower envelope

$$g^-_{u_0}(x) = \min_{[x,x_0]} g(x) \tag{4.263}$$

is traversed. This means that for monotonic input variations the elementary hysteresis operator $\hat{\gamma}_g u(t)$ is defined as follows:

$$\hat{\gamma}_g u(t) = \begin{cases} x^+(t), & \text{if } u(t) \text{ is monotonically increased,} \\ x^-(t), & \text{if } u(t) \text{ is monotonically decreased.} \end{cases} \tag{4.264}$$

Here $x^+(t)$ and $x^-(t)$ are the solutions of the following equations, respectively:

$$g^+_{u_0}(x^+(t)) = u(t) \ , \tag{4.265}$$

$$g^-_{u_0}(x^-(t)) = u(t) \ . \tag{4.266}$$

Since upper $g^+_{u_0}(x)$ and lower $g^-_{u_0}(x)$ envelopes usually have "horizontal" parts parallel to the x-axis, solutions of equations (4.265) and (4.266) may not be unique for some values of $u(t)$. This difficulty can be removed by using minimal and maximal solutions of equations (4.265) and (4.266), respectively:

$$x^+(t) = \min\left\{x : g^+_{u_0}(x) = u(t)\right\} , \tag{4.267}$$

$$x^-(t) = \max\left\{x : g^-_{u_0}(x) = u(t)\right\} . \tag{4.268}$$

The elementary operator $\hat{\gamma}_g u(t)$ has been so far defined for monotonic input variations. This definition can be extended to the case of piece-wise monotonic inputs by consecutively applying the definition (4.264) for each time interval of monotonic variation of $u(t)$. The ambiguity of choosing x_0 in equation (4.261) can be removed if it is agreed that the evolution is

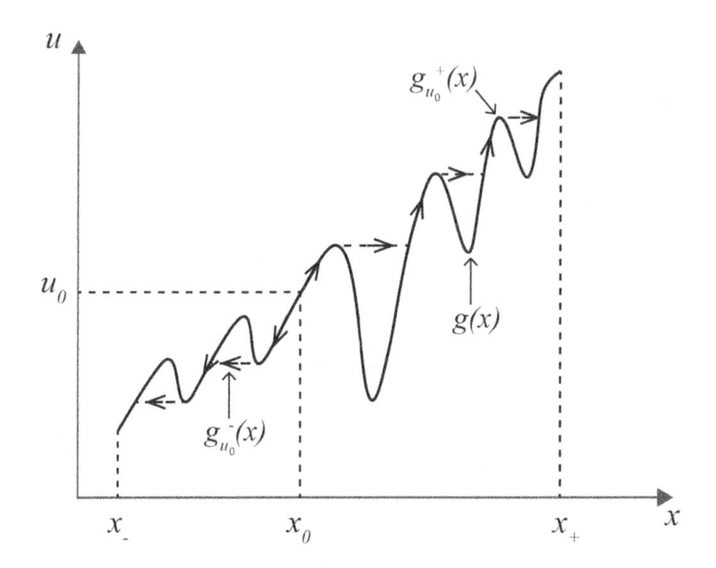

Fig. 4.20

started from the state x_- (or x_+) of negative (or positive) saturation. The given definition of elementary hysteresis operator $\hat{\gamma}_g u(t)$ is illustrated by Fig. 4.21. It is clear that elementary operator $\hat{\gamma}_g u(t)$ is rate-independent. This is because the output value $x(t)$ depends only on the current value of input $u(t)$ and the past history of input variations but does not depend on the rate of input variations. It is also clear that the operator $\hat{\gamma}_g u(t)$ has local memory. This is because the simultaneous specification of output and input uniquely defines the state of elementary hysteretic nonlinearity $\hat{\gamma}_g u(t)$. Finally, it is clear that the operator $\hat{\gamma}_g u(t)$ exhibits "the erasure" property. In a way, the erasure property can be regarded as a consequence of local memory. It is important to note that not all parts of $g(x)$ are accessible. For instance, part A shown in Fig. 4.21 is not accessible. This part of $g(x)$ will not be traversed for any input variations. In this sense, the same elementary hysteresis operator $\hat{\gamma}_g u(t)$ is defined on the equivalence class of functions $g(x)$ with the same accessible parts.

Now, consider some set G of generating functions $g(x)$ and some measure $\mu(g)$ defined on this set. Then the functional (path) integration model of hysteresis can be formally defined as follows:

$$f(t) = \int_G \hat{\gamma}_g u(t) d\mu(g) \ . \tag{4.269}$$

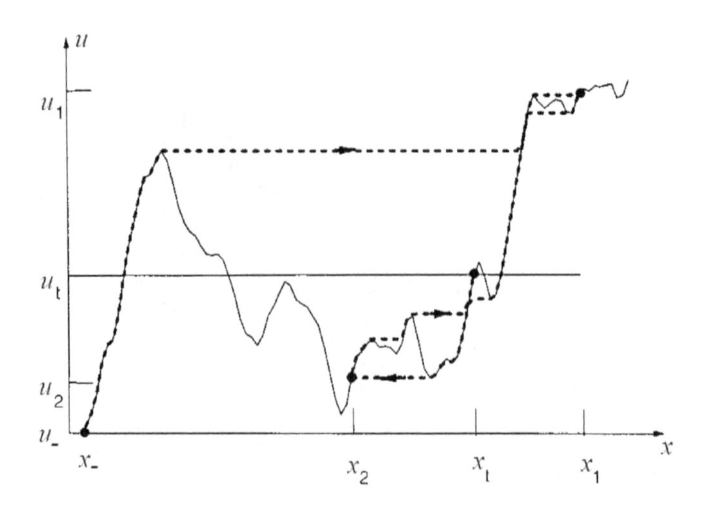

Fig. 4.21

The above model is quite general. Its structure depends on the measure $\mu(g)$ introduced on the set G. Next, we demonstrate that the classical Preisach model is a particular case of the path integration model (4.269). To this end, consider the subset G_p of G that consists of functions with two vertical parts $(x_- = -1, u \leq \alpha)$ and $(x_+ = 1, u \geq \beta)$ separated by inaccessible parts $\lambda(x)$ with $\beta < \lambda(x) < \alpha$ (see Fig. 4.22). It is clear that for such functions

$$\hat{\gamma}_g u(t) = \hat{\gamma}_{\alpha\beta} u(t), \quad \text{for } g(x) \in \Lambda_{\alpha\beta} , \tag{4.270}$$

where $\Lambda_{\alpha\beta}$ is the equivalence class of functions from G_p that have the same values of α and β. Now, consider the measure $\mu(g)$ that is concentrated on the subset G_p. Since G_p is the union of nonintersecting equivalence classes $\Lambda_{\alpha\beta}$, the model (4.269) can be written as follows:

$$f(t) = \iint\limits_{\alpha \geq \beta} \left(\int\limits_{\Lambda_{\alpha\beta}} \hat{\gamma}_g u(t) d\mu_{\alpha\beta}(g) \right) d\alpha d\beta , \tag{4.271}$$

where $\mu_{\alpha\beta}(g)$ are the measures on the equivalence classes $\Lambda_{\alpha\beta}$ induced by the measure $\mu(g)$ on G_p.

By using (4.270) in (4.271), we obtain

$$\int\limits_{\Lambda_{\alpha\beta}} \hat{\gamma}_g u(t) d\mu_{\alpha\beta}(g) = \left(\int\limits_{\Lambda_{\alpha\beta}} d\mu_{\alpha\beta}(g) \right) \hat{\gamma}_{\alpha\beta} u(t) = \mu(\alpha, \beta) \hat{\gamma}_{\alpha\beta} u(t) , \tag{4.272}$$

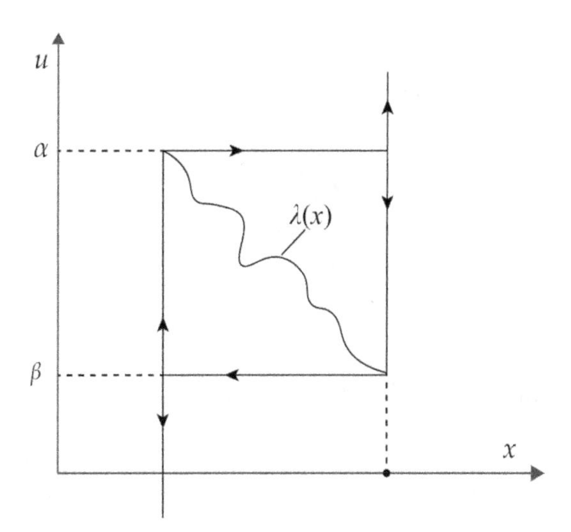

Fig. 4.22

where the following notation is introduced

$$\mu(\alpha,\beta)=\int\limits_{\Lambda_{\alpha\beta}} d\mu_{\alpha\beta}(g)\ . \tag{4.273}$$

By substituting (4.272) into (4.273), we end up with the classical Preisach model

$$f(t)=\iint\limits_{\alpha\geq\beta}\mu(\alpha,\beta)\hat{\gamma}_{\alpha\beta}u(t)d\alpha d\beta\ . \tag{4.274}$$

In the case when vertical parts in Fig. 4.22 are replaced by curved paths (see Fig. 4.23), the corresponding elementary hysteresis operator $\hat{\gamma}_g u(t)$ can be represented as follows:

$$x(t)=\frac{v^{+}\left(u(t)\right)-v^{-}\left(u(t)\right)}{2}\hat{\gamma}_{\alpha\beta}u(t)+\frac{v^{+}\left(u(t)\right)-v^{-}\left(u(t)\right)}{2}\ , \tag{4.275}$$

where $v^{+}(u)$ and $v^{-}(u)$ are inverses of $g^{+}(x)$ and $g^{-}(x)$, respectively.

By choosing measure $\mu(g)$ concentrated on the set of functions shown in Fig. 4.23 and literally repeating the same line of reasoning as before, it can be demonstrated that the path integration model (4.269) is reduced to the Preisach model with the input dependent measure (see Chapter 2).

It has been demonstrated above that the path integration model (4.269) is reduced to the classical Preisach model if the measure $\mu(g)$ is concentrated on functions $g(x)$ such that $\hat{\gamma}_g u(t)=\hat{\gamma}_{\alpha\beta}u(t)$. Below, it will be shown

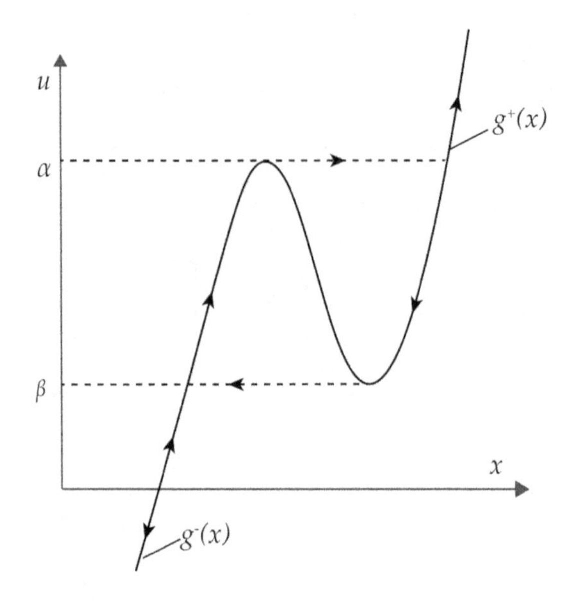

Fig. 4.23

that this reduction is also possible in the cases when the measure $\mu(g)$ is concentrated on functions $g(x)$ such that $\hat{\gamma}_g u(t) \neq \hat{\gamma}_{\alpha\beta} u(t)$. This will further emphasize the generality of the classical Preisach model.

In general, it is not immediately obvious how to generate measure on the functional set G and how to carry out functional integration in (4.269), in other words, how to compute output $f(t)$. In turns out that the above difficulties can be appreciably circumvented if the set G is interpreted as a set of samples of a stochastic diffusion process, which is the Markovian process with continuous samples generated by the Itô stochastic differential equation

$$dg_x = b\big(g_x, x\big)dx + \sigma\big(g_x, x\big)dW_x \ . \tag{4.276}$$

Here x must be construed as fictitious "stochastic" time that must not be confused with real physical time t.

In the above case, the measure $\mu(g)$ is the stochastic measure that, in principle, can be generated by using the transition probability density function for the process g_x. However, there is no need to do this because, as it will be demonstrated below, the output $f(t)$ can be interpreted as an average level-crossing (stochastic) time. As a result, the mathematical machinery developed for the solution of level-crossing (exit) problems can

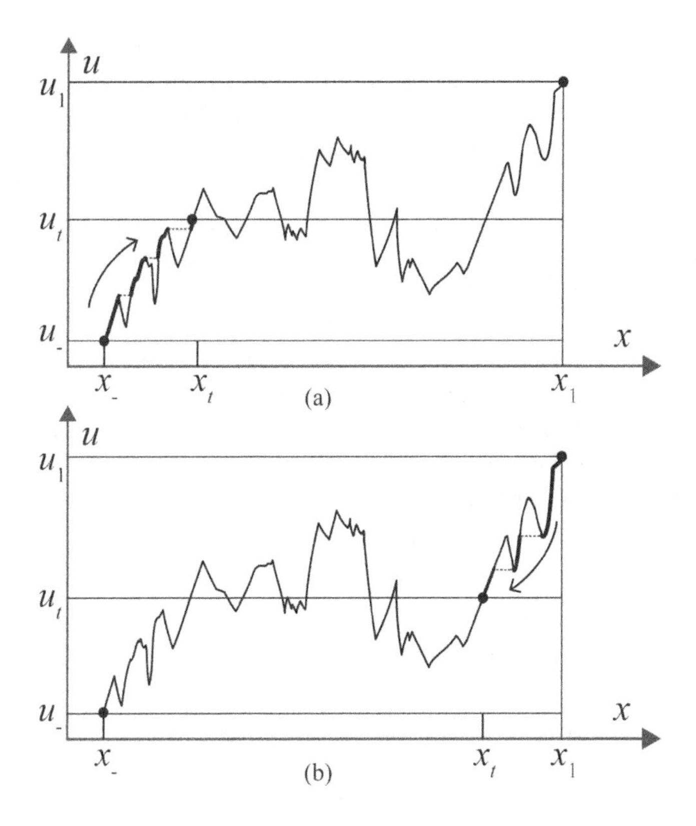

Fig. 4.24

be extensively used for the output calculations of functional integration type models (4.269).

First, we shall discuss the meaning of $\hat{\gamma}_g u(t)$ when the generating function $g(x)$ is a sample of diffusion stochastic process. This meaning is different for monotonically increasing and monotonically decreasing inputs. To illustrate this, let us consider Fig. 4.24 where a particular sample $g(x)$ of diffusion stochastic process that starts from the negative saturation value u_- is shown. It is clear from this figure and the definition of $\hat{\gamma}_g u(t)$ that for monotonically increasing input $u(t)$ the elementary operator $\hat{\gamma}_g u(t)$ has the meaning of the *first* level-crossing time, where the level is equal to the current value of input $u(t)$. This time is a random variable and, consequently, the output of the functional integration model (4.269) is equal to the *average value of the first level-crossing time.* This is true for any value of input until $u(t)$ reaches some maximum value u_1. It is clear from Fig. 4.24 and the definition of $\hat{\gamma}_g u(t)$ that for the subsequent monotonic decrease of input $u(t)$ the elementary operator $\hat{\gamma}_g u(t)$ has the meaning of the *last* level-crossing time, where the level is equal to the current input value $u(t)$. More precisely, this is the last time of crossing the level $u(t)$ before the first time of crossing the level u_1. This last level-crossing time is also a random variable. Thus, for monotonically decreasing input, the output of the functional integration model (4.269) is equal to the *average value of the last level-crossing time*. It is this difference in the meaning of output values of the path integration model (4.269) corresponding to monotonically increasing and decreasing inputs $u(t)$ that results in hysteresis.

Next, we shall present the mathematical formalism that supports the statements outlined above. Let $T(\alpha, x_\alpha|\beta, x_\beta)$ be the notation for the probability density of the first crossing time x_α of the level α under the condition that the sample of stochastic process crossed the level $\beta < \alpha$ at the time x_β. It is clear that

$$\int_{x_\beta}^{\infty} T\left(\alpha, x_\alpha \middle| \beta, x_\beta\right) dx_\alpha = 1 \,. \tag{4.277}$$

It is apparent that the probability densities $p_\alpha(x_\alpha)$ of x_α and $p_\beta(x_\beta)$ of x_β are related by the expression

$$p_\alpha(x_\alpha) = \int_0^{x_\alpha} T\left(\alpha, x_\alpha \middle| \beta, x_\beta\right) p_\beta(x_\beta) dx_\beta \,. \tag{4.278}$$

Consider the set G of all samples of the diffusion process g_x that satisfy the condition (4.260). Let us analyze mathematically how the output of the path integration model (4.269) changes when the input u_t is increased from u_- to some maximum value u_1 and then is decreased to some minimum value u_2. During the monotonic input increase the elementary operator $x_t = \hat{\gamma}_g u(t)$ has the meaning of the first time of crossing the level u_t. By using the notations $p_\beta(x_\beta) = p_u(x_-)$ and $p_\alpha(x_\alpha) = p_u(x_t)$, according to (4.278) we find

$$p_{u_t}(x_t) = \int_0^{x_t} T\left(u_t, x_t \middle| u_-, x_-\right) p_{u_-}(x_-) dx_- \,. \tag{4.279}$$

The probability density function $p_{u_-}(x_-)$ must be chosen as the part of the characterization of the initial state of lower saturation. For instance, it can be chosen as $\delta(x - x_-)$. After that, equation (4.279) permits one to compute the unknown probability density $p_{u_t}(x_t)$ provided that the first time level-crossing problem has been preliminarily solved and the function $T(u_t, x_t | u_-, x_-)$ has been found. By using the probability density $p_{u_t}(x_t)$, the output value of the path integration model (4.269) can be computed as follows:

$$f(u_t) = \int_0^\infty x_t p_{u_t}(x_t) dx_t \, . \tag{4.280}$$

Formulas (4.279) and (4.280) can be used to compute $p_{u_t}(x_t)$ and $f(u_t)$ for all values of u_t between u_- and u_1. In this way, the ascending branch of the major loop can be computed. For $u_t = u_1$, we have

$$p_{u_1}(x_1) = \int_0^{x_1} T\left(u_1, x_1 | u_-, x_-\right) p_{u_-}(x_-) dx_- \, . \tag{4.281}$$

Next, consider the monotonic decrease of input from u_1 to u_2. For this input variation, the elementary operator $x_t = \hat{\gamma}_g u(t)$ has the meaning of the last time of crossing the level u_t before the level u_1 is reached for the first time. This means that the probability density $p_{u_t}(x_t)$ of the last level-crossing time x_t satisfies the integral equation

$$p_{u_1}(x_1) = \int_0^{x_1} T\left(u_1, x_1 | u_t, x_t\right) p_{u_t}(x_t) dx_t \, . \tag{4.282}$$

This integral equation can be (in principle) solved for any value of u_t between u_1 and u_2. In this way, $p_{u_t}(x_t)$ can be found and used in formula (4.280) for the calculation of the output value $f(u_t)$ along the descending branch attached to the previous ascending branch at the point $u_t = u_1$. After $p_{u_2}(x_2)$ is found by solving integral equation

$$p_{u_1}(x_1) = \int_0^{x_1} T\left(u_1, x_1 | u_2, x_2\right) p_{u_2}(x_2) dx_2 \, , \tag{4.283}$$

it can be used in formulas

$$p_{u_t}(x_t) = \int_0^{x_t} T\left(u_t, x_t | u_2, x_2\right) p_{u_2}(x_2) dx_2 \, , \tag{4.284}$$

$$p_{u_3}(x_3) = \int_0^{x_3} T\left(u_3, x_3 | u_2, x_2\right) p_{u_2}(x_2) dx_2 \tag{4.285}$$

for computations of $p_{u_t}(x_t)$ and $p_{u_3}(x_3)$ for the third hysteresis branch when input $u(t)$ is monotonically increased from u_2 to u_3. Similarly, $p_{u_3}(x_3)$ can be used in the integral equations

$$p_{u_3}(x_3) = \int_0^{x_3} T\left(u_3, x_3 \middle| u_t, x_t\right) p_{u_t}(x_t) dx_t \ , \tag{4.286}$$

$$p_{u_3}(x_3) = \int_0^{x_3} T\left(u_3, x_3 \middle| u_4, x_4\right) p_{u_4}(x_4) dx_4 \tag{4.287}$$

for computations of $p_{u_t}(x_t)$ and $p_{u_4}(x_4)$ for the fourth hysteresis branch when input $u(t)$ is monotonically decreased from u_3 to u_4. It is clear that the computations described above can be recursively used to find any branch of hysteresis described by the path integration model (4.269) with stochastic measure.

It is important to note that in the case when $u_3 = u_1$ the probability densities $p_{u_3}(x_3)$ and $p_{u_t}(x_t)$ coincide. This directly follows from the coincidence equations (4.283) and (4.285) for the above case. The coincidence of $p_{u_3}(x_3)$ and $p_{u_1}(x_1)$ for $u_3 = u_1$ implies the validity of the "erasure" property for the path integration model. This fact can also be deduced from the validity of "erasure" property for each elementary hysteresis operator $\hat{\gamma}_g u(t)$.

Now, consider a particular case when the stochastic process g_x is homogeneous (translationally invariant) with respect to "stochastic time" x. Such a process is described by the Itô stochastic differential equation

$$dg_x = b(g_x)dx + \sigma(g_x)dW_x \ . \tag{4.288}$$

Due to the translational invariance, the conditional first time level-crossing probability density $T\left(\alpha, x_\alpha \middle| \beta, x_\beta\right)$ has the property:

$$T\left(\alpha, x_\alpha \middle| \beta, x_\beta\right) = T\left(\alpha, x_\alpha - x_\beta \middle| \beta, 0\right) \ . \tag{4.289}$$

Next, we shall use this property to compute the expressions for ascending $f^+(u_t)$ and descending $f^-(u_t)$ branches of hysteresis loops formed when the input $u(t)$ is monotonically increased from some minimum value u_{2k} to some maximum value u_{2k+1} and then is monotonically decreased back to u_{2k}. For the calculation of $f^+(u_t)$, formulas similar (4.280) and (4.284) are appropriate. This leads to the expression:

$$\begin{aligned} f^+(u_t) &= \int_0^\infty x_t p_{u_t}(x_t)dx_t \\ &= \int_0^\infty x_t \left(\int_0^{x_t} T\left(u_t, x_t - x_{2k} \middle| u_{2k}, 0\right) p_{u_{2k}}(x_{2k})dx_{2k} \right) dx_t \ . \end{aligned} \tag{4.290}$$

By using Fig. 4.25, the above double integral can be transformed as follows:

$$\begin{aligned} f^+(u_t) &= \int_0^\infty \left(\int_{x_{2k}}^\infty x_t T\left(u_t, x_t - x_{2k} \middle| u_{2k}, 0\right) dx_t \right) p_{u_{2k}}(x_{2k})dx_{2k} \\ &= \int_0^\infty \left(\int_{x_{2k}}^\infty (x_t - x_{2k}) T\left(u_t, x_t - x_{2k} \middle| u_{2k}, 0\right) dx_t \right) p_{u_{2k}}(x_{2k})dx_{2k} \\ &+ \int_0^\infty \left(\int_{x_{2k}}^\infty T\left(u_t, x_t - x_{2k} \middle| u_{2k}, 0\right) dx_t \right) x_{2k} p_{u_{2k}}(x_{2k})dx_{2k} \ . \end{aligned} \tag{4.291}$$

By using the change of variables

$$z = x_t - x_{2k} \ , \tag{4.292}$$

from formula (4.291) we find:

$$\begin{aligned} f^+(u_t) &= \int_0^\infty \left(\int_0^\infty T\left(u_t, z \middle| u_{2k}, 0\right) dz \right) x_{2k} p_{u_{2k}}(x_{2k})dx_{2k} \\ &+ \int_0^\infty \left(\int_0^\infty z T\left(u_t, z \middle| u_{2k}, 0\right) dz \right) p_{u_{2k}}(x_{2k})dx_{2k} \ . \end{aligned} \tag{4.293}$$

By using formulas (4.277) and (4.280) as well as the normalization condition

$$\int_0^\infty p_{u_{2k}}(x_{2k})dx_{2k} = 1 \tag{4.294}$$

in the second integral, from (4.293) we find

$$f^+(u_t) = f(u_{2k}) + F(u_t, u_{2k}) \ , \tag{4.295}$$

where

$$F(u_t, u_{2k}) = \int_0^\infty z T\left(u_t, z \middle| u_{2k}, 0\right) dz \ . \tag{4.296}$$

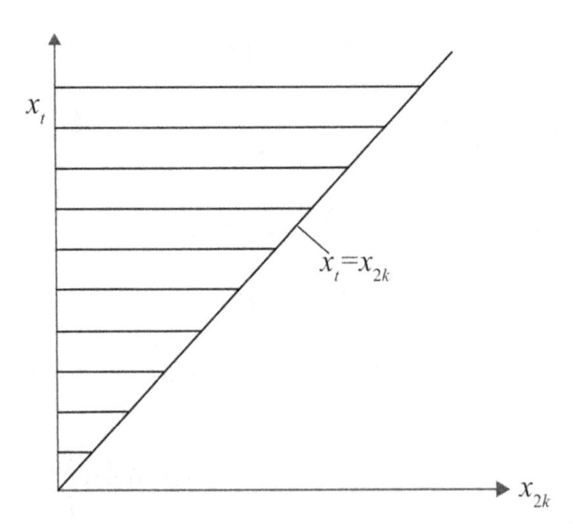

Fig. 4.25

It is clear from formula (4.295) that the current value of output on the ascending branch is determined only by the current value of input u_t and the last minimum value u_{2k}. We shall next establish a similar result for the descending branch $f^-(u_t)$ of the hysteresis loop. According to (4.280) and (4.286) we have

$$\begin{aligned} f(u_{2k+1}) &= \int_0^\infty x_{2k+1} p_{u_{2k+1}}(x_{2k+1}) dx_{2k+1} \\ &= \int_0^\infty x_{2k+1} \left(\int_0^{x_{2k+1}} T\left(u_{2k+1}, x_{2k+1} \middle| u_t, x_t\right) p_{u_t}(x_t) dx_t \right) dx_{2k+1} \\ &= \int_0^\infty x_{2k+1} \left(\int_0^{x_{2k+1}} T\left(u_{2k+1}, x_{2k+1} - x_t \middle| u_t, 0\right) p_{u_t}(x_t) dx_t \right) dx_{2k+1} \, . \end{aligned} \tag{4.297}$$

By using Fig. 4.26, the last double integral can be transformed as follows:

$$f(u_{2k+1}) = \int_0^\infty \left(\int_{x_t}^\infty x_{2k+1} T\left(u_{2k+1}, x_{2k+1} - x_t \middle| u_t, 0\right) dx_{2k+1} \right) p_{u_t}(x_t) dx_t \, . \tag{4.298}$$

By using the change of variables

$$z = x_{2k+1} - x_t \, , \tag{4.299}$$

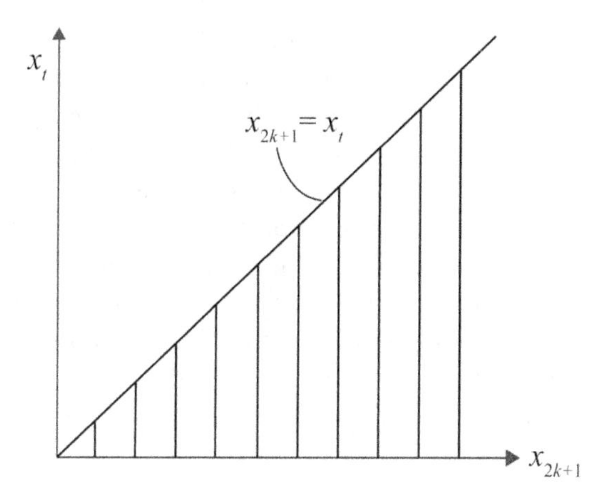

Fig. 4.26

from formula (4.298) we derive

$$\begin{aligned} f(u_{2k+1}) = & \int_0^\infty \left(\int_0^\infty zT\left(u_{2k+1}, z \middle| u_t, 0\right) dz \right) p_{u_t}(x_t) dx_t \\ & + \int_0^\infty \left(\int_0^\infty T\left(u_{2k+1}, z \middle| u_t, 0\right) dz \right) x_t p_{u_t}(x_t) dx_t \ . \end{aligned} \tag{4.300}$$

Now, by using the same reasoning that was used to simplify formula (4.293), we obtain

$$f(u_{2k+1}) = F\left(u_{2k+1}, u_t\right) + f^-(u_t) \ , \tag{4.301}$$

which leads to

$$f^-(u_t) = f(u_{2k+1}) - F\left(u_{2k+1}, u_t\right) \ . \tag{4.302}$$

Formulas (4.295) and (4.302) show that the shapes of generic ascending and descending branches of a minor hysteresis loop are the same regardless of the past input history. The past history is reflected in the values of $f(u_{2k})$ and $f(u_{2k+1})$. In other words, the minor hysteresis loops corresponding to different past histories are congruent. Since the erasure property and the congruency of minor loops (formed for the same back- and-forth input variations) represent the necessary and sufficient conditions for the description of hysteresis by the Preisach model, we conclude that *the path integration model* (4.269) *with the stochastic measure corresponding to the homogeneous diffusion process is equivalent to the Preisach model.*

It is clear from the previous discussion that the output calculations for the path integration model can be performed if the function $T(\alpha, x_\alpha|\beta, x_\beta)$ is known. This function can be computed by solving the exit problem for the stochastic process defined by equation (4.276). This, in turn, requires the solution of initial-boundary value problems for the backward Kolmogorov equation similar to those discussed in Section 4.3. In particular, by using the mathematical machinery of the exit problem, the closed form expressions can be derived for the weight function $\mu(\alpha, \beta)$ of the Preisach model which is equivalent to the path integration model (4.269) with the stochastic measure generated by the process (4.288). Below, we present the final results; the mathematical details of the derivation can be found in the paper [20]. Consider the function

$$\psi(g) = \exp\left(-2\int_0^g \frac{b(g')}{\sigma^2(g')}dg'\right) , \tag{4.303}$$

then the function $F(\alpha, \beta)$ from (4.296) and $\mu(\alpha, \beta)$ can be computed as follows:

$$F(\alpha, \beta) = \frac{2}{K_{\alpha\beta}}\int_\beta^\alpha \left(\int_\beta^g \psi(g')dg'\right)\left(\int_g^\alpha \psi(g')dg'\right)\frac{dg}{\sigma^2(g)\psi(g)} , \tag{4.304}$$

$$\mu(\alpha, \beta) = \frac{\psi(\alpha)\psi(\beta)}{K^2_{\alpha\beta}}F(\alpha, \beta) , \tag{4.305}$$

where

$$K_{\alpha\beta} = \int_\beta^\alpha \psi(g)dg . \tag{4.306}$$

As examples, consider the following cases:

(1) g_x is the Wiener process ($b = 0, \sigma = 1$). Then $\psi(g) = 1$, $K_{\alpha\beta} = \alpha - \beta$ and

$$\mu(\alpha, \beta) = \frac{1}{3}, \quad F(\alpha, \beta) = \frac{1}{3}(\alpha - \beta)^2 . \tag{4.307}$$

Thus, the Preisach weight function is simply a constant and all hysteresis branches are parabolic (see Fig. 4.27).

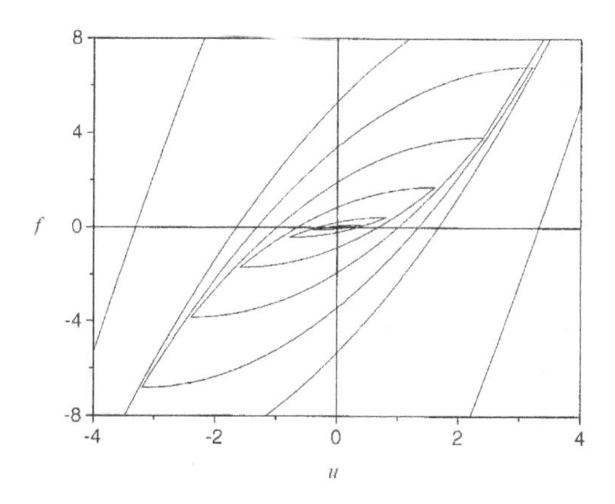

Fig. 4.27

(2) g_x is the diffusion process with constant drift $[b(g) = 1/(2\chi), (\chi > 0),\ \sigma = 1]$. In this case we have

$$\psi(g) = e^{-g/\chi}\ , \tag{4.308}$$

$$K_{\alpha\beta} = e^{-\beta/\chi} - e^{-\alpha/\chi}\ , \tag{4.309}$$

$$\mu(\alpha,\beta) = \frac{\frac{\alpha-\beta}{2\chi}\coth\left(\frac{\alpha-\beta}{2\chi}\right) - 1}{\sinh^2\left(\frac{\alpha-\beta}{2\chi}\right)}\ , \tag{4.310}$$

$$F(\alpha,\beta) = 4\left[\left(\frac{\alpha-\beta}{2\chi}\right)\coth\left(\frac{\alpha-\beta}{2\chi}\right) - 1\right]\ . \tag{4.311}$$

Typical hysteresis branches computed for this case are shown in Fig. 4.28.

(3) g_x is the Ornstein-Uhlenbeck process ($b(g) = -g/\chi$, $\sigma = 1$). In this case,

$$\psi(g) = e^{g^2/\chi}\ , \tag{4.312}$$

$\mu(\alpha,\beta)$ and $F(\alpha,\beta)$ are obtained by inserting the last expression in the formulas (4.304)–(4.306).

The described functional (path) integration model (4.269) admits the following physical interpretation. It is known that hysteresis is due to the existence of multiple metastable states in the system free energy $F(X)$

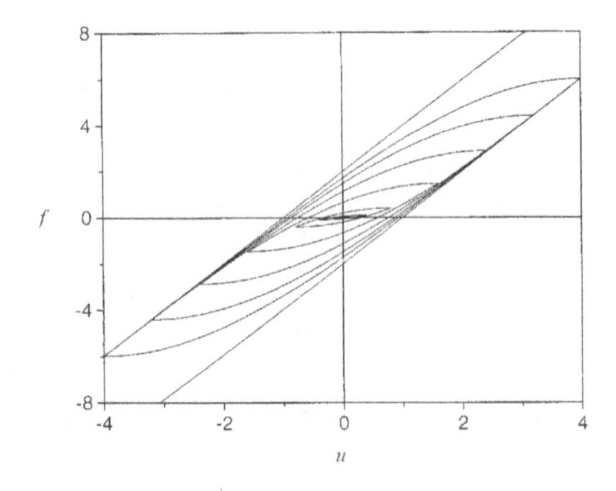

Fig. 4.28

(the temperature dependence is tacitly understood), which means that the system may be trapped in individual metastable states for long times.

Consider a simple case where the state variable X is a scalar quantity and the relevant free energy in the presence of the external magnetic field H is $\Phi(X;H) = F(X) - HX$. The metastable states available to the system are represented by Φ-minima with respect to X for which $\partial\Phi/\partial X = 0$ and $\partial^2\Phi/\partial X^2 > 0$. When H is changed with time, the number and properties of these minima are modified by the variation of the term $-HX$. The consequence is that previously stable states are made unstable by the field action and the system moves to other metastable states through a sequence of (Barkhausen) jumps. Because the condition $\partial\Phi/\partial X = 0$ is equivalent to $H = \partial F/\partial X$ one can analyze the problem by using the field representation shown in Fig. 4.29. The response of the system, expressed in terms of $H(X)$, is obtained by traversing the upper and lower envelopes of $\partial F/\partial X$ for increasing and decreasing H, respectively. From the physical viewpoint, this construction amounts to assuming that the system, once made unstable by the action of the external field, jumps to the nearest available energy minimum, which means that this excludes dynamic effects that could aid the system to reach more distant minima. It is clear from the above description that $\partial F/\partial X$ and H are similar to the generating functional $g(x)$ and input $u(t)$, respectively, within the framework of the function (path) integration model (4.269). The functional integration model itself can be interpreted as the average hysteresis response of a statistical ensemble of independent (elementary) systems evolving in random free energy landscape. This

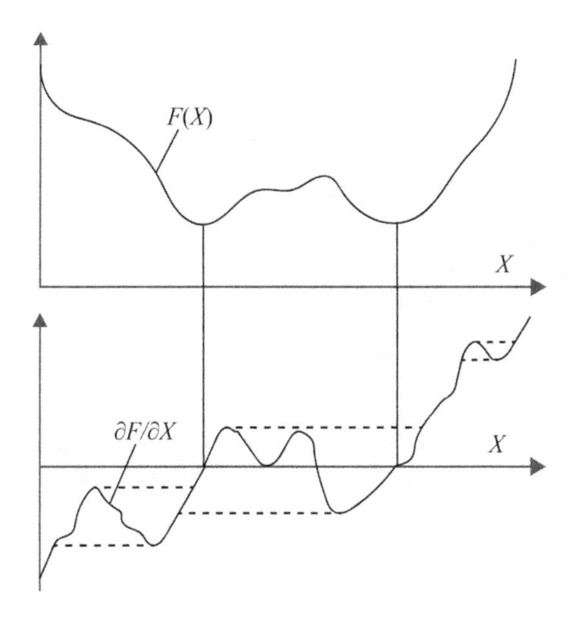

Fig. 4.29

interpretation can be of importance in applications where randomness due to structural disorders plays a key role in the appearance of hysteretic effects. A particularly important example is the motion of magnetic domain walls in ferromagnets, where various forms of structural disorder (point defects, dislocations, gain boundaries, etc.) are responsible for the random character of $\partial F/\partial X$. There are classical papers in the literature, [21] and [22], where the domain wall picture has been applied to the prediction of coercivity and magnetization curve shapes, starting from some assumption $F(X)$. Equations (4.303)–(4.306) provide a general solution for the case where the process $\partial F/\partial X$ is Markovian, continuous, and homogeneous. In particular, the proven equivalence of Markovian disorder to the Preisach model gives a sound statistical interpretation of the latter.

References

[1] C. W. Gardiner, "Handbook of stochastic methods for physics, chemistry and the natural sciences," Springer Verlag, Berlin, 1982.
[2] W. A. Gardner, "Introduction to Random Processes," Macmillan, New York, 1986.
[3] P. C. Bressloff, "Stochastic Processes in Cell Biology," Springer, 2014.

[4] I. Mayergoyz, "Mathematical Models of Hysteresis and Their Applications," Academic Press (an imprint of Elsevier), 2003.
[5] I. D. Mayergoyz and C. E. Korman, "Preisach model with stochastic input as a model for viscosity," Journal of Applied Physics, Vol. 69 (4), pp. 2128-2134, 1991.
[6] I. D. Mayergoyz and C. E. Korman, "On a new approach to the modeling of viscosity in hysteretic systems," IEEE Transactions on Magnetics, Vol. 27 (6), pp. 4766-4768, 1991.
[7] C. E. Korman and I. D. Mayergoyz, "The input dependent Preisach model with stochastic input as a model for aftereffect," IEEE Transactions on Magnetics, Vol. 30 (6), pp. 4368-4370, 1994.
[8] I. D. Mayergoyz and C. E. Korman, "The Preisach model with stochastic input as a model for aftereffect," Journal of Applied Physics, Vol. 75, pp. 5478-5480, 1994.
[9] C. E. Korman and I. D. Mayergoyz, "Preisach model driven by stochastic inputs as a model for aftereffect," IEEE Transactions on Magnetics, Vol. 32 (5), pp. 4204-4209, 1996.
[10] C. E. Korman and I. D. Mayergoyz, "Review of Preisach type models driven by stochastic inputs as a model for after-effect," Physica B, Vol. 233 (4), pp. 381-389, 1997.
[11] M. E. Freidlin and A. D. Wentzell, "Diffusion Processes on Graphs and the Averaging Principle," The Annals of Probability, Vol. 21, No. 4, pp. 2215-2245, 1993.
[12] M. I. Freidlin, I. D. Mayergoyz and R. Pfeiffer, "Noise in hysteretic systems and stochastic processes on graphs," Physical Review E, Vol. 62, No. 2, pp. 1850-1855, 2000.
[13] C. E. Korman and I. D. Mayergoyz, "Semiconductor noise in the framework of semiclassical transport," Phys. Rev. B, Vol. 54 (24), pp. 17620-17627, 1996.
[14] I. D. Mayergoyz and M. Dimian, "Analysis of spectral noise density of hysteretic systems driven by stochastic processes," Journal of Applied Physics, Vol. 93, pp. 6826-6828, 2003.
[15] M. Dimian and I. D. Mayergoyz, "Spectral density analysis of nonlinear hysteretic systems," Phys. Rev. E, Vol. 70, 046124, 2004.
[16] S. Schubert and G. Radons, "Preisach models of hysteresis driven by Markovian input processes," Phys. Rev. E, Vol. 96, 022117, 2017.
[17] G. Radons, "Hysteresis-Induced Long-Time Tails," Phys. Rev. Lett., Vol. 100, 240602, 2008.
[18] G. Radons, "Spectral properties of the Preisach hysteresis model with random input. I. General results," Phys. Rev. E, Vol. 77, 061133, 2008.
[19] G. Radons, "Spectral properties of the Preisach hysteresis model with random input. II. Universality classes for symmetric elementary loops," Phys. Rev. E, Vol. 77, 061134, 2008.
[20] G. Bertotti, I. D. Mayergoyz, V. Basso and A. Magni, "Functional integration approach to hysteresis," Phys. Rev. E, Vol. 60 (2), pp. 1428-1440, 1999.

[21] L. Néel, "Théories des lois d'aimantation de Lord Rayleigh," Cahiers de physique, Vol. 12, pp. 1-20, 1942.
[22] H. Kronmuller, "Magnetic Hysteresis in Novel Magnetic Materials," (edited by Hadjipanayis), Vol. 85, Kluwer, Dordrecht, 1997.

Index

CPSIA information can be obtained
at www.ICGtesting.com
Printed in the USA
BVHW072324200819
556373BV00005B/8/P

9 789811 209505